W0051423

Advances in Controlled Clinical Inhalation Studies

ILSI Monographs

Carcinogenicity:
The Design, Analysis, and Interpretation of Long-Term Animal Studies
H.C. Grice and J.L. Ciminera, Editors
1988. 279 pp. ISBN 0-387-18301-9

Inhalation Toxicology: The Design and Interpretation of Inhalation
Studies and Their Use in Risk Assessment
U. Mohr, Editor-in-Chief
D.L. Dungworth, G. Kimmerle, J. Lewkowski, R.O. McClellan, W. Stöber
1988. 318 pp. ISBN 0-387-17822-8

Radionuclides in the Food Chain
M.D. Carter, Editor-in-Chief
J.H. Harley, G.D. Schmidt, G. Silini, Editors
1988. 518 pp. ISBN 0-387-19511-4

Assessment of Inhalation Hazards:
Integration and Extrapolation Using Diverse Data
U. Mohr, Editor-in-Chief
D.V. Bates, D.L. Dungworth, P.N. Lee, R.O. McClellan, F.J.C. Roe, Editors
1989. 382 pp. ISBN 3-540-50952-6

Advances in Controlled Clinical Inhalation Studies
U. Mohr, Editor-in-Chief
D.V. Bates, H. Fabel, M.J. Utell, Editors
1993. 442 pp. ISBN 3-540-54958-7

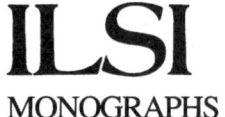

ILSI
MONOGRAPHS

Sponsored by
the International
Life Sciences Institute

U. Mohr
Editor-in-Chief

Advances in Controlled Clinical Inhalation Studies

D. V. Bates   H. Fabel   M. J. Utell
Editors

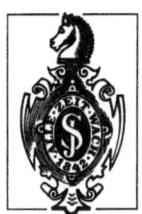

Springer-Verlag
Berlin Heidelberg New York
London Paris Tokyo
Hong Kong Barcelona
Budapest

Ulrich Mohr, Prof. Dr. med.
Medizinische Hochschule Hannover, Institut für Experimentelle Pathologie, Konstanty-Gutschow-Straße 8, 3000 Hannover 61, FRG

David V. Bates, M.D., F.R.C.P., F.R.C.P.C., F.A.C.P., F.R.S.C.
University of British Columbia, Dept. Health and Epidemiology, 5804 Fairview Crescent, Mather Building, Vancouver, BC, Canada V6T 1W5

H. Fabel, Prof. Dr. med.
Medizinische Hochschule Hannover, Abteilung Pneumologie, Konstanty-Gutschow-Straße 8, 3000 Hannover 61, FRG

Mark J. Utell, M.D.
Professor of Medicine and Environmental Medicine, Pulmonary and Critical Care Unit, University of Rochester Medical Center, 601 Elmwood Avenue, Rochester, NY 14642, USA

With 101 Figures

ISBN-13:978-3-642-77178-1   e-ISBN-13:978-3-642-77176-7
DOI: 10.1007/978-3-642-77176-7

This work is subject to copyright. All rights are reserved, whether the whole or part of the material is concerned, specifically the rights of translation, reprinting, reuse of illustrations, recitation, broadcasting, reproduction on microfilm or in any other way, and storage in data banks. Duplication of this publication or parts thereof is permitted only under the provisions of the German Copyright Law of September 9, 1965, in its current version, and permission for use must always be obtained from Springer-Verlag. Violations are liable for prosecution under the German Copyright Law.

© Springer-Verlag Berlin Heidelberg 1993
Softcover reprint of the hardcover 1st edition   1993

The use of general descriptive names, registered names, trademarks, etc. in this publication does not imply, even in the absence of a specific statement, that such names are exempt from the relevant protective laws and regulations and therefore free for general use.

Product liability: The publishers cannot guarantee the accuracy of any information about dosage and application contained in this book. In every individual case the user must check such information by consulting the relevant literature.

Typesetting: Best-set Typesetter Ltd., Hong Kong
23/3145-5 4 3 2 1 0 – Printed on acid-free paper

Series Foreword

The International Life Sciences Institute (ILSI), a nonprofit, public foundation, was established in 1978 to advance the sciences of nutrition, toxicology, and food safety. ILSI promotes the resolution of health and safety issues in these areas by sponsoring research, conferences, publications, and educational programs. Through ILSI's programs, scientists from government, academia, and industry unite their efforts to resolve issues of critical importance to the public.

As part of its commitment to understanding and resolving health and safety issues, ILSI is pleased to sponsor this series of monographs that consolidates new scientific knowledge, defines research needs, and provides a background for the effective application of scientific advances in toxicology and food safety.

Alex Malaspina
President
International Life Sciences Institute

Contents

Contributors*

ABEL, U.   185
ADLKOFER, F.   387
ANGERER, J.   387

BARBER, R.W.   357
BATES, D.V.   **3**
BECKER, S.   169
BEHRENDT, H.   323
BEN-JEBRIA, A.   309
BERNSTEIN, O.   109
BROMBERG, P.A.   169, **235**
BRUCKMANN, P.   317
BUCK, M.   **9**

CALZIA, E.   377
CONZE, C.   387

DEVLIN, R.B.   169
DRENK, F.   327

FABEL, H.   159
FLEISCHER, W.   411
FRAMPTON, M.W.   **199**
FREEMAN, N.C.G.   285

GINCHEVA, N.   297
GLASER, U.   185

HACKNEY, J.D.   **135**
HADNAGY, W.   323, 393
HAMMERMAIER, A.   411
HANLEY, Q.S.   109
HAZUCHA, M.J.   **247**
HEINRICH, U.   185, 209, 327
HERMENAU, H.   345

HEYDER, J.   **103**
HIGENBOTTAM, T.W.   357
HOLLÄNDER, W.   **123**
HOWLETT, C.T., JR.   303
HRISTEVA, V.   373
HU, S.C.   309
HUBER, A.   377

ISLAM, M.S.   365

JAEGER, H.   411
JÖRRES, R.   151

KAPPOS, A.D.   **317**
KIELL, A.   323
KLINGEBIEL, R.   **209, 337**
KNOPP, D.   **345**
KOCH, W.   **57**
KOENIG, J.Q.   109
KOREN, H.S.   **169**
KOSS, G.   317
KREFT, A.   185

LAMBERT, W.E.   95
LARSON, T.V.   **109**
LEVSEN, K.   **43**
LINN, W.S.   135
LIOY, P.J.   **31, 285**
LIPPMANN, M.   **69**
LÜTHE, N.   185

MAGNUSSEN, H.   **151**
MCKEE, D.J.   **269**
MEYER, M.   **347, 377**
MOHAMMED, S.P.   **357**

---

* The numbers after the names refer to the contribution title page, where the author's complete address can be found. Numbers in bold indicate senior authors.

Part I
Symposium Presentation

The Emergence of Controlled Human Exposure Studies

D.V. BATES

University of British Columbia, Dept. Health and Epidemiology, 5804 Fairview Crescent, Mather Building, Vancouver, BC, Canada V6T 1Z3

Introduction

It is a great pleasure to take part once again in a symposium in Hanover and a special privilege to have been asked to start off this interesting discussion. My task is to trace where we have been in controlled exposure studies, that is, to provide a context within which our present understanding can be viewed. This has not proved easy, and I should warn you that I may well have missed some historically important references; if so, I hope that you will point them out to me.

1895: Haldane's Experiments on Himself

I think there is little doubt that these experiments represent the first comprehensive studies of the effects of human exposure to a toxic gas. The 1895 paper is remarkable in many respects. Haldane wanted to relate the build-up of COHb in the blood to subjective symptoms. He describes the breathing circuit. Pure CO was added to the breathing line from a flask by displacement by water at a constant rate. An empty glass in the circuit contained a mouse, which he could observe at the same time as he breathed the gas. A dry bellows gasmeter recorded his ventilation. He noted symptoms (and watched the mouse), and blood samples were taken for later analysis.

In experiment II, he noted at 90s of breathing, "mouse panting;" after 13 min, "mouse remains on its side when put there." A specimen of Haldane's blood was 23% saturated, and he noted, "no symptoms yet." In experiment VII, he reached 49% saturation and had difficulty walking across the room as he was very unsteady. He described hyperpnea on effort, "but this was not much noticed, as the other symptoms were so much more prominent." At this point he "said over the German numerals correctly up to 25." I hope that neurobehavioral toxicologists will note this.

U. Mohr et al. (Eds.)
Advances in Controlled Clinical
Inhalation Studies
© Springer-Verlag Berlin Heidelberg 1993

From 1895 to 1964

After Haldane's experiments, there is a long gap. Of course, a number of investigators from about 1910 onwards were breathing different concentrations of CO_2 to determine the effect on ventilation and to elucidate the control of breathing. In 1935 Haldane and Priestley in their textbook of respiration described Paul Bert's early experiments on decompression and illustrated the steel chamber which he built for these studies. I looked up Findeisen's famous 1935 paper on particle deposition to see whether or not he had any human data. His paper was based on knowledge of the geometry of the human bronchial tree and applied theoretical physics to predict the deposition of particles of different sizes. He did not do any experiments, as far as I can tell, to confirm his predictions (which have proved, I believe, remarkably accurate). His paper in *Pflugers Archiv* contains two references only, both to papers by A. Einstein in a physics journal in 1905 and 1906. The advantage of being a pioneer is that one does not have to clutter up a paper with a bibliography.

In 1943, Henderson and Haggard at Harvard published their book on noxious gases. They extended Haldane's work on CO and noted occupational experience of accidental exposure to gases such as ammonia, chlorine, and nitrogen dioxide. Their monograph does not contain data from controlled exposure studies.

From 1964 to 1980

I published a paper in 1964 on the effects of breathing ozone through a mouthpiece (Young et al.). Before I start describing these and other studies which I initiated, I should warn you of a recent quotation from the *New York Review of Books*: "Autobiography is, of course, the highest form of fiction."

I had been interested in ozone since 1954, when the possibility of contamination by ozone in the cabin of the Comet aircraft, which flew higher than other planes, had been raised. I had access to the data on the ozone layer, first collected I believe as a result of rocket firings in Germany during the war. I knew that the American Conference of Governmental Industrial Hygienists in 1960 had set a standard for ozone exposure (of 0.1 ppm), but this was not based on human data. We had done an experiment in 1962 on a DC-8 (the first delivered to Air Canada) which showed that ozone levels when the aircraft was above 30 000 feet were probably between 0.3 and 0.4 ppm and were higher in the cockpit than at the rear of the passenger cabin (Young et al. 1962). The following year I studied a small group of welders who had been exposed to ozone and found that they had normal lung function (Young et al. 1963). In 1964 we reported that 0.6–0.8 ppm of ozone when breathed for 2 h at rest had measureable effects on vital capacity, FEV 0.75 × 40, and diffusing capacity (Young et al. 1964).

It was at this point that I realised that human exposures should include exercise data, and I had an opportunity in 1967 to build a Plexiglas chamber for this purpose. In 1969 Goldsmith and Nadel published their paper on ozone breathing, and in 1972 we published a paper on the effects of 0.75 ppm of ozone, including exercise data from three subjects (Bates et al. 1972). All 10 subjects in this study were physicians or assistants. We noted symptoms and drew attention to variability of response among the subjects, one of whom showed on response at all. We also noted the fall in maximal inspiratory pressure as an early effect of ozone, a phenomenon now documented in detail (Hazucha et al. 1989).

In 1975 Pepys and Hutchcroft published their paper on "Bronchial provocation tests in etiologic diagnosis and analysis of asthma," and launched the intensive study of airway reactivity. This work led also to the development of non-specific tests using histamine or mecholyl.

By 1978 a number of human exposure chambers had been built, and in that year, the US Environmental Protection Agency published a report on a symposium held to discuss the development of controlled human exposures. This represents an important watershed. The symposium contained a detailed paper by Lippmann on aerosol generation and measurement, and I noted the tardy development of human exposure experiments after major pollution episodes more than 25 years earlier. I also ventured to look forward and, if I may be permitted to quote myself, said:

In the case of sulphur dioxide, for instance, we do not know precisely the range of individual variablity, or the aassociation of a high sensitivity to sulphur dioxide as measured by changes in airway resistance, to other thresholds of sensitivity as measured by the inhalation of mecholyl or histamine. We do not have a precise quantitation of the effect of mouth or nose breathing in an atmosphere of SO_2 on the development of changes in airway resistance. We do not know whether a two-hour exposure on one day will influence the response in a given individual in succeeding days. We do not know whether the acute response to sulphur dioxide is any different in individuals who live and work in relatively high concentrations of this gas, and, in general, we have very little acute laboratory data to put alongside our guesses of its chronic effects.

It was 2 years later in 1980 that Sheppard and his colleagues clearly established that asthmatics were more sensitive to SO_2 than other people. I still think it remarkable that there was a gap of 28 years between the London smog disaster, in which SO_2 levels exceeded 1 ppm in some locations (HMSO 1954), and detailed controlled exposure data on its effects.

Modern Developments

Since 1980 there have been so many developments and refinements in the field of controlled human exposure that it is difficult to know where to begin describing them. I believe that the experiments in Aarhus in Denmark pioneered by Molhave and colleagues, starting in about 1985 (Molhave 1985), represent a distinct step forward in the use of controlled human exposure to mixtures of hydrocarbons. Their recent paper on the effects of *n*-decane is a model of such experiments (Kjaergaard et al. 1989).

In 1987 Hazucha summarized data on the effect of different concentrations of ozone on the FEV_1 during 2-h exposures with intermittent exercise. Considering that there is significant variation in individual response between normal subjects, there was very satisfactory concordance between the results from several different laboratories. The reasons for the individual variation (most recently documented again by Horstman and his colleagues at Chapel Hill; McDonnell et al. 1991) remain one of the most important unexplained phenomena in relation to ozone.

Another major development has been the increase in sophistication of outcome measurements. The effect of ozone on airway reactivity and on lung permeability and, most particularly, the use of bronchial lavage to measure the onset of an inflammatory response all represent important steps forward from simple dependence on the FEV_1 as an indicator of effect.

We are just getting to the stage of learning the effects of exposure to one pollutant on the response to another, e.g., that ozone increases the subsequent response to SO_2 in asthmatics (Koenig et al. 1990). We are developing a much more sophisticated understanding of probable patterns of pollutant exposure in the general population. For example, in the northeast of North America in the summer, children playing out of doors encounter intermittent high peaks of ozone and sulfuric acid aerosol, sometimes simultaneously and sometimes one pollutant at a high concentration on one day and the other at a high concentration the next (Spengler et al. 1990).

We have witnessed the major impact which controlled human exposure studies have on the determination of safe levels for public exposure to O_3, SO_2, and NO_2, a topic to be addressed in this symposium. There is , in my opinion, no doubt that this trend will continue.

Conclusion

At the beginning, I warned you that I might well have missed significant early work on controlled human exposures, and I hope you will add to my knowledge of this field by drawing my attention to contributions I have omitted. This span of work over the past 100 years well illustrates the crescendo of scientific work in our generation, since major discoveries have really only occurred in the past 30 years. With the body of work now considerable and the questions no less urgent, we may look forward to great advances in the future.

In 1978, as I have mentioned, I drew attention to the questions ahead of us; I will not attempt that now, but by the end of this symposium, we should all have been able to get a glimpse of what the future may hold.

References

American Conference of Governmental Industrial Hygienists (1960) Threshold limit values for 1960. Arch Environ Health 1:140–148

Bates DV, Bell GM, Burnham CD, Hazucha M, Mantha J, Pengelly LD, Silverman F (1972) Short-term effects of ozone on the lung. J Appl Physiol 32:176–181

Findeisen W (1935) Uber das Absetzen kleiner, in der Luft suspendierter Teilchen in der menschlichen Lunge bei der Atmung. Pfluger's Arch 236:367–379

Goldsmith JR, Nadel JA (1969) Experimental exposure of human subjects to ozone. J Air Pollu Control Assoc 19:329–330

Haldane J (1895) The action of carbonic oxide on man. J Physiol 18:430–462

Haldane, JS, Priestley JG (1935) Respiration, 2nd edn. Oxford University Press, New York

Hazucha M (1987) Relationship between ozone exposure and pulmonary function changes. J Appl Physiol 62:1671–1680

Hazucha M, Bates DV, Bromberg P. (1989) Mechanism of action of ozone on the human lung. J Appl Physiol 67:1535–1541

Henderson Y, Haggard HW (1943) Noxious gases. Reinhold, New York

Hmso (Her Majesty's Stationery Office) (1954) Mortality and morbidity during the London fog of December 1952. HMSO, London (Report no 95 on Public Health and Medical subjects)

Kjaergaard S, Molhave L, Pedersen OF (1989) Human reactions to indoor air pollutants: n-decane. Environ Int 15:473–482

Koenig JQ, Covert DS, Hanley QS, van Belle G, Pierson WE (1990) Prior exposure to ozone potentiates subsequent response to sulfur dioxide in adolescent asthmatic subjects. Am Rev Respir Dis 141:377–380

Molhave L (1985) Volatile organic compounds as indoor air pollutants. In: Gammasge RB, Kaye SV (eds) Indoor air and human health. Lewis, Chelsea, pp 403–414

Pepys J, Hutchcroft BJ (1975) Bronchial provocation tests in etiologic diagnosis and analysis of asthma. Am Rev Respir Dis 112:829–859

Sheppard D, Wong WG, Uehara CF, Nadel JA, Boushey HA (1980) Lower threshold and greater bronchomotor responsiveness of asthmatic subjects to sulfur dioxide. Am Rev Respir Dis 122:873–878

Spengler JD, Brauer M, Koutrakis P (1990) Acid air and health. Environ Sci Technol 24:946–956

US Environmental Protection Agency (1978) Methodologies and protocols in clinical research: Evaluating environmental effects in man. US Environmental protection Agency, Research Triangle Park NC (EPA-600/9-78-008)

Young WA, Shaw DB, Bates DV (1962) Presence of ozone in aircraft flying at 35 000 feet. Aerosp Med 33:311–318

Young WA, Shaw DB, Bates DV (1963) Pulmonary function in welders exposed to ozone. Arch Environ Health 7:337–340

Young WA, Shaw DB, Bates DV (1964) Effect of low concentrations of ozone on pulmonary function in man. J Appl Physiol 19:765–768

McDonnell WF, Kehrl HR, Abdul-Salaam S, Ives PJ, Folinsbee LJ, Devlin RB, O'Neil JJ, Horstman DH (1991) Respiratory response of humans exposed to low levels of ozone for 6.6 hours. Arch Environ Health 46:145–150

References

Section 1. The Outdoor Environment in Europe

Trend of Air Quality in North Rhine-Westphalia (Rhine-Ruhr Area) During the Past 20 Years

M. Buck

Landesamt für Immissionsschutz des Landes Nordrhein-Westfalen, Wallneyer Straße 6, W-4300 Essen 1, FRG

At the beginning of the 1960s, sulfur dioxide and dustfall were still indicators, even more than that, they were the synonyms for air pollution. The variations of the ambient concentrations of these substances over the last 3 decades in the urban-industrialized Rhine-Ruhr area are shown in Figs. 1 and 2.

The sharp decline of the SO_2 concentration to about 15% of that in 1964 was due to the following measures:

- In the 1960s the emitting plants were modernized. By tearing down old plants and implementing new technological processes low in emissions, the ambient concentrations dropped noticeably.
- The "high-stack" policy of the 1970s shifted the SO_2 emission to greater distances, leading to a regional reduction of the ambient concentration.
- The steep decrease in ambient SO_2 in the following years was due to the desulfurization of fuels and to the rigid requirements of reducing emissions by flue gas cleaning, which led to a large-scale reduction of SO_2 pollution to about one-seventh the concentration of 30 years ago. The achieved level of approx. $30\,\mu g/m^3$ lies below the ambient air quality standard recommended by the EEC of $40-60\,\mu g/m^3$ and tends towards values lower than the $30\,\mu g/m^3$ recommended by the WHO for the protection of vegetation.

Fig. 3 shows the changes of the ambient concentrations that have taken place over the past 25 years in the form of the frequency distribution of the annual averages for small areas of the size of $1\,km^2$. It can be seen that in the Rhine-Ruhr area spanning approximately $5000\,km^2$ the upper level of present day air pollution ends where the lower level began 25 years ago [1].

No concentrations in excess of the German air quality standards occur nowadays. The SO_2 level in the Rhine-Ruhr area is expected to sink further to the extent that the SO_2, emitted in the former German Democratic Republic and in other eastern European countries will be reduced, which

U. Mohr et al. (Eds.)
Advances in Controlled Clinical
Inhalation Studies
© Springer-Verlag Berlin Heidelberg 1993

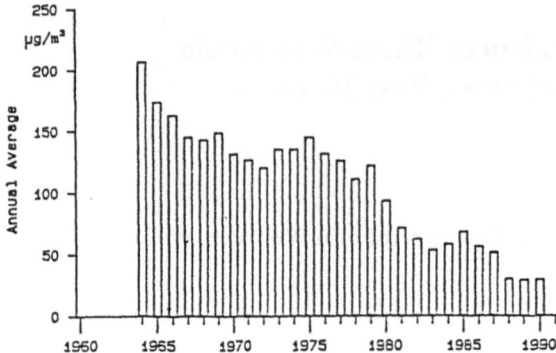

Fig. 1. Variation of sulfur dioxide concentration in Rhine-Ruhr area

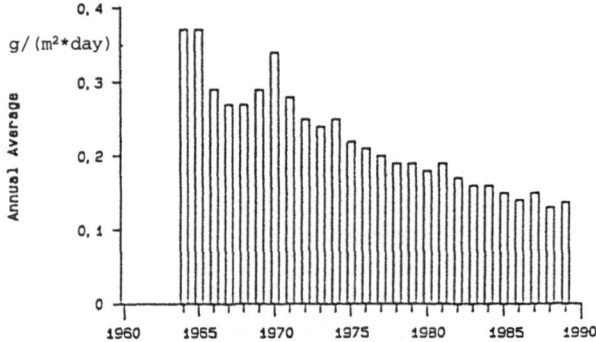

Fig. 2. Variation of dustfall concentration in Rhine-Ruhr area

will have an impact on East-West transport of SO_2. Thus, SO_2 will cease to be a significant indicator of air pollution.

The same is true for dustfall. As with SO_2, it dropped considerably over the past 25 years to a level one-third of the initial value in 1964. Here, too, reductions were due to industrial modernization at the outset, followed immediately by rigidly enforced dust precipitation, whose efficiency improved following technological progress [2].

The dust components lead and cadmium also declined significantly. As with suspended particulate matter, their levels dropped more than the dustfall total. This means dustfall became low in heavy metals due to the efficiency of the respective emission-reducing measures (Figs. 4, 5).

In the greater area of Duisburg, which traditionally has been the center of the basic metal industries, the levels of lead and cadmium laid down in air quality standards are still being exceeded in the vicinity of these plants. As the applied measurement method inherently includes resuspended dust to a greater or lesser extent in the deposited dust, measured data do not necessarily reflect the level of present dust emissions by industrial plants;

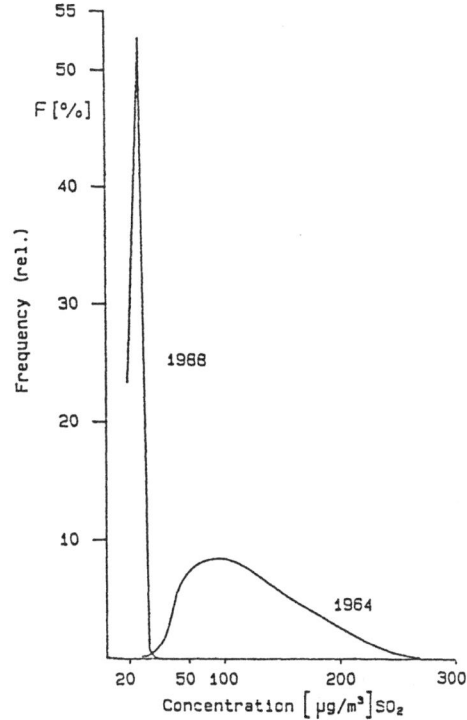

Fig. 3. Changes of ambient SO_2 concentration by frequency distribution of annual averages for small areas $(1 \, km^2)$

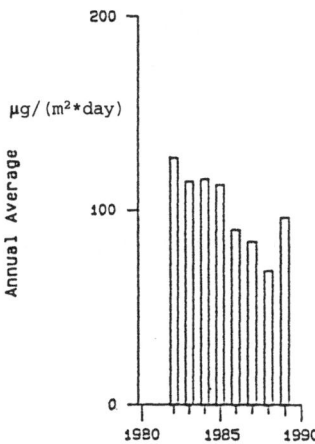

Fig. 4. Variation of lead deposition in Rhine-Ruhr area

heavy metal contaminated soils, for example, are an important emission source as well.

With regard to suspended particulate matter, which has been systematically measured since 1970, the average concentration amounts today to about one-third of that 2 decades ago (Fig. 6). A similar but more pro-

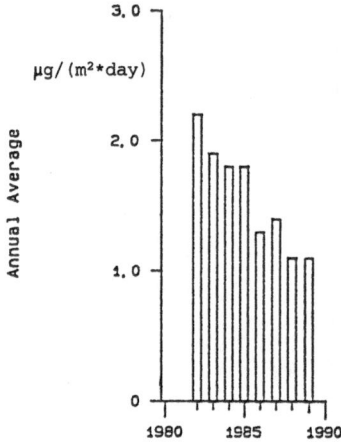

Fig. 5. Variation of cadmium deposition in Rhine-Ruhr area

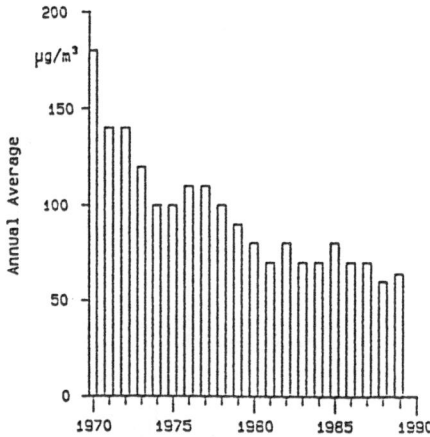

Fig. 6. Variation of total suspended particulate matter in Rhine-Ruhr area

nounced declining trend is observed with lead and cadmium aerosols. The concentrations of both substances declined to one-sixth of the initial measurements, while during the same period of time (1974–1989), the concentration of suspended particulate matter dropped only to half the original amount (Figs. 7, 8). The lead and cadmium compounds diminished in aerosols to a similar extent as in dustfall. No values exceeding the national or EEC air quality standards for suspended particulate matter and heavy metal aerosols have been observed, with the exception of in the immediate vicinity of heavy metal smelters.

The ambient CO concentration has remained almost unchanged for about 10 years at approx. $1\,mg/m^3$. It fluctuates about this value in

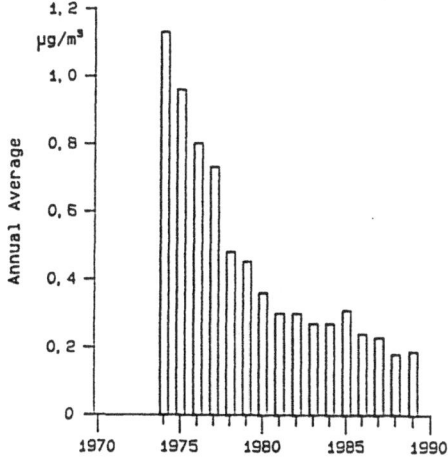

Fig. 7. Variation of lead content in total suspended particulate matter

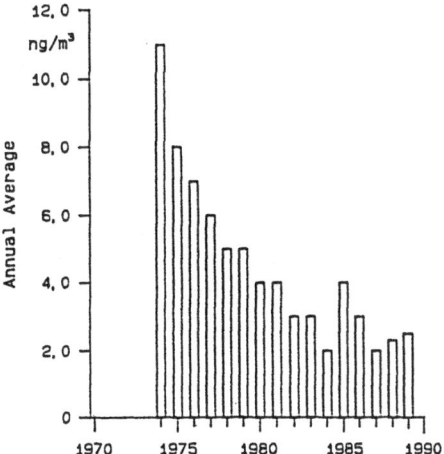

Fig. 8. Variation of cadmium content in total suspended particulate matter

accordance with the annual meteorological variations (Fig. 9). This finding agrees with the temporal development of CO emissions, which have not been reduced as much as, for example, those of SO_2 because they are less harmful – even under smog conditions, no hazardous CO levels are reached. Road vehicle emissions will experience a marked reduction only once most cars in operation are equipped with a three-way catalyst [3].

Comparably with CO, the NO and NO_2 levels remained at the annual average levels of the 1960s of 40–50 $\mu g/m^3$. The reason for this stagnation lies in the higher emissions from an increased road traffic, which offset the reductions of emissions by optimizing the combustion processes of stationary

14   M. Buck

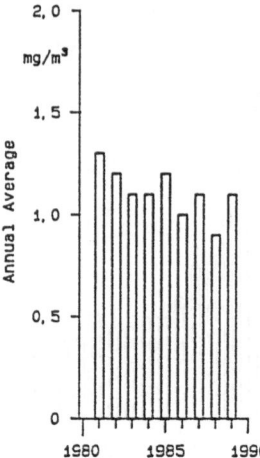

Fig. 9. Variation of carbon monoxide level in Rhine-Ruhr area

sources over the past 2 decades. Significant reductions in emissions and declining ambient concentrations can only be expected once denitrification of power plant flue gases and road vehicle exhausts has become fully effective. A declining trend of NO and NO_2 in ambient air should become noticeable by the mid-1990s. The fluctuations of the annual averages of NO and NO_2, shown in Figs. 10 and 11, are mostly due to meteorological influences.

For NO_2, which is formed in the atmosphere by a photo-chemical reaction from emitted NO, it can be said that, although its annual averages are somewhat below the recommended EEC standard of $50 \mu g/m^3$, the 98-percentiles of the short-term values (1-h averages) exceed at certain points close to road traffic the recommended value of $135 \mu g/m^3$. The EEC air

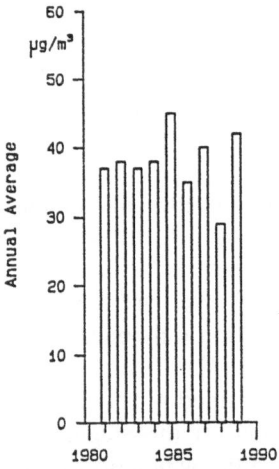

Fig. 10. Variation of nitrogen oxide level in Rhine-Ruhr area

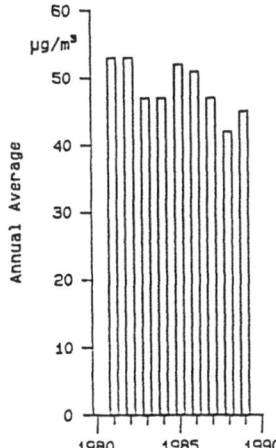

Fig. 11. Variation of nitrogen dioxide
level in Rhine-Ruhr area

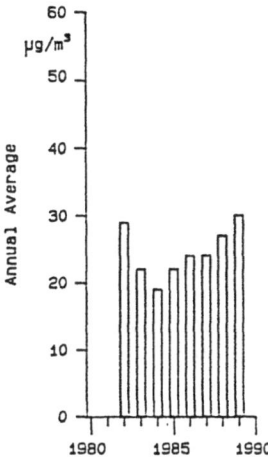

Fig. 12. Variation of ozone level in Rhine-Ruhr area

quality standard of 200 μg/m^3, which agrees with the national standard, however, is not reached [3].

Rigorous reductions of NO$_x$ are needed also because of the function of NO and NO$_2$ as precursors of photochemical ozone production. Short-term ozone concentrations during atmospheric high-pressure conditions in summer have reached a critical level. The mean atmospheric ozone concentration is on a steady rise. This trend becomes apparent from Fig. 12. Since in urban-industrialized areas there is enough NO available during the night for ozone destruction so that the ozone level drops sharply, it becomes enriched in the more remote rural areas over a longer period of time because of the relatively low NO level there. As a consequence, the annual average ozone concentrations in rural areas are more than twice as high as

Table 1. Concentration of air pollutants in different areas (annual average for 1989)

Compound	Traffic impacted location ("hot spot")	Urban-industralized area (Rhine-Ruhr area)	Rural area ("background")
Benzo[a]pyrene (ng/m^3)	5.8	2.8	0.5
Suspended particulates (TSP) (μg/m^3)	81	62	34
Pb (μg/m^3)	0.4	0.2	<0.05
SO$_2$ (μg/m^3)	40	29	13
NO (μg/m^3)	168	42	5
NO$_2$ (μg/m^3)	64	45	16
O$_3$ (μg/m^3)	15	30	65
Benzene (μg/m^3)	31	5	1
Diesel soot[a]	10–20	3–5	<1
CO (mg/m^3)	3.6	1.1	<0.5
Dustfall g/(m$^2 \cdot$ d)		0.13	<0.03

[a] Unpublished results (1990).

in urban areas (Table 1). In this respect, ozone forms an exception among air pollutants.

On sunny days of the months May to September, the hourly ozone concentrations reach levels of up to 400 μg/m^3, and the recommended German air quality standard of 120 μg/m^3 is frequently exceeded. As far as the territory of the "original" FRG is concerned, the population is asked to give up voluntarily straining outdoor physical activities as soon as the 2-h average of 180 μg/m^3 is exceeded [4].

As for other air pollutants, such as organic or carcinogenic substances, only shorter measurement series are available.

In Figs. 13 and 14, the temporal variations of benzo[a]pyrene and benzene are illustrated as an example. Not shown are the average concentrations of benzo[a]pyrene in the Rhine-Ruhr area of about 25 years ago. They amounted to approx. 25–75 ng/m^3 and were 10–30 times as high as today. The sharp decrease of the benzo[a]pyrene and other polylyclic aromatic hydrocarbons (PAH) concentrations up to the 1970s is primarily due to the conversion of coal-fired domestic heating systems to oil or gas. In the following years, the reduction of the number of coking plants as well as the modernization of the remaining plants played a role. There is evidence that the present concentration of PAH in ambient air is caused by road vehicle traffic and that, together with the meteorologically induced fluctuations, it will balance out to about 1–2 ng/m^3 in urban areas.

For benzene, no trend is discernible [5]. No air quality standards have been set for the two carcinogens because no scientifically founded no-effect levels can be given.

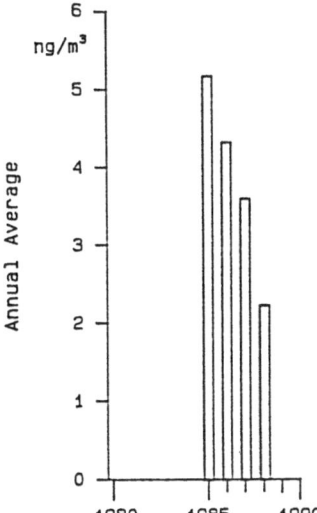

Fig. 13. Variation of benzo[*a*]pyrene content in total suspended particulate matter

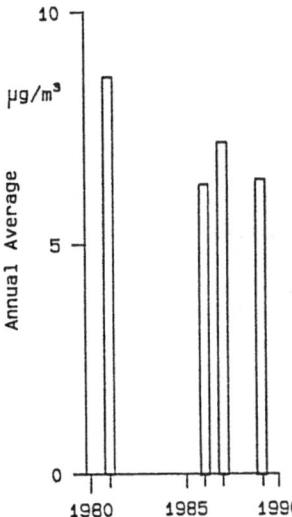

Fig. 14. Variation of benzene level in Rhine-Ruhr area

Table 1 provides a survey of the concentrations of air pollutants in various areas and shows the importance of road vehicle traffic as a source of air pollutants.

Tables 2–4 list current concentrations of various organic substances in ambient air. These are selected substances, which assumed importance for various reasons and which have been measured systematically since 1988. Conclusions about trends are, quite understandably, not yet possible. They can only be drawn after several years.

Table 2. Concentration of dioxins in ambient air [annual average in 1989 (fg/m^3)] [6]

Compound	Urban-industrialized area (Rhine-Ruhr area)	Rural area ("background")
2,3,7,8-TCDD	5–10	<1
2,3,7,8-TCDF	50–300	<10
PCDD+PCDF	5000–20 000	<1000
Toxicity equivalency factor		
BGA (Germany)	100–300	<20
NATO (CCMS)	150–350	<30

Abbreviations: TCDD, tetrachloro-*p*-dibenzodioxin; TCDF, tetrachloro-*p*-dibenzo-furan; PCDD, polychlorinated dioxins; PCDF, polychlorinated furans; BGA, Bundesgesundheitsamt (German Federal Office of Health); CCMS, Committee on the Challenges of Modern Society.

Table 3. Concentration of organic air pollutants[a] [annual average in 1989 (µg/m^3)]

Compound	Traffic impacted location ("hot spot")	Urban-industrialized area (Rhine-Ruhr area)	Rural area ("background")
Volatile organic compounds			
Hexane	10–15	2–5	<0.5
Benzene	20–40	5–7	1
Toluene	50–100	5–20	<2
Xylenes	50–100	2–20	<1
Ethyltoluene	20–40	2–10	<0.5
Aldehydes			
Formaldehyde	5–10	2–6	<1
Acetaldehyde	–	2–5	<1
Benzaldehyde	–	<1	<0.2

[a] Selection from more than 25 compounds subject to routine air quality monitoring.

A critical evaluation of the present air quality as it has been described led to the following results and strategies for future air quality monitoring:

1. The "clean-up" of the Rhine-Ruhr area, in former years termed the nation's black spot, is largely complete.
2. Air pollutants originating from road vehicles predominate and determine the amount and type of air pollution. Thus, air pollution in the Rhine-Ruhr area is no longer different from other urbanized, road vehicle traffic impacted, densely populated areas such as Frankfurt, Munich, Hamburg, Stuttgart, or Berlin.
3. Because of the political developments in 1990, which led to the unification of the former GDR on 3 October with the FRG, areas have to be

Table 4. Concentration of chlorinated hydrocarbons in ambient air[a] [annual average in 1989 ($\mu g/m^3$)]

Compound	Vicinity of dry cleaning shops or plants	Urban-industrialized area	Rural area ("background")
Dibromomethane	0.02–0.1	<0.1	<0.02
Trichloromethane	0.2–0.4	0.1–0.3	<0.1
Tetrachloromethane	0.6–0.7	0.4–0.8	<0.5
1,2-Dichloroethane	0.5–3	0.5–1	<1
1,1,1-Trichloromethane	1–15	1–3	<1
1,1,2-Trichloroethene	0.5–10	0.5–3	<0.3
Tetrachloroethene	5–1000	1–5	<0.5
Chlorobenzene	0.2	0.2	<0.2
Dichlorobenzenes	0.2	0.2–0.5	<0.2
Hexachlorobenzene	<0.3	<0.3	<0.05

[a] Selection from more than 20 compounds subject to routine air quality monitoring.

taken into consideration which are, in comparison with the "original" FRG, extremely polluted. Type and concentration level of air pollution in these new areas of the FRG correspond to those prevailing 30 years ago in the Rhine-Ruhr area. This has become apparent from data on the concentrations of SO_2 and other substances found in secret archives of the former GDR.

4. In these areas, many measures will be required over the next few years to bring air quality to the level we have in the Rhine-Ruhr area and the remaining area of the "original" FRG.

5. In the "original" areas, the following subjects have assumed priority:
   - Measurement, evaluation, and reduction of carcinogenic and highly toxic substances
   - Measurement and evaluation of anthropogenic ozone and reduction of its precursors nitrogen oxides and organic substances
   - Study of the development of substances exerting an influence on the climate and taking steps to reduce them
   - Stepping up measurement and evaluation of the deposition of lipophilic and persistent substances such as, for instance, chlorinated organic components and study of pathways (emission – atmosphere – deposition – soil – vegetation – animal – man)

6. With regard to comparability of the conditions of air quality and to applied air pollution control strategies in Europe, it can be roughly said that
   - in Western European countries they are similar to those in the "original" FRG
   - in Eastern European countries they are roughly similar to those in the former GDR

- in Southern European countries such as Greece or Spain they resemble the "original" FRG and the Western European countries as far as air pollution control strategies are concerned. The air quality, however, seems to be as insufficient as in Eastern European countries, at least as far as densely populated and industrialized areas are concerned.

References

1. Buck M, Ixfeld H, Ellermann K (1989) Bericht über die Ergebnisse der diskontinuierlichen Schwefeldioxid- und Mehrkomponenten-Messungen im Rhein-Ruhr-Gebiet für die Zeit vom 1.1.1981–31.12.1988. Schriftenreihe der Landesanstalt für Immissionsschutz, NRW, Essen (1989) 67:69–91 Cornelsen Schwann-Giradet, Düsseldorf
2. Manns H, Buck M (1990) Überwachungsstrategien für nicht-radioaktive Luft- schadstoffe. In: Proceedings der DAtF-Fachtagung: Schadstoffemissionen bei der Energiegewinnung, 24–25 Oct 1990, Bonn. Deutsches Atomforum, Bonn
3. Pfeffer H-U, Külske S, Beier R (1989) Ergebnisse aus dem Telemetrischen Immissionsmeßnetz TEMES in Nordrhein-Westfalen – TEMES-Jahresbericht 1989. Landesanstalt für Immissionsschutz, Nordrhein-Westfalen, Essen
4. Pfeffer H-U (1989) Immissionsbelastung durch Ozon in Nordrhein-Westfalen. In: Tätigkeitsbericht der Landesanstalt für Immissionsschutz 1989. Landesanstalt für Immissionsschutz, Nordrhein-Westfalen, Essen, pp 55–60
5. Buck M, Ellermann K (1988) Die Immissionsbelastung durch Benzol in Nordrhein-Westfalen. Landesanstalt für Immissionsschutz, Nordrhein-Westfalen, Essen (LIS-Bericht no. 82) (ISSN 0720-8499)
6. Kirschmer P (1990) Die Dioxin-Immissionsbelastung in Nordrhein-Westfalen. In: Tätigkeitsbericht der Landesanstalt für Immissionsschutz, Nordrhein-Westfalen 1990. Landesanstalt für Immissionsschutz, Nordrhein-Westfalen, Essen, pp 51–54 (ISSN 0931-5497)

Air Pollution in the Former German Democratic Republic: Consequences for Health Control

B. THRIENE

Landeshygieneinstitut Magdeburg, Wallonerberg 2–3, PF 1748, O-3010 Magdeburg, FRG

Introduction

The current problems for the natural environment and the continuing environmental burdens on humans are a cause for concern among the population in the former GDR. The report on the environment of the GDR published by the Ministry for the Environment, Nature Conservation, Energy, and Reactor Safety (Institut für Umweltschutz Berlin 1990), the reports by the State Hygiene Inspectorate of the Ministry for Health in the fields of air, water, and ground hygiene and local noise protection (Ministerium für Gesundheitswesen Berlin 1990) as well as the reports on the environment by the former counties edited by the County Hygiene Inspectorates and/or the State Inspectorates for the Environment (Bezirkshygieneinspektion und -institut Magdeburg 1990; Rat des Bezirkes Halle 1990) disclosed data and information on the state of the natural environment and hinted at possible links with health problems – these were the first data made public to the people of the GDR after 10 years of secrecy.

Two legal provisions were published in the law gazette of the GDR in November 1989 which made the disclosure of data on the environment possible and fixed the requirements for triggering smog alarms (Gesetzblatt 1989a,b). These regulations were a general demand by the grass-roots movement and took into account the urgent need for information on the state of the environment in the GDR.

Air Pollution

The environment in the GDR was considerably damaged by the structure of its source of energy, which is unique in the world. The country fulfilled 70% of its primary energy consumption by the extraction of 320 million tonnes of raw lignite; oil and natural gas amounted to 12% and 10%, respectively. As

U. Mohr et al. (Eds.)
Advances in Controlled Clinioal
Inhalation Studies
© Springer-Verlag Berlin Heidelberg 1993

a result, since the oil crisis in the early 1970s there has been a continuous increase in sulfur dioxide and dust emissions in the GDR, which included emissions from households and residential areas because of the strategy of replacing coke and gas by lignite. While, until recently, the GDR worked for the purpose of international treaties on the basis of an SO_2 emission of 4 million tons (a figure from 1978!), a peak of 5.6 million tons was reached in 1987. In addition to this, there were 2.3 million tons of dust.

The State Hygiene Inspectorate responsible for the monitoring and control of immissions states that because of wrong decisions in energy, location, and structural policy and a growing discrepancy between ecology and economy, no improvements in the air hygiene situation had been achieved in the past decade. Only the mild winters of 1988 and 1989 eased the situation to some degree.

With reference to the area of the country of 108 333 km^2 and a population of 16.709 million, pollutant emissions in 1989 were 5.2 million tons SO_2, 2.0 million tons dust, and 0.7 million tons NO_x. The large territorial variations in pollution are shown in Table 1. Hence, the GDR was by far the leader among European countries with regard to SO_2 and dust emission per inhabitant and year at 316 kg and 125 kg, respectively. The emission density for SO_2 was 49 tons/km^2 and for dust, 19 tons/km^2. These data led to an

Table 1. Pollutant emissions in the GDR by county (1989) (according to figures from the County Inspectorates for the Environment)

County	Area (km^2)	Inhabitants (×1000)	SO_2 (1000 tons)	Dust (1000 ktons)
Rostock	7075	902	66	43
Schwerin	8672	592	71	32
Neubrandenburg	10948	620	58	40
Potsdam	12568	1121	114	56
Frankfurt (Oder)	7186	707	127	116
Cottbus	8262	883	1368	436
Magdeburg	11526	1252	180	133
Halle	8771	1791	1054	446
Erfurt	7349	1236	221	119
Gera	4004	741	167	53
Suhl	3856	550	106	38
Dresden	6738	1776	396	216
Leipzig	4966	1378	954	225
Karl-Marx-Stadt	6009	1876	304	100
Berlin (East)	403	1284	70	27
GDR	108333	16709	5256	2018

unacceptably high immission load for 36.6% of the population for SO_2 and 26.3% for dust, which gave evidence that the legally prescribed maximum immission concentrations (MIC values) were exceeded in the land register areas over the calendar year. In the counties of Halle, Karl-Marx-Stadt, and Leipzig, as much as 73.3%, 76.5%, and 87%, respectively, of the population were subjected to an unacceptably high SO_2 load; 2%, 9.6%, and 27.7% of the citizens, respectively, received an SO_2 load level of 5 (very seriously overloaded). In these cases, the figures were 2.5 times higher than the MIC value of 0.15 mg of SO_2/m^3 on an arithmetic mean!

Table 2 gives an extract from the MIC and TIL (technical immission limit) values for the GDR. For pollutants with a carcinogenic effect, TIL values have been laid down, as according to the WHO medically justified threshold values cannot be established (Gesetzblatt 1987a,b).

The trend towards higher values for other pollutants continued in the big cities of the GDR, as can be seen from those recorded for NO_x (708 000 tonnes, 300 000 tonnes of which are emitted by motor vehicles). Pollution by CO, phenol, and H_2S exceeded the limit values in the city centers as a result of motor traffic and domestic heating. In the vicinity of the lignite processing plants in the counties of Leipzig and Cottubs, pollution level 5 occurred (Böhlen, Espenhain, Schwarze Pumpe), and a considerable odor nuisance was caused over an extensive area.

In 1989, the Meteorological Service measured the highest daily mean

Table 2. Maximum immission concentration (MIC) values of selected pollutants

	MIC_S (mg/m³)	MIC_L (mg/m³)
Ammonia	0.2	0.004
Asbestos[a]	0.005	–
Benzene[a]	0.3	0.1
Cadmium and its compounds calculated as Cd	–	0.00005
Chlorine	0.1	0.03
Gaseous F compounds (HF, SiF_4) calculated as F	0.02	0.005
Carbon monoxide	5.0	3.0
Phenol	0.01	0.003
Sulfur dioxide	0.5	0.15
Hydrogen sulfide	0.015	0.008
Dust (nontoxic)	0.5	0.15
Nitrogen oxides calculated as NO_2	0.1	0.04
Tetrachloroethane[a]	0.5	0.06

Source: Gesetzblatt (1987a).
[a] TIL values.
MIC_S, short-term; MIC_L, long-term limit.

value for ozone on Mount Fichtelberg at $0.196\,mg/m^3$ and in the town of Meiningen at $0.171\,mg/m^3$ (Institut für Umweltschutz Berlin 1990). In the summer of 1990, the guide or warning value for ozone of $0.180\,mg/m^3$, set by the Conference of the Federal Ministers for the Environment, was frequently exceeded in the centers of the big cities for a period of several hours a day. The major cause was the massive increase in traffic after the opening of the borders and the purchase of cheap second-hand cars without catalyst technology.

Moreover, there is also a considerable air pollution load in the areas around the chemical combines in the center of the country at Bitterfeld, Leuna, and Merseburg, the metallurgical works of the Mansfeld combine (nonferrous metals), locations of iron metallurgy, as well as plants of the lime and cement industries, viscose staple fiber and artificial silk manufacture, and the asbestos cement industry, which all have a more local effect.

The emissions described have in the past frequently led to smog episodes in the conurbations of the GDR. Until the political turnaround in November 1989, smog was not a public topic in the GDR. The Environmental Data Order was a decisive prerequisite for the Smog Order passed in November 1989 (Gesetzblatt 1989a,b). Similarities to the Orders of the Federal States existed in the three smog levels and in the trigger criteria for SO_2 as well as the determination of 20 smog danger areas.

The inhabitants of the affected areas were informed through the local press and regional programs of the broadcasting services about the alarm levels as well as the current and anticipated levels of pollution. Recommendations on how to act under smog conditions were part of this information. Special public information and advisory services were set up in health offices but also in outpatient departments and local authorities and announced via the media (Thriene 1991).

Although the Smog Order of the former GDR from 2 November 1989 is outdated, a new one on the basis of the model draft for a smog order (Conference of Ministers for the Environment 1984) cannot be put into practice in the short term, as the prerequisites in the field of organisation and instrumentation are still lacking and will only be available for the entire territory in 1991/92. Consequently, the smog levels and behavioral recommendations of the old Smog Order are applicable and binding in the form of a transitional order on smog (Gesetz- und Verordnungsblatt für das Land Sachsen-Anhalt 1990).

The New Energy Policy

Due to the fact that the smog conditions in the cities of the former GDR were mainly caused by decentralized fireplaces, domestic heating, and small industries, the centralization of heat supply, rational application of energy, and optimum availability of low-emission energy sources are, therefore, also demanded by the Public Health Service as an urgent requirement for prophylactic health care.

The government of the GDR had adopted a new energy policy which aimed to reduce the energy demand by a change in the structure of energy sources and the abolition of subsidies, i.e., a new price and tariff system. Among the measures planned were a reduction of lignite production and an increase in coal and coke imports as well as increasing natural gas imports. This not only included the completion of the 4000-MW nuclear power station at Stendal and the increased use of renewable energy sources, but also thermal insulation programs for pipelines and buildings, energy-saving household appliances, and waste heat recovery, which had to form part of a policy of saving energy.

Through the use of gas and district heating, the number of coal-heated dwellings in the East German federal states is to be substantially reduced from the current 65%. However, first of all the simplest technical requirements for temperature control in dwellings and public buildings must be provided in order to counteract the squandering of energy. In addition, there is the closure of carbo-chemical, chlorine gas, and carbide production works enforced by the citizens as well as the installation of boilers in which raw lignite is burned by the circulated fluidized bed principle, as well as the fundamental movement towards power-heat coupling (at present only 5%) which will lead to an appreciable reduction in emissions. In 1990, the closure of plants and the general decline in production had the greatest share in this reduction.

The New Legal Situation

At the end of May 1990, the joint environmental commission of the two German states drew up the outline of a basic law on the environment to harmonize the legal provisions of environmental protection. In the legislative intent of the law (Gesetzblatt 1990) passed in the People's Chamber at the end of June, reference was made to the fact that the environmental union between the two German states aimed at in the Treaty of 18 May 1990 on the creation of a monetary, economic and social union between the GDR and the FRG, will be characterized by the basic idea of a comprehensive protection of man and environment, effective environmental safeguards, and the guarantee of an environmental compatibility test for projects. To the areas of immission control, nuclear safety and radiation protection, water and waste management, legislation for chemicals, nature conservation and care of the countryside, as well as an environmental compatibility test, the law contains appropriate harmonization regulations which were to facilitate the rapid adoption of the most important parts of the environmental legislation of the FRG in the GDR. The existing regulations of the FRG have been applicable since 1 July 1990 when the treaty came into effect and became law for the territory of the GDR from 3 October 1990 with the accession of the GDR in accordance with article 23 of the Constitution; these regulations were specified in two annexes to the law.

Epidemiological Environmental Research – A Task for the Health Service

With the restoration of the 5 new Federal States to the territory of the FRG and the formation of Regional Institutes for Hygiene and Regional Authorities for Environmental Protection, health-related and technical environmental protection will be separated and reorganized, although very relevant arguments speak against this, such as the unity of measurement and assessment or the possible examination – despite the technical limitations in the Institutes for Hygiene – of biological, chemical, and physical parameters including radioactivity of air, water, ground, foodstuffs, etc. Likewise, the teamwork by doctors, chemists, physicists, biologists, and technicians would be at its best under these conditions. Thus, the new approach to a complex supervision of the environment and health under the responsibility of several ministries is, at present, endangered rather than free to develop naturally after the political turnaround and requires a higher level of co-ordination and cooperation.

In 1990, inter-German working groups agreed upon immediate environment-related epidemiological investigations in the five new Bundes-länder (Federal States). Projects for research and development (health survey, environmental survey) have been presented to the respective minis-tries and in some cases have already begun with priority studies (Bitterfeld).

The development of efficient environment-related epidemiological research brings with it a powerful apparatus for prophylactic medicine and the early detection of illness, which must be set up as an attractive medical discipline and encouraged as such. Thus, epidemiological cross-sectional and longitudinal studies would be very useful to furnish proof of the exposure-effect relationship between SO_2 and other air pollutants and damage to health at various locations. The state of health of the population and especially of risk groups can be examined and compared with values as-certained in the original Bundesländer.

The life expectancy of the people presents the most important indicator of the state of health (Table 3).

The GDR increased the mean life expectancy by 6.2 years for men and 8.4 years for women in 1989 as compared with 1952, but still took place 17 with 69.5 years for men and place 18 for women with 75.4 years in 1985 among a listing of 24 European countries (FRG: place 12 with 71.3 years for men and place 11 for women with 78.1 years). The stagnation in the life expectancy of men even brought the GDR down to place 22 for the age group of 65-year-olds (Kant 1988; Statistisches Jahrbuch der DDR 1990). This development commenced for men only after 1975; before this date the

Table 3. Development of life expectancy in the GDR from 1952–1989

Life expectancy from age (years)	1952	1960	1970	1980	1985	1989	Increase (years)
Male							
0	63.9	66.5	68.1	68.7	69.5	70.1	+6.2
1	67.3	68.5	68.5	68.7	69.3	69.8	+2.5
15	54.9	55.4	55.1	55.1	55.7	56.1	+1.2
45	27.6	27.7	27.4	27.3	27.8	28.1	+0.5
65	12.6	12.4	11.9	12.1	12.4	12.9	+0.3
Female							
0	68.0	71.4	73.3	74.6	75.4	76.4	+8.4
1	70.7	72.7	73.5	74.4	75.1	75.8	+5.1
15	58.0	59.6	60.0	60.7	61.4	62.1	+4.1
45	30.3	31.2	31.3	31.9	32.5	33.1	+2.8
65	13.8	14.3	14.4	14.9	15.3	15.9	+2.1

GDR even had higher life expectancy figures. The lead in life expectancy in the FGR amounted to 2.3 years for men and 2.9 years for women in 1987.

If we frankly discuss the causes today, then the overall social conditions play a decisive role. Because of the better circumstances than in the original FRG as far as the number of road deaths is concerned, and because of a strictly organized program of vaccination eliminating children's diseases to a large extent, and the infant mortality rate being roughly comparable with that in the FRG, the problems of overfeeding and false nutrition as well as failure to cope with stress gain in importance. The high degree of employment among women, eagerness to watch Western TV programs, as well as the lack of facilities to satisfy leisure needs limited well-known forms of communication, mass physical recreation, etc.

At the same time, the living conditions of elderly people are a crucial factor. Suicide rates twice as high as in the FRG draw attention to the social factors of quality of life and the living environment; they are an expression of social stagnation and social isolation, the latter being an aspect of mass housing construction and poor socioeconomic conditions. Wiesner draws attention to the additional factor of lack of religious or personal commitment and, consequently, a lack of strong and sound convictions and resulting activity patterns (Wiesner 1990).

So-called avoidable deaths from cardiovascular diseases, hypertension, respiratory tract infections, carcinomas, and appendicitis, among others, were 4.6 times more frequent in the GDR than in the FRG. This fact alludes to the quality of medical care, including possibilities for the extensive use of diagnostic, and therapeutic facilities, and in this connection especially the advanced equipment and the availability of pharmaceuticals, various materials, benefit services, etc., that is to say, possibilities for therapeutic intervention for the prevention of mortality in these cases.

In this respect, the contribution by environmental pollution can be speculated on; however, no comprehensive scientific statement can be made so far. Investigations made by Thielebeule and Grindel (1991) in children's groups in the Bitterfeld area revealed double the rate for respiratory tract illnesses than in the county of Halle. They found for blood test results, FEV, vital capacity, and bone growth, among others, significant deviations from groups in control areas which could be positively influenced for the long term by convalescence stays in clean air areas. However, the life expectancy for men in Bitterfeld takes 5th place among 23 districts of the county of Halle, and the cancer rate is no higher there than it is in Rostock or Wismar. Does this mean that workers in the chemical industry form a special group of the population? Are health criteria instrumental to the choice of location and occupation? Are health and social surroundings of large companies and conurbations perhaps more favorable than the atmosphere in the villages? The backwardness of the latter in development compared with the original Bundesländer meets with less notice than is the case with cities, but which is perhaps even greater? In any case, there existed noticeable differences in life expectancy between the counties (Table 4), and the rural areas of the north have had the worse position for years compared with the conurbations of the central and southern areas (Statistisches Jahrbuch der DDR 1990).

Examinations made by Bredel and Herbarth (1989) in Leipzig point to an influence of air pollution on mortality as well as on diseases of the respiratory tracts and cardiovascular system. Smog in Leipzig was a

Table 4. Life expectancy in the GDR by county 1988/1989

Counties	Men (years)	Women (years)
Rostock	69.13	76.23
Schwerin	68.8	76.41
Neubrandenburg	68.27	75.99
Potsdam	69.67	75.89
Frankfurt/Oder	69.08	75.83
Cottbus	69.33	75.81
Magdeburg	69.40	75.50
Halle	69.66	76.11
Erfurt	70.24	75.97
Gera	71.11	76.54
Suhl	69.81	75.64
Dresden	70.90	77.11
Leipzig	70.42	76.44
Karl-Marx-Stadt	70.68	76.52
Berlin (East)	71.19	76.24
GDR	70.03	76.23

perennial topic in winter, with the pollutant loads verging on that of the London smog catastrophe of 1952. Comparison of the daily mean death rate during smog periods with those of the previous and following periods showed an appreciable increase in overall mortality with the known delay of about 1 day. However, disruptive incidences which interfer with medical examinations such as the vigors of the weather and virus circulation are also commonly realized. It is still wishful thinking that one can detect significant exposure-effect relationships between air pollutants and health impairment.

Moreover, reference should be made to investigations carried out in Magdeburg in the 1980s during longer smog episodes. In these cases a relative increase could always be observed in cardiovascular and respiratory tract diseases needing emergency medical attention, whereby the weekly course of activity by the emergency doctors is marked by a rise at the weekends due to medical practices being closed on Saturdays and Sundays. Influenza epidemics also appear to be much more dramatic. Therefore, investigations should focus predominantly on high-risk groups and should be oriented to the eastern part of the FRG. As it is difficult with the present concentration of pollutants in the original FRG states to furnish definite proof of any health damage caused by smog, values from more polluted areas in the former GDR could be drawn on for comparison to support existing theses (M. Csicsaky, personal communication).

A cooperative relationship between the Medical Institute for Environmental Hygiene at Düsseldorf University and the State Hygiene Institute in Magdeburg has enabled cross-sectional and longitudinal studies for the year 1990/1991, aiming to quantify the correlation between air pollution and health problems among some 4000 children and 100 people with previous health impairments living in Magdeburg, Wernigerode, Halle, and Leipzig compared with a control area in the Altmark region. The results will be soon available. Participation of the people approached was over 90%. In my opinion, this is our big and, perhaps, last chance to use the territory of the former GDR with currently still high environmental pollution loads for an incontestable statement on their relevance to health.

Alongside illness and death, another aspect should be assessed or taken into consideration. In the case of long-term effects of environmental factors on the organism, the latter's abilities for regulation can be pathologically distorted. This applies to the nervous system, functions of the immune system, lung cleansing mechanism, etc. Data collected point to special demands on the mechanism for adaptation, ranging from tolerance through depression to stimulation. In most cases, only the physiological range of the clinical parameters is exhausted. However, as at the present state of knowledge these changes can not often yet be interpreted, they must be considered – as is the case when substantiating limiting or guide line values – as a consequence of exceeding these limits and must not meet with acceptance of any kind.

30   B. Thriene: Air Pollution in the Former German Democratic Republic

References

Bezirks-Hygieneinspektion und -institut Magdeburg (1990) Umwelthygienischer Jahresbericht des Bezirkes Magdeburg 1989
Bredel H, Herbarth O (1989) Epidemiologische Untersuchungen zur akuten Wirkung von Luftverunreinigungen. Schriftenr Gesundh Umwelt 5(3):10 Forschungsinstitut für Hygiene und Mikrobiologie, Bad Elster
Gesetzblatt (1987a) Erste Durchführungsbestimmung zur Fünften Durchführungs- verordnung zum Landeskulturgesetz – Reinhaltung der Luft – Begrenzung, Überwachung und Kontrolle der Immissionen vom 12.2.1987. Gesetzblatt I no. 7:56
Gesetzblatt (1987b) Fünfte Durchführungsverordnung zum Landeskulturgesetz – Reinhaltung der Luft – vom 12.2.1987. Gesetzblatt I no. 7:51
Gesetzblatt (1989a) Verordnung über Umweltdaten vom 13.11.1989. Gesetzblatt I no. 22:241
Gesetzblatt (1989b) Vierte Durchführungsbestimmung zur Fünften Durchführungs- verordnung zum Landeskulturgesetz – Reinhaltung der Luft – Smogordnung vom 2.11.1989. Gesetzblatt I no. 21:239
Gesetzblatt (1990) Umweltrahmengesetz der DDR vom 29.6.1990. Gesetzblatt I no. 42:649
Gesetz- und Verordnungsblatt für das Land Sachsen-Anhalt (1990) Smog- Übergangsverordnung vom 17.12.1990 Gesetz- und Verordnungsblatt für das Land Sachsen-Anhalt no. 1
Institut für Umweltschutz Berlin (ed) (1990) Umweltbericht der DDR. Visuell, Berlin
Kant H (1988) Zur Lebenserwartung in Europa – Fakten, Tendenzen, Ziele. Z ges Hyg 34:442
Ministerium für Gesundheitswesen Berlin (1990) Berichte der Staatlichen Hygieneinspektion über die Situation auf den Gebieten der Lufthygiene, Wasserhygiene, Bodenhygiene, kommunalen Lärmbelastung und -bekämpfung 1989 in der DDR
Rat des Bezirkes Halle (1990) Umweltbericht des Bezirkes Halle 1989
Statistisches Jahrbuch der DDR (1990) Haufe, Berlin
Thielebeule U, Grindel B (1991) Sofortprogramm Bitterfeld – Versuch einer komplexen Einschätzung des Gesundheitszustandes einer extrem umweltbelasteten Bevölkerung. Frühjahrstagung der Deutschen Gesellschaft für Hygiene und Mikrobiologie, Berlin, 14–15 March 1991
Thriene B (1991) Die lufthygienische Situation in der DDR – Situation und Erfordernisse. Öff Gesundheitswes 53:54
Wiesner GE (1990) Zur Gesundheitslage der beiden Bevölkerungsteile DDR und BRD – ein Ausdruck sozialer Ungleichheit? In: Thiele W (ed) Das Gesundheitswesen der DDR: Aufbruch oder Einbruch? Asgard, Sankt Augustin

The Outdoor Environment in North America

Exposure to Oxidant Gases and Acidic Particles in the United States

P. J. Lioy

Robert Wood Johnson Medical School, Univ. of Med. & Dentistry of New Jersey,
Dept. of Environmental and Community Med., 675 Hoes Lane, Piscataway, NJ
08854-5635, USA

Introduction

Primary public health issues associated with air pollution in the United
States involve ozone (and other oxidants), toxic organic substances, and
possibly acidic particles. The precursor pollutant sources are common for
oxidants and acid aerosols, and each can accumulate in urban and rural
areas. National Ambient Air Quality Standards (NAAQS) presently exist
for ozone (O_3), the nitrogen oxides, carbon monoxide, particulate matter,
sulfur dioxide, and lead. There are none for sulfuric acid, even though there
is a World Health Organization (WHO) (1985) guideline for that substance.
The US EPA (1988) is evaluating the need for a standard. Other oxidant
gases, such as formaldehyde (HCHO) and nitric acid (HNO_3), do not have
standards. The WHO (1985), however, has guidelines for HCHO.

There are two types of atmospheric conditions associated with the
accumulation of acidic species and oxidant gases (US EPA 1985, 1988). The
first is defined as photochemical air pollution. It occurs in and downwind of
urban areas during the summertime and produces high concentrations of O_3
(peaks ranging from 200 to 500 ppb), and virtually all oxidant gases and
acidic aerosol can be found (Cleveland et al. 1976; Cobourn and Husar
1982; Martinez and Singh 1979; Paul et al. 1987; Tuazon et al. 1981; US
PEA 1985; Vukovich and Fishman 1982; Wolff and Lioy 1980; Wolff et al.
1982). The second type is known as a reducing sulfurous atmospheric smog
(Lodge 1969; Waller and Lawther 1957). In the USA we rarely see sulfurous
smog today, but this type of episode highlighted the need for regulations on
soft coal use in the early 1950s in London, UK, and in Donora, Pennsylvania
(US EPA 1988). Today, sulfurous smog is possible in industrialized parts of
the world, such as eastern Europe and China, that use high-sulfur coal as
the primary fuel. A summary of the characteristics of these types of air
pollution is found in Table 1.

The exposure patterns for individuals or the general population will be
different for each type of episode since they occur during different times of

U. Mohr et al. (Eds.)
Advances in Controlled Clinical
Inhalation Studies
© Springer-Verlag Berlin Heidelberg 1993

Table 1. Characteristics of sulfurous smog and photochemical air pollution

Item	Sulfurous smog	Photochemical air pollution
Primary emissions	SO_2, soot from coal burning	NO_x, nonmethane hydrocarbons from automobiles, etc.
Dominant mechanisms	Liquid droplet and catalytic	Photochemistry and liquid droplet
Major secondary products	H_2SO_4 and neutralized sulfate salts, organic particles, carbon, sulfonic acid, CO	Ozone, nitric acid, H_2SO_4 and salts, aldehydes, organic particles, HONO
Temperature	Cool (<55°F)	Hot (>75°F)
Relative humidity	High, usually fog	Usually low in California, varies in eastern USA
Inversion	Radiation (ground, nocturnal)	Subsidence (high pressure system)
Pollution peaks	Early morning and overnight	Afternoon and evening

the year and reflect a variety of activity patterns, e.g. outdoor exercise, vacations, and school (Lioy and Dyba 1988; Lippmann 1989; Mage et al. 1985; Paul et al. 1987). The highest exposures are anticipated during photochemical air pollution episodes, since people spend more time outdoors during the summer. The fall or winter are conducive to producing sulfurous episodes. These exposures depend upon the duration of outdoor activities and outdoor air penetration into structures (Yocum 1982).

The following features these two types of outdoor air pollution. The potential population exposure during episodes will be examined both in terms of the magnitude of the concentrations and the length of time during which the population would experience high concentrations of oxidant gases and/or acidic species.

Photochemical Air Pollution: Oxidant Gases and Acidic Particles

Ozone

The mechanisms of ozone and other oxidant formation have been identified in laboratory chamber studies and in simulation modeling (Atkinson and Lloyd 1984; Finlayson-Pitts and Pitts 1976; Graedel et al. 1976; Jeffries et al. 1981; US EPA 1985). Formation is initiated by the NO_2 sunlight reaction (λ 320 nm) after sunrise. The reactant species in photochemical air pollution include nitrogen oxides and nonmethane hydrocarbons (NMHC). Each will react with various compounds and free radical species according to the type of compounds emitted into the atmosphere. The sources of NMHC are motor vehicles, large and small stationary sources, commercial activities, and personal products. The main classes are the alkenes, alkanes, alkynes, and aromatics (Finlayson-Pitts and Pitts 1976). Individual compounds will have different rates of reaction with oxidizing materials in the atmosphere, although as a class the alkenes (olefins) are the most reactive compounds. The sources of nitrogen oxides include various types of combustion: automobile, trucks, and stationary sources, i.e., power plants (US EPA 1985).

The formation of photochemical air pollution is closely coupled with meteorology. The nature of O_3 accumulation is highly dependent upon (a) concentration of O_3 precursors leaving a source area, (b) induction time, (c) turbulent mixing, (d) wind speed and wind direction, (e) depletion of reactants and products during transport, (f) injection of new emissions along the trajectory of an air mass, and (g) local and synoptic weather conditions.

Oxidants formed in the atmosphere have the potential for polluting areas at great distances downwind from the precursor pollutant sources (Cleveland et al. 1976; Finlayson-Pitts and Pitts 1976; Jeffries et al. 1981). They can accumulate to high levels downwind in suburban and rural areas. Little NO_2 is necessary to continue the cycle in a photochemically reactive atmosphere. Therefore, the compounds can be transported and accumulate over large areas. This is based in part on the daily emissions of nitrogen oxides by automobile and truck traffic on interstate highways across the eastern USA (US EPA 1985; Wolff et al. 1982; Wolff and Lioy 1980). A virtual "ozone river" was described from the Gulf coast through to the Northeast during 1977 when many monitors recorded daily maximum levels of $O_3 > 100$ ppb on 1 or more days (Wolff and Lioy 1980). The transport of oxidants to different urban and rural areas will, in fact, range from urban to synoptic scale (Table 2) (US EPA 1985). The extent of accumulation of oxidant species can range from <10 km to thousands of km during a particular photochemical smog episode.

Ozone Exposure

Paul et al. (1987) used the features of mesoscale O_3 and oxidant production to estimate human exposure within urban locations in the USA. Incremental, microenvironmental exposure is determined by the equation:

$$E_k = \sum_{j=1}^{n} C_{ij} t_{jk}$$

where E_k is exposure of k_{th} individual, C_{ij} is the concentration of the i_{th} species at times t_j, and t_{jk}, is the time of the j_{th} exposure for the k_{th} individual.

Their results showed that on any given day in urbanized areas 13 million moderately exercising people could be affected by O_3 above the NAAQS

34   P.J. Lioy

Table 2. Transport regimes associated with summertime ozone accumulation

Regime	Characteristics
Urban scale	Occurs in most large urban areas (Los Angeles, New York, Houston, St. Louis, etc.)
	Simple advection of photochemically reactive air and local wind patterns
	O_3 and oxidants found after 1 or 2 h
	Maximum concentrations 20 miles from precursor emissions area
Mesoscale scale	Development of urban plume
	Includes O_3, oxidants, and precursors
	Sea breeze and overnight transport (Los Angeles basin, Washington to Boston corridor)
	O_3 and oxidants extend 100–200 miles, and the area can include thousands of square miles
Synoptic scale	Widespread increases in ozone above 100 ppb
	Generally occurs with slow moving, high-pressure, or anticyclone systems; weak winds and stable surface layers
	Includes from 1000 to >100 000 square miles

Adapted from text in US EPA Criteria Document (Ozone, 1985, vol. II).

(120 ppb for 1 h) for at least 1 h. Exercising is emphasized since the most significant transient O_3 health effects are associated with exercising individuals (Folinsbee et al. 1988; Lioy et al. 1985; Lippmann 1989; McDonnell et al. 1983). The extent of the O_3 problem is significant since 101 metropolitan areas were in violation of the NAAQS in 1988 (US EPA 1990).

In addition to the high 1-h O_3 peak, Lioy and Dyba (1988), Berglund et al. (1988), and Rombout et al. (1986) have shown that because of the nature of O_3 production and transport, O_3 will accumulate to levels that can be in excess of the NAAQS or at least in excess of 100 ppb for multiple hours during the day. In some cases, the concentrations will be above 100 ppb for at least 8 h, which is significant, since this exposure is above the occupational Threshold Limit Value (TLV). The preceding suggests that people who exercise or participate in outdoor activities have many opportunities to be exposed to single or multiple hours of higher levels of O_3 and other oxidants during the day. This concept is not typical of the traditional approaches of air pollution identification, exposure, and control. A traditional strategy would assume that the highest exposures occur near the source and during peak emission periods. Traditional air pollution includes volatile organic compounds and carbon monoxide.

High concentrations of O_3 can persist for 2–21 days depending upon the particular location (US EAP 1985). Fig. 1 shows a 3-day episode at Montague, Massachusetts, when O_3 was above the NAAQS for a number of hours during the day and evening and above the 8-h TLV each day (Martinez and Singh 1979).

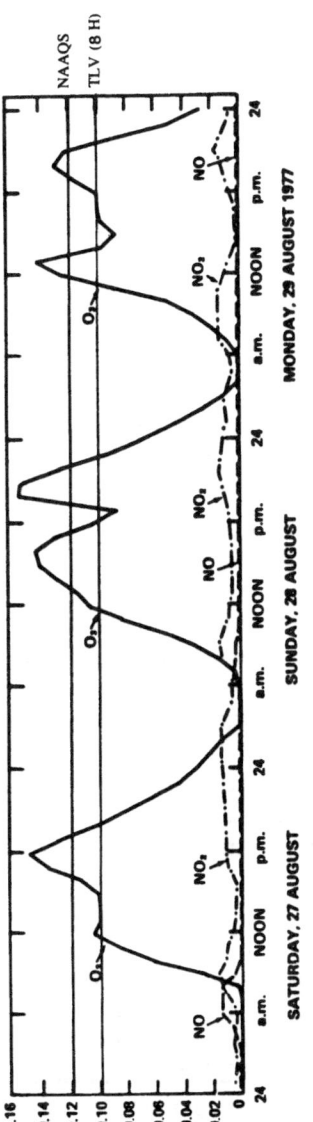

Fig. 1. Three-day sequence of hourly ozone concentrations at Montague, Massachusetts. SURE station showing locally generated midday peaks and transported late peaks. (Adapted from Martinez and Singh 1979)

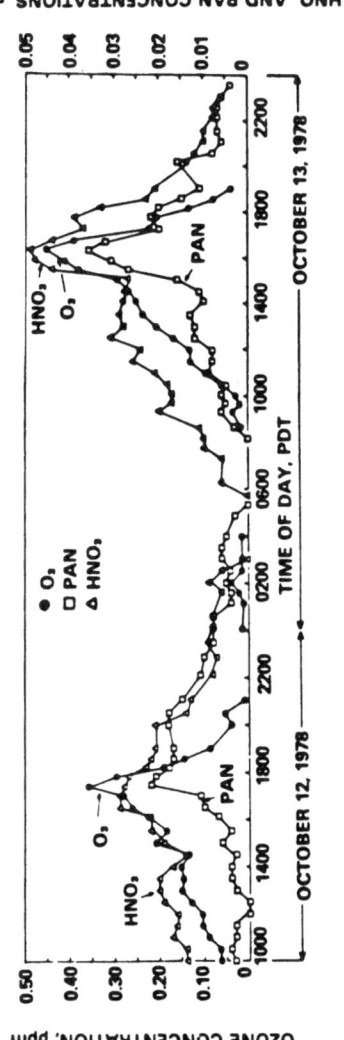

Fig. 2. Diurnal profiles of ozone and PAN at Claremont, California, October 12 and 13, 1978, 2 days of a midday smog episode. (Reproduced with permission from Tuazon et al. 1981)

Exposure/dose calculations were completed by Lioy and Dyba (1989) for 4 consecutive days in Mendham, New Jersey, with O_3 concentrations above 100 ppb for at least 8 h each day. The estimated dose delivered to a typical summer camper was based on activities and their duration and estimates of the minute ventilation and deposition of O_3 in the lung. The results were compared with a dose estimate for adult volunteers who participated in 6.6 h of moderate exercise at 120 ppb O_3 and indicated that a camper received about the same dose as the volunteers (Folinsbee et al. 1988).

Other Oxidants

Other components of photochemical air pollution include NO_2, aldehydes, peroxyacetyl nitrate (PAN), and HNO_3. Except for NO_2, only limited data are available on the presence of these compounds in the atmosphere. PAN and aldehydes usually have much lower values than O_3 (Spicer et al. 1983, Tuazon et al. 1981; US EPA 1985). The PAN/O_3 ratio ranges from 0.01 to 0.20 (US EPA 1985). Aldehydes average 50 ppb, with HCHO being the most abundant compound; however, aldehyde concentrations >100 ppb can occur with indoor emissions from particle board and insulation (Samet et al. 1988). HNO_3 concentrations have only recently been measured reliably, but the limited data suggest that peaks of greater than 50 ppb can occur (US EPA 1988). In some cases, it appears that PAN and HNO_3 follow the diurnal O_3 cycle, but the concentrations persist into the evening (Fig. 2) (Tuazon et al. 1981). The concentrations of PAN measured in rural areas appear to be quite low, suggesting that higher population exposures will occur closer to the sources of precursor compounds.

One area with short-term high NO_2 levels is the Los Angeles basin. The peak concentrations of NO_2 occur during the morning and the late afternoon and range from 100 to 800 ppb (US EPA 1985). The outdoor peaks occur at a different time of day than those of O_3 and other oxidants. Recent work on indoor air pollution, however, indicates that annual and peak NO_3 exposures to most individuals are primarily associated with indoor emissions of NO_2 from gas stoves and other combustion sources (Yocum 1982).

Acid Sulfates

Acid sulfates are produced from the oxidation of SO_2. This occurs primarily at an SO_2 homogeneous oxidation rate of 1.5%/h (Calvert and Stockwell 1983), but the rate can increase substantially for liquid droplet reactions in fog (Gillani et al. 1981, 1983). The species sulfuric acid, ammonium bisulfate, and ammonium sulfate have been measured at a number of locations in North America using different analytical methods (US EPA 1988).

Acidic and neutralized species can range in concentration from 0 to $50\,\mu g/m^3$ at a particular location or at a number of locations simultaneously (Appel et al. 1982; Cadle 1985; Cobourn et al. 1982; Ellestad 1980; Lioy and Lippmann 1986; Lioy et al. 1980, 1987; Lyons and Olsson 1972; Pierson et al. 1980; Tanner and Marlow 1977; Tanner et al. 1981; US EPA 1988; Waldman et al. 1990; Wolff et al. 1982). Some of the highest levels have been observed in Glasgow, Illinois, downwind of the St. Louis, Missouri, urban plume ($39\,\mu g/m^3$ average for 12 h), in Dunsville, Ontario, Canada, ($46\,\mu g/m^3$ for 4 h), in Highpoint, New Jersey ($>10\,\mu g/m^3$ for 6 h over consecutive days), in the Allegheny Mountains, Pennsylvania ($30\,\mu g/m^3$), in the Laurel Mountains, Pennsylvania ($42\,\mu g/m^3$), and in Uniontown, Pennsylvania ($39.4\,\mu g/m^3$); all are downwind of the regional SO_2 emissions from coal-fired power plants in the eastern USA (Lioy et al. 1980; Pierson et al. 1980; Raizenne et al. 1989; Tanner and Marlow 1977; Spengler et al. 1990). These acid sulfates are found primarily in the fine particle size range ($<2.5\,\mu m$ in diameter).

Summertime acidic sulfate levels can increase to above $20\,\mu g/m^3$ for an hour or so, or it can be sustained at relatively high concentrations (10–$20\,\mu g/m^3$) for 6–24 h at one or more sites. Studies have shown that acid sulfates are produced during the initial phase of a photochemical air pollution episode but are neutralized to $(NH_4)_2SO_4$ by local ground level ammonia emissions (Cobourn and Husar 1982; Morandi et al. 1983). Depending upon the physical and/or chemical processes of neutralization and production in the atmosphere, however, the acid concentrations can vary from day to day.

Acid Sulfate Exposure

Our knowledge of acidic sulfate exposure is not as clearly defined as for O_3, since there are no routine monitoring networks (US EPA 1988). However, the available data are consistent in suggesting that in the summer acidic sulfates can achieve concentrations and exposures [($\mu g/m^3$) per h] which are similar to those shown to have effects on mucociliary clearance in the lungs of clinical volunteers and/or animals (Koenig et al. 1983; Lippmann 1985; Schlesinger 1985; Gearhart and Schlesinger, 1989; Schlesinger et al. 1983; US EPA 1988). Clinical effects at H_2SO_4 levels of $100\,\mu g/m^3$) per h have shown that exposures longer than 1 h will enhance, not just add to, the effect (Spektor et al. 1989; US EPA 1988). Lioy and Waldman (1989) and Spengler et al. (1989) have estimated that local population exposures during specific summertime episodes can reach above $300\,\mu g/m^3$ per h. Spengler et al. (1989) estimated the acid sulfate dose inhaled by the campers at Dunsville, Ontario, during an episode and calculated values similar to those inhaled during clinical studies (Koenig et al. 1983; US EPA 1985).

Speizer (1989) has shown that the annual average hydrogen ion concentrations are correlated with the prevalence of bronchitis rates for 10–12-year-old children in four cities of Harvard's six-city study (Kingston, Tennessee; Steubenville, Ohio; St. Louis, Missouri; Portage, Wisconsin). The peak annual average was approximately only $1.8\,\mu g/m^3$ (as H_2SO_4). Spengler et al. (1989) showed that the peaks occurred during the summertime in each city.

Sulfurous Smog Episodes

There are qualitative and quantitative analyses (Commins and Waller 1967; Lodge 1969; US EPA 1988; Waller and Lawther 1957) of conditions that existed when soft, high-sulfur coal was burned in London from the 13th century through the 1950s. Control measures to reduce the emissions of SO_2 and particulate matter were, however, not introduced until after the December 1952 episode, when an estimated 4000 people died. Ito and Thurston (1987) retrieved acidic sulfate data measured in the London area during the late 1950s, 1960s, and early 1970s, which was after the smoke control order of 1954. They observed that during this interval the annual acid sulfate concentration averaged above $10\,\mu g/m^3$, with relatively few peaks $>20\,\mu g/m^3$. These annual averages exceeded those in the Harvard six cities by greater than a factor of five (Speizer 1989). It can be expected that the levels were higher in 1952.

The mechanisms of acidic sulfate formation in the winter are quite different from those in the summer. Laboratory and theoretical studies have suggested that sulfuric acid is produced by the catalytic reaction of SO_2 with a transition element (e.g., manganese) in the presence of fog. The magnitude of the H_2SO_4 concentrations are coupled to SO_2 emissions from coal-burning for space heating, oil-burning for space heating, high-sulfur oil-burning for space heating, and local industrial processes. Increases of acid sulfates in the wintertime and the late fall will be associated with atmospheric inversions (radiative), since there is usually fog formation and the concurrent build-up of SO_2 and soot in the atmosphere. Liquid droplet chemistry enhances the oxidation of SO_2 to H_2SO_4 at rates higher than 5%/h SO_2 oxidation. The area affected will probably be more limited than in the summertime, since only micro- and mesoscale plumes develop.

Relatively few measurements have been made of the acidic aerosol concentration present in urban and rural areas during the winter. The measurements available in the USA show that the frequency of acidic sulfate events is reduced and their duration much shorter ($<6\,h$) than in summer. The average concentrations are also much lower, but the peak values can exceed $30\,\mu g/m^3$ (Cobourn and Husar 1982; Spengler et al. 1989; EPA 1990). Data collected in 6 cities found no daily H_2SO_4 level above $5\,\mu g/m^3$ during the winter for 1986–1987 (Spengler et al. 1990). Future studies need to be conducted in high-sulfur coal-burning countries to obtain a better understanding of the accumulation of wintertime H_2SO_4. Exposures would be from the outdoors and the penetration of fine particle acid sulfate indoors (60%–70% of fine particles penetrate indoors) (Yocum 1982).

Conclusion

Levels of O_3 and acidic particle species in North America are primarily dependent upon the presence of photochemical air pollution. There is evidence, however, that exposures may occur during the winter in areas which use high-sulfur fuel. At the present time, concerns in the USA about exposure to these species should be directed toward the outdoor activity patterns during summertime photochemical air pollution episodes.

The O_3 dose that can be inhaled by active children in summer camps are within 50% (Lioy and Dyba 1989) and 25% (Mage et al. 1985) of the dose that has produced clinically significant decrements in pulmonary function and increased the symptoms in adults after 6.6 h exposure in a given day (Folinsbee et al. 1988).

Lioy and Dyba (1989) indicate that O_3 concentrations can peak any time between 12 noon and 6 p.m., and the 8-h average peak above 100 ppb can occur anywhere from 12 noon until 8 p.m. Acid sulfate exposures have been estimated for 6-, 12-, and 24-h samples by the EPA issues paper (1988), Lioy and Waldman (1989), and Spengler et al. (1989). The results suggest that outdoor exposures occur which are similar to those affecting mucociliary clearance in humans and animals (Samet et al. 1988; Schlesinger 1985).

In any particular instance, the actual magnitude of the acidic species exposure will be highly dependent upon the availability of ammonia for neutralization (Larson et al. 1978). It has been estimated that large quantities of ammonia are emitted in the midwestern USA and decrease toward the more populated areas in the east (US EPA 1988). However, in an urban environment, intense neutralization will occur because of the presence of neutralizing species derived from human and animal excrements and industrial activities. Recent work in Wuhan, China, has shown that the high ammonia content can mitigate the accumulation of H_2SO_4 even in a location that uses a high-sulfur coal (Waldman et al. 1991). Noting the emission strength of neutralizing species will increase our ability to predict where high acid particle exposures can occur.

Acknowledgements. I wish to thank Mrs. Arlene Bicknell and Mrs. Malti Patel for typing this manuscript. Major sections of this manuscript are reprinted with permission from Annual Reviews Inc., Palo Alto, California. This work was supported in part by NIEHS Center grant no. ESO5022.

References

Appel BR, Hoffer EM, Tokiwa Y, Kothny EL (1982) Measurement of sulfuric acid and particulate strong acidity in the Los Angeles basin. Atmos Environ 16: 589–593

Atkinson R, Lloyd AC (1984) Evaluation of kinetic and mechanistic data for modeling of photochemical smog. J Phys Chem Ref Data 13:315–444

Berglund RL, Dittenhoefer AC, Ellis HM, Watts BJ, Hansen JL (1988) Evaluation of the stringency of alternate forms of a national ambient air quality standard for ozone. TR-12 Acid and Waste Management Association, Pittsburgh, pp 343–369

Cadle SH (1985) Seasonal variations in nitric acid, nitrate, strong aerosol acidity and ammonia in an urban area. Atmos Environ 19:181–188

Calvert JG, Stockwell WR (1983) Acid generation in the troposphere by gas-phase chemistry. Environ Sci Technol 17:428a–43a

Cleveland WS, Kleiner B, McRae JE, Warner JL (1976) Photochemical air pollution: transport from New York City area into Connecticut and Massachusetts. Science 191:179–181

Cobourn WG, Husar RB (1982) Diurnal and seasonal patterns of particulate sulfur and sulfuric acid in St Louis, July 1977–June 1978. Atmos Environ 16:1441–1450

Commins BT, Waller RE (1967) Observations from a ten-year study of pollution at a site in the city of London. Atmos Environ 1:49–68

Ellestad TG (1980) Aerosol composition of urban plumes passing over a rural monitoring site. Ann NY Acad Sci 338:202–218

Finlayson-Pitts BJ, Pitts JN Jr (1976) Photochemistry of the polluted atmosphere. Science 192:111–119

Folinsbee LJ, McDonnell WF, Horstman DH (1988) Pulmonary function and symptom responses after 6.6 hour exposure to 0.12 ppm ozone with moderate exercise. J Air Pollut Control Assoc 38:28–35

Gearhart JM, Schlesinger RB (1989) Sulfuric acid induced changes in the physiology and structure of the tracheobronchial airways. Environ Health Perspect 79: 127–137

Gillani NV, Kohli S, Wilson WE (1981) Gas-to-particle conversion of sulfur in power plant plumes – I. Parameterization of the conversion rate for dry moderately polluted ambient conditions. Atmos Environ 15:2293–2313

Gillani NV, Colby JA, Wilson WE (1983) Gas-to-particle conversion of sulfur in power plant plumes. III. Parameterization of plume-cloud interaction. Atmos Environ 17:1753–13

Graedel TE, Farrow LA, Weber TA (1976) Kinetic studies of the photochemistry of the urban atmosphere. Atmos Environ 10:1095–1116

Ito K, Thurston GD (1987) The estimation of London England aerosol exposures from historical visibility records. Proceedings of the 80th International Air Pollution Control Association (APCA) Annual Meeting, Pittsburgh, p 422

Jeffries HE, Sexton KG, Salmi CN (1981) Effects of chemistry and meteorology on ozone calculations using simple trajectory models and the EKMA procedure. US Environmental Protection Agency (USEPA), Research Triangle Park NC (EPA-450/4-81-034)

Koenig JQ, Pierson WE, Horike M (1983) The effects of inhaled sulfuric acid on pulmonary function in adolescent asthmatics. Am Rev Respir Dis 128:221–225

Larson TV, Covert DS, Frank R (1978) Respiratory NH$_3$: a possible defense against inhaled acid sulfate compounds In: Folinsbee LF et al. (eds) Environmental stress: individual human adaptations. Academic, New York, pp 91–99

Lioy PJ, Dyba RV (1989) Tropospheric ozone: the dynamics of human exposure. Toxicol Ind Health 5:493–504

Lioy PJ, Lippmann M (1986) Measurement of exposure to acidic sulfur aerosols. In: Lee SD, Schneider T, Grant LD, Verkerk PJ (eds) Aerosols: research risk assessment and control strategies. Lewis, Chelsea, pp 743–752

Lioy PJ, Waldman JM (1989) Acidic sulfate aerosols: characterization and exposure. Environ Health Perspect 79:15–34

Lioy PJ (1989) Expose to oxidants and acids. Ann Rev Public Health 10:69–84

Lioy PJ, Samson PJ, Tanner RL, Leaderer BP, Minnich T, Lyons W (1980) The distribution and transport of sulfate "species" in the New York metropolitan area during the 1977 summer aerosol study. Atmos Environ 14:1391–1407

Lioy PJ, Vollmuth TA, Lippmann M (1985) Persistence of peak flow decrement in children following ozone exposures exceeding the NAAQS. J Air Pollut Control Assoc 35:1068–1071

Lioy PJ, Spektor D, Thurston G, Citak K, Lippmann M et al. (1987) The design considerations for ozone and acid aerosol exposure and health investigations: the Fairview Lake summer camp-photochemical smog case study. Environ Int 13:271–283

Lippmann M (1985) Airborne acidity: estimates of exposure and human effects. Environ Health Perspect 63:63–70

Lippmann M (1989) Effects of ozone on respiratory function and structure. Annu Rev Public Health 10:49–68

Lodge JP Jr (1969) Selections of the smoke of London Two Prophecies. Maxwell, Elmsford

Lyons WA, Olsson LE (1972) Mesoscale air pollution transport in the Chicago lake breeze. J Air Pollut Control Assoc 22:876–881

Mage DT, Raizenne M, Spengler J (1985) The assessment of individual human exposures to ozone in a health study. In: Lee SD (ed) Trans APCA 4:238–249

Martinez JR, Singh HB (1979) Survey of the role of NO in nonurban ozone formation. USEPA (US Environmental Protection Agency) Research Triangle Park (EPA report #EPA-450/4-79-035)

McDonnell WF, Horstman DH, Hazucha MJ, Seal E, Haak ED et al. (1983) Pulmonary effects of ozone exposure during exercise: dose response characteristics. J Appl Physiol 54:1345–1352

Morandi MT, Kneip TJ, Cobourn WG, Husar R, Lioy PJ (1983) The measurement of H_2SO_4 and other sulfate species at Tuxedo NY with a thermal analysis flame photometric detector and simultaneously collected quartz filter samples. Atmos Environ 17:843–848

Paul RA, Biller WF, McCurdy T (1987) National estimates of population exposure to ozone. Proceedings of the 80th International Air Pollution Control Association (APCA) Annual Meeting, Pittsburgh, pp 87–427

Pierson WR, Brachaczek WW, Truex TJ, Butler JW, Korniski TJ (1980) Ambient sulfate measurements on Allegheny Mountain and the question of atmospheric sulfate in the northeastern US. Ann NY Acad Sci 338:145–173

Raizenne ME, Stern B, Burnett PT, Franklin CA, Spengler JD (1989) Acute Pulmonary function responses to ambient acid aerosol exposures. Environ Health Perspect 79:129–186

Rombout PJ, Lioy PJ, Goldstein BG (1986) Rationale for an 8-hour ozone standard. J Air Pollut Control Assoc 36:913–917

Samet JM, Marbury MC, Spengler JD (1988) Health effects and sources of indoor air pollution, part II. Am Rev Respir Dis 137:221–242

Schlesinger RB (1985) Effects of inhaled acids on respiratory tract defense mechanisms. Environ Health Perspect 63:25–38

Schlesinger RB, Naumann BD, Chen LC (1983) Physiological and histological alterations in bronchial mucociliary clearance system of rabbits following intermittent oral and nasal inhalation of sulfuric acid mist. J Toxicol Environ Health 12:441–465

Speizer FE (1989) Studies of acid aerosols in six cities and in a new multicity investigation; design issues. Environ Health Perspect 79:69–72

Spektor DM, Yen BM, Lippmann M (1989) Effect of concentration and cumulative exposure of inhaled sulfuric acid on tracheobronchial particle clearane in healthy humans. Environ Health Perspect 79:167–172

Spengler JD, Keeler GJ, Koutrakis P, Raizenne ME (1989) Exposures to acid aerosols. Environ Health Perspect 79:48–52

Spengler JD, Brauer M, Koutrakis P (1990) Acid air and health. Environ Sci Technol 24:946–955

Spicer CW, Holdren MW, Keigley GW (1983) The ubiquity of peroxyacetyl nitrate in the continental boundary layer. Atmos Environ 17:1055–1058

Tanner RL, Marlow WH (1977) Size discrimination and chemical composition of ambient airborne sulfate particles by diffusion sampling. Atmos Environ 11:1143–1150

Tanner RL, Leaderer BP, Spengler JD (1981) Acidity of atmospheric aerosols: a summary of data concerning their chemical nature and amounts of acid. Environ Sci Technol 15:1150–1153

Tuazon EC, Winer AM, Pitts JN Jr (1981) Trace pollutant concentrations in a multiday smog epidose in the California South Coast Air Basin by long path Fourier transformation infrared spectrometry. Environ Sci Technol 15:1232–1237

US EPA (Environmental Protection Agency) (1985) Air quality criteria for ozone and other photochemical oxidants, vols I–IV ECAO, Research Triangle Park NC (EPA-600/8-84-20b)

US EPA (Environmental Protection Agency) (1990) Acid aerosols issue paper. USEPA, Research Triangle Park NC (EPA report #EPA-600/8-88-005A)

US EPA (Environmental Protection Agency) (1990) National air quality emissions trends report (1988). (EPA Office of Air Quality Planning and Standards #EPA-450/4-90-002 March 1990)

Vukovich FM, Fishman J (1986) The climatology of summertime ozone and sulfur dioxide (1977–1981). Atmos Environ 20:2423–2433

Waldman JM, Lioy PJ, Thurston G, Lippmann M (1990) Analyses of spatial and temporal patterns in sulfate aerosol acidity and neutralization within a metropolitan area. Atmos Environ 24B:115–126

Waldman JD, Lioy PJ, Zelenka M, Jing L, Lin YN, He QC, Qian ZM, Chapman R, Wilson WE (1991) Wintertime measurements of aerosol acidity and trace elements in Wuhan A City in Central China. Atmos Environ 24B: (in press)

Waller RE, Lawther PJ (1957) Further observations on London fog. Br Med J 4:1473–1475

Wolff GT, Lioy PJ (1980) Development of an ozone river associated with synoptic scale episodes in the eastern United States. Environ Sci Technol 14:1257–1260

Wolff GT, Kelly NA, Ferman MA (1982) Source regions of summertime ozone and haze episodes in the eastern United States. Water Air Soil Pollut 18:65–81

World Health Organization (1985) World Health Organization Working Group on air quality guidelines for major urban air pollutants. WHO, Bilthoven, pp 14–19

Yocum JE (1982) Indoor-outdoor air quality relationships: a critical review. J Air Pollut Control Assoc 32:500–520

Section 2. Indoor Air: Home and Workplace

Investigation of Indoor Air Pollution Sources in Climate Chambers: Emissions from Textile Floor Coverings

S. Sollinger[1] and K. Levsen[2]

[1] Akzo Research Laboratories, W-8753 Obernburg, FRG
[2] Fraunhofer-Institut für Toxikologie und Aerosolforschung, Nikolai-Fuchs-Straße 1, W-3000 Hannover 61, FRG

Introduction

While the pollution of both outdoor and occupational atmospheres by chemicals has received considerable attention for many years, it is only recently that scientists have become aware that non-occupational indoor air is also contaminated by a large variety of inorganic and in particular organic compounds, the concentrations of which frequently exceed those of outdoor air by a factor of up to 10 (Seifert 1987; Hawthorne et al. 1986; Repace 1982). Many indoor air pollutants have been identified and quantified in numerous field studies (Yocom 1982; Lebret et al. 1986; Krause et al. 1987). The sometimes high concentrations of indoor air compounds and the fact that people spend most of their time (19–22 h) (Sexton and Hayward 1987) indoors may lead to the health effects, or at least to the irritations, which have been referred to as the "sick building syndrome" (Molhave et al. 1991).

There are many sources which may contribute to the contamination of indoor air, especially by organic compounds. Emissions from building materials are of particular importance. As these different materials often emit, at least in part, the same compounds, the sources of indoor air pollution cannot be identified unequivocally by field studies. Test chamber studies of building materials have been employed for source identification (Wanner and Kuhn 1986; Wallace et al. 1987; Matthews 1987). Climate chambers used for measuring formaldehyde released from particle-board are now manufactured commercially and will be standardized in the near future. These chambers are, however, not suited for measuring so-called "volatile organic compounds" (VOCs).

We have set up two types of climate chambers, the performance of which has been tested extensively. These chambers have been used to study the emissions from textile floor coverings. In this paper investigations under static conditions are reported.

U. Mohr et al. (Eds.)
Advances in Controlled Clinical
Inhalation Studies
© Springer-Verlag Berlin Heidelberg 1993

Climate Chambers

Two different climate chambers have been developed, a small glass chamber and a medium-sized stainless steel chamber. The latter was constructed by a commercial manufacturer (Weiss Umwelttechnik) according to our requirements.

The small chamber, with a volume of 33 l, is made of Duran glass and can be placed in a hot air cabinet allowing thermostatization at temperatures ranging from 23.5° to 70°C (tolerance ±1°C) (Sollinger et al. 1992). The chamber can be opened by a lid which is pressed air-tight onto the chamber. Nitrogen, further purified by passing it through charcoal, Tenax TA (Chrompack), and Carbosieve S II (Restek) adsorbents was used as purge gas. The nitrogen can be humidified by organic-free water (Millipore), thus allowing the variation of humidity (0% and 10%–90%; tolerance = 2%). To reduce the background of the chamber (see above) it can be heated up to 200°C while purging it with purified nitrogen. Especially for dynamic experiments (not reported here) the chamber is equipped with a fan to allow a thorough mixing of the atmosphere.

The medium-sized chamber, with a net volume of 1000 l, is made of stainless steel that is electropolished (Sollinger et al. 1991). The chamber can be thermostatized at temperatures of 20°–60°C (tolerance ±0.5°C) using indirect heating via a heated glycol solution pumped through heat exchange tubes arranged around the surfaces of the outer walls. The humidity can be varied from 30% to 80% (tolerance ±3%) using the dew point principle. Special care was taken to avoid the use of plastic materials, with the exception of the door insulation, for which special degassed silicon rubber was used. The atmosphere is mixed using a fan and two air-conduction plates. The chamber is purged by compressed air purified by passing it through charcoal. To reduce memory effects the chamber can be heated up to 200°C with the aid of an additional heating system.

Analytical Methods

Samples were collected on stainless steel adsorption tubes filled with Tenax TA and Carbosieve S II. When Carbosieve S II is used the gaseous sample is dried by passing it through a Nafion tube mounted coaxially in a stainless steel tube with the ring-gap between the two tubes is purged by helium. Memory effects by this Nafion tube consist of n-pentane and isobutane. Both are emitted from this Nafion material.

The compounds trapped in the adsorption tube are thermally desorbed into a GC/MS system (Hewlett-Packard 5970) using a modified "thermal desorption cold trap injector" from Chrompack (modifications are described in Sollinger et al. 1992). In this unit the desorbing compounds are first cryofocused in a capillary kept at −100°C before the final flash desorption into the gas chromatograph. The gas chromatograph (Hewlett-Packard 5890 II) is equipped with a thick film capillary (Rtx-Volatiles, Restek) and an additional cooling system which allows temperatures below 0°C to be reached. The electron impact mass spectrometer is operated under full scan conditions for peak identification and under "multiple ion detection" for quantification. Quantification is achieved by using the method of external or internal standard; in the latter, toluene-d_8 is injected onto the adsorption tube prior to desorption.

Performance of the Chambers

Recoveries

To evaluate the overall method, including sampling and analysis, recovery experiments were carried out. For this, 15 compounds which were previously identified as emissions originating from textile floor coverings were introduced into the preconditioned climate chambers at concentrations typically found in the quantification experiment of a typical carpet. For this investigation the chamber was kept at 200°C to minimize wall effects. When the small chamber was used, a solution of the compounds in n-pentane was first injected onto Tenax. After removing the solvent by purging at 60°C for 6 min (which does not lead to a loss of the other adsorbed compounds) the compounds were desorbed at 280°C into the chamber. This method allows the introduction of small amounts of organic compounds without the introduction of an excess of solvent. The volume of the second stainless steel chamber ($1\,m^3$) is sufficiently large to allow direct injection of the compounds without the use of solvents. The recoveries for the small chamber are shown in Fig. 1 (mean of at least four separate measurements, standard deviation 10%–15%). Fig. 1 demonstrates that the recovery is close to 100%, with the exception of aniline. The high recoveries demonstrate the overall reliability of the experimental setup.

Blanks

Initial blank values of the small and particularly the medium-sized chamber were reduced step by step by heating the chamber up to 200°C under a stream of purified nitrogen or compressed air for several days. In the case of the small glass chamber the blank value of toluene is below the detection limit (below 5–10 ppt). It was more difficult to achieve low blanks with the $1\,m^3$ stainless steel chamber. Finally, chamber blanks, i.e. of m/p-xylene, were below 0.5 ng/l.

recovery [%]

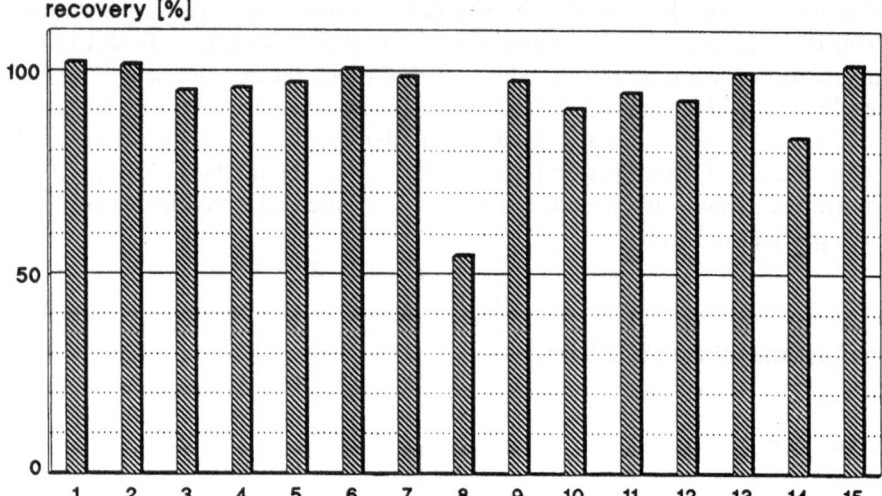

Fig. 1. Recovery of 15 organic compounds from the climate chamber. *1*, Toluene; *2*, ethylbenzene; *3*, nonane; *4*, styrene; *5*, cumene; *6*, 1,3-trimethylbenzene; *7*, 2-ethyltoluene; *8*, aniline; *9*, *p*-cymene; *10*, 1,4-dichlorobenzene; *11*, *n*-dodecane; *12*, *n*-tridecane; *13*, benzothiazole; *14*, *n*-hexadecane; *15*, 2,6-di-*tert*-butyl-4-methylphenol

Detection Limits

The detection limit (defined as S/N = 3) was determined for the small glass chamber by injecting 0.3–0.5 ng of 25 compounds found as emissions from textile floor coverings onto Tenax and subsequent thermal desorption into the GC/MS system. Detection limits vary strongly from compound to compound and range from 18 pg for toluene to 340 pg for *n*-hexanal. As a volume of 10 l can be sampled by the Tenax method without breakthrough, this corresponds to a detection limit varying from 0.4 to 2.9 ppt.

Air Mixing Within the Chamber

Sampling and modeling of dynamic experiments require a well-mixed gaseous phase within the test chamber. To study the performance of the mixing device methane was used as tracer. The residence time distribution of this tracer was recorded using a flame ionization detector. Thorough mixing within the test chamber leads to the residence time distribution curve of an ideal, continuously stirred tank reactor, described by the equation:

$$c_{\text{out}} = c_o e^{-\tau/s} = c_o e^{-\tau n}$$

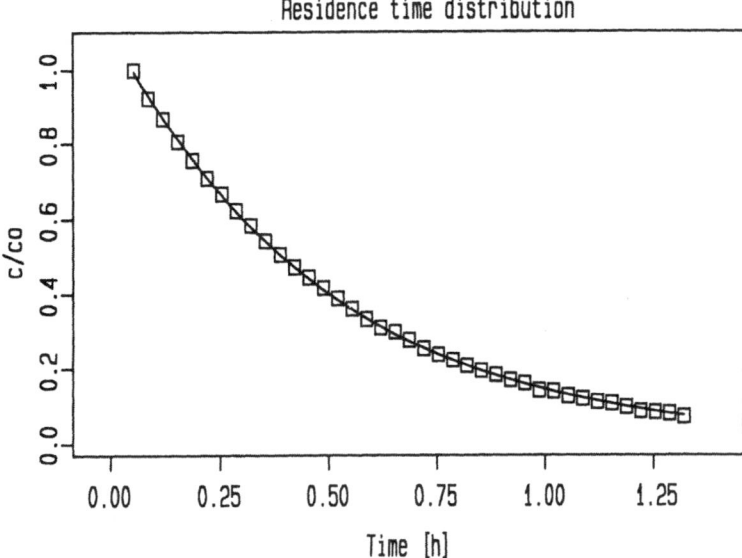

Fig. 2. Residence time distribution

where c_{out} is the concentration of methane at the outlet of the chamber, c_0 is the initial concentration of methane, τ is the mean residence time and n is the number of air exchanges.

Fig. 2 shows the theoretical residence time distribution curve (solid line) as compared to the actually measured curve (squares) for an air exchange of $2\,h^{-1}$.

Wall Effects

Wall effects were determined for both chambers using the procedure described for the recovery experiment. However, in this case the chamber was kept at three distinct temperatures (21°, 40°, and 61.5°C in the small glass chamber; 23°, 40°, and 60°C in the larger stainless steel chamber). The results of ten compounds are shown for the two chambers in Fig. 3. While volatile compounds such as toluene and most alkyl benzenes are almost quantitatively recovered at all temperatures from both chambers, demonstrating that for these compounds wall effects are of minor importance, the recovery is low for polar compounds and compounds of low volatility. Thus, for instance, in the case of the small glass chamber 2,6-di-*tert*-butyl-4-methylphenol was recovered to only 35% at a chamber temperature of 61.5°C. The recovery decreases dramatically when the temperature is lowered, reaching 8% at 21°C. Thus, the wall represents an important sink for compounds of low volatility, which must be kept in mind when dynamic

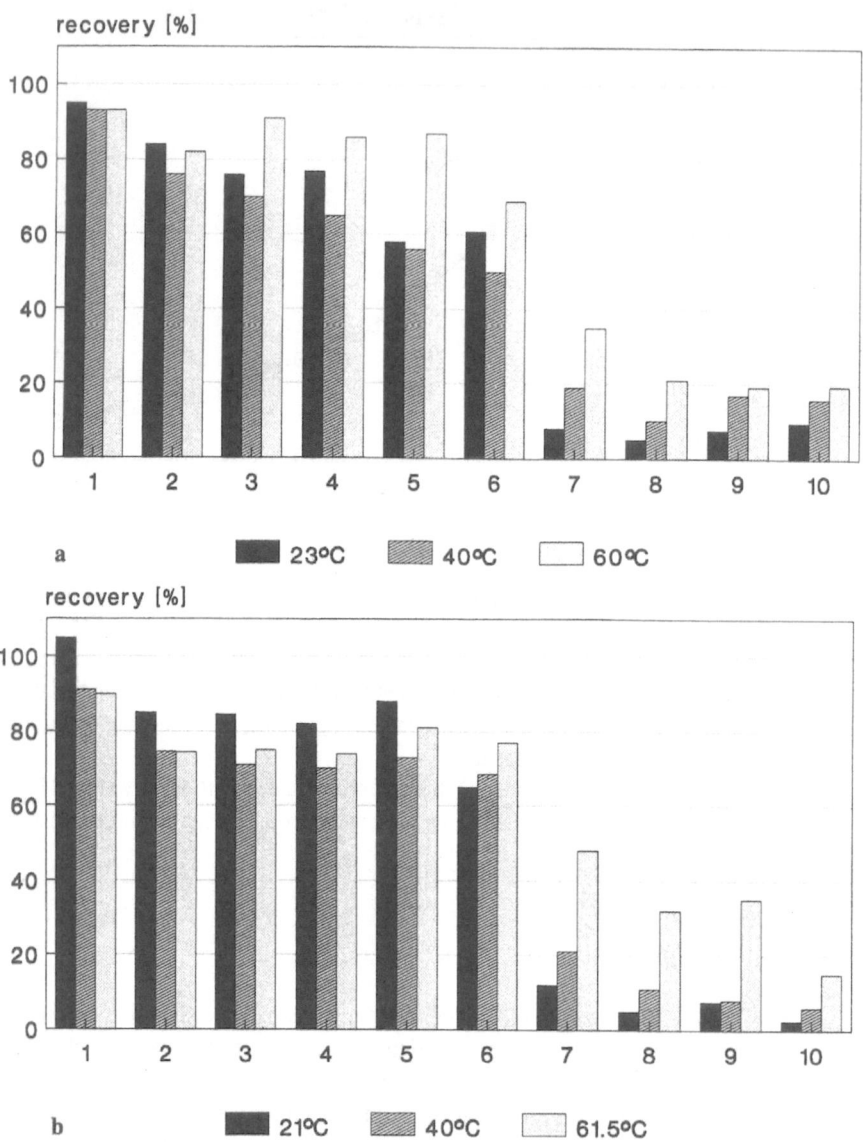

Fig. 3a,b. Wall effects in the test chambers for ten compounds **a** Stainless steel chamber. **b** Glass chamber. *1*, Toluene; *2*, styrene; *3*, 1,3,5-trimethylbenzene; *4*, 2-ethyltoluene; *5*, 1,4-dichlorobenzene; *6*, 1,3-diethylbenzene; *7*, *n*-tridecane; *8*, *n*-tetradecane; *9*, 2,6-di-*tert*-butyl-4-methylphenol; *10*, *n*-hexadecane

chamber experiments are carried out. In a real indoor environment not only the walls but also the surface of the furniture as well as the pile of the carpet itself represent sinks for compounds of low volatility which may be reemitted over extended periods. As the wall effects for both chambers have been investigated under almost identical conditions, Figs. 3 and 4 can be compared directly. Surprisingly, wall effects are of the same order of magnitude although the wall material and particularly the volume differ significantly. This may be explained by the fact that the surface-to-volume ratio is similar in the two chambers ($12 \, \mathrm{m}^{-1}$ for the $1 \, \mathrm{m}^3$ chamber, $16 \, \mathrm{m}^{-1}$ for the 331 chamber). The surface of the additional air conduction plates in the stainless steel chamber lead to the surprisingly high value of the surface-to-volume ratio. The observation that the wall effects are independent of wall material may be explained by the fact that water is present in the chamber in excess as compared to the organic compounds. The water molecules cover the complete surface of the chamber.

Emissions from Textile Floor Coverings

Compound Spectrum Emitted from Textile Floor Coverings

Ten textile floor coverings, seven provided with a styrene-butadiene rubber backing, one with a polyurethane backing, and two with a textile backing were under investigation. Textile floor coverings with backings of styrene butadiene rubber (SBR) are used most frequently in Germany. All emissions were studied under equilibrium conditions, i.e., with zero air exchange. To this end a piece of carpet was transferred into the chamber and allowed to equilibrate for at least $24 \, \mathrm{h}$.

From all carpets, 95 compounds have been identified. These are listed in Table 1, grouped according to the compound classes. They include 25 branched and unbranched alkanes and cycloalkanes, 5 alkenes, 36 alkylbenzenes, 5 phenols, 3 alkanoles, 7 aldehydes and ketones, both aliphatic and aromatic amines, chlorobenzenes, and several other compounds among which carbon disulfide and benzothiazole deserve particular attention.

The origin of several compounds or compound classes is well understood. Thus, it is likely that the large number of alkylbenzenes are impurities of the styrene monomer. 4-Phenylcyclohexene is formed by Diels-Alder reaction during the polymerization of styrene and butadiene. For the vulcanization of the rubber backing at low temperatures, vulcanization accelerators are added to the styrene-butadiene latex. Benzothiazole is found as an emission product. Derivates of this compound (e.g., 2-mercaptobenzothiazole, Zn-2-mercaptobenzothiazole, dibenzothiazyl-disulfide) are known as such accelerators. Dithiocarbamates are known as other types of vulcanization accelerators. The manufacturing process of the SBR-backing includes an acidification step which converts the dithiocarbamates into their corresponding free acids, which themselves are instable and decompose to alkyldiamines and carbondisulfide (Scröder and Klingenberger 1988). Indeed, carbondisulfide is found in emissions from SBR-backed carpets. Several other

Table 1. Identified volatile organic compounds released from textile floor covering

Alkanes

n-Hexane	n-Decane	n-Tetradecane
n-Heptane	n-Undecane	n-Pentadecane
n-Octane	n-Dodecane	n-Hexadecane
n-Nonane	n-Tridecane	n-Heptadecane
Cyclohexane	Diethylcyclohexane	i-Dodecanes
Methylhexane	Methyloctane	i-Tridecanes
Ethylcyclohexane	Methylnonane	i-Octane
Methylcyclohexane	Dimethylheptane	Octahydro-4,7-methano-¹H-indene

Alkenes

n-Dodecene	n-Tetradecene	Trimeric isobutenes
n-Tridecene	Octen	

Alkylbenzenes

Toluene, Styrene	2-Ethyltoluene	2-Isopropyltoluene
	3-Ethyltoluene	3-Isopropyltoluene
1,2-Dimethylbenzene	4-Ethyltoluene	4-Isopropyltoluene
1,3-Dimethylbenzene		2-Propyltoluene
1,4-Dimethylbenzene	n-Butylbenzene	3-Propyltoluene
Ethylbenzene	i-Butylbenzene	4-Propyltoluene
	sec-Butylbenzene	
i-Propylbenzene	1,2,3,4-Tetramethylbenzene	1,2-Diisopropylbenzene
n-Propylbenzene	1,2,3,5-Tetramethylbenzene	1,3-Diisopropylbenzene
1,2,4-Trimethylbenzene	1,2,4,5-Tetramethylbenzene	1,4-Diisopropylbenzene
1,2,3-Trimethylbenzene	1,2-Diethylbenzene	
1,3,5-Trimethylbenzene	1,3-Diethylbenzene	1,3,5-Triisopropylbenzene
	1,4-Diethylbenzene	4-Phenylcyclohexene
	Ethyldimethylbenzene	Diisobutenyltoluene

Phenoles

Diisopropylphenoles
2,6-Di-tert-butyl-4-methylphenol
2,6-Dimethylphenol
2,4,6-Tri-tert-butylphenol
2,6-Di-tert-butyl-4-methoxyphenol

Alkanoles

2-Propanol
1,2-Propandiol

2-Ethylhexanol

Aldehydes/ketones

2-Butanone
Hexanal
Cyclopentanone
Cyclohexanone

Methylhexanone
2-Cyclohexen-1-one
2,6-Di-tert-butyl-p-quinone

Amines

Diethylamine
Dimethylquinoline
Diphenylamine
1,2-Dihydro-2,2,4-trimethylquinoline

N,N-Dimethylformamide

Other aromatics

1,3-Dichlorbenzene
1,4-Dichlorbenzene
1,2,4-Trichlorbenzene

Naphthalene

Others

Carbon disulfide
Benzothiazole
Tetrahydrofurane
Diisooctylphtalate
Butyl acetate

Table 2. Concentration of volatile organic compounds released from a tufted textile floor covering with styrene butadiene rubber backing under equilibrium conditions

	23°C (ng/l)	40°C (ng/l)
Toluene	491 ± 24	330 ± 30
Hexanal	13.4 ± 1.0	25.1 ± 3.0
Ethylbenzene	68.9 ± 5.9	44.3 ± 4.0
n-Nonane	14.6 ± 0.9	10.9 ± 1.1
m,p-Xylene	112 ± 7	85.1 ± 7.2
Styrene	5.6 ± 0.6	7.6 ± 0.6
Cumene	21.1 ± 1.5	12.1 ± 1.3
1,3,5-Trimethylbenzene	6.7 ± 0.5	9.9 ± 0.9
2-Ethyltoluene	ND	9.2 ± 1.2
Aniline	27.6 ± 1.6	87.3 ± 6.8
2-Ethylhexanol	14.2 ± 0.7	36.0 ± 4.4
p-Cymene	5.8 ± 0.6	13.6 ± 0.6
1,4-Dichlorobenzene	45.9 ± 3.7	83.3 ± 8.2
1,3-Diethylbenzene	4.2 ± 0.2	4.8 ± 0.5
n-Dodecane	5.6 ± 0.3	21.1 ± 3.2
n-Tridecane	1.9 ± 0.1	6.2 ± 0.7
Benzothiazole	6.7 ± 1.4	30.5 ± 3.7
n-Tetradecane	2.2 ± 0.2	10.2 ± 1.5
2,6-Di-tert-butyl-4-methylphenol	1.8 ± 0.4	10.3 ± 0.9
n-Hexadecane	2.4 ± 0.4	2.8 ± 0.5

Mean of at least five separate determinations. ND, Not determined.

compounds, known as aging retardants, are found as emission products, i.e., diphenylamine, 1,2-dihydro-2,2,4-trimethylchinoline, dimethylchinoline, and 2,6-di-tert-butyl-4-methylphenol. The major compounds emitted from a textile floor covering with SBR backing have been quantified in cases where reference compounds were available. Quantitative data for 23° and 40°C and a humidity of 45% are summarized in Table 2. The most abundant compound emitted is a trimeric isobutene. Isobutene is a major impurity of the butadiene used in the polymerization process. Further dominating compounds emitted from the carpet are: toluene, $8700 \mu/m^3$; ethylbenzene, $100 \mu g/m^3$; m/p-xylene, $100 \mu g/m^3$; diethylamine and aniline, $40 \mu g/m^3$; benzothiazole, $13 \mu g/m^3$; 4-phenylcyclohexene and 2,6-di-tert-butyl-4-methylphenol, 3 µg/l (concentrations at 23°C and 45% relative humidity).

Temperature Dependence

The temperature dependence of the emissions was studied by determining the equilibrium concentrations at 23°, 30°, 40°, 50.5°, 61°, and 71°C. The concentration for two temperatures are shown in Table 2. Figure 4 illustrates the temperature dependence of four compounds of different volatility and polarity. Figure 4a demonstrates that styrene (a relatively volatile com-

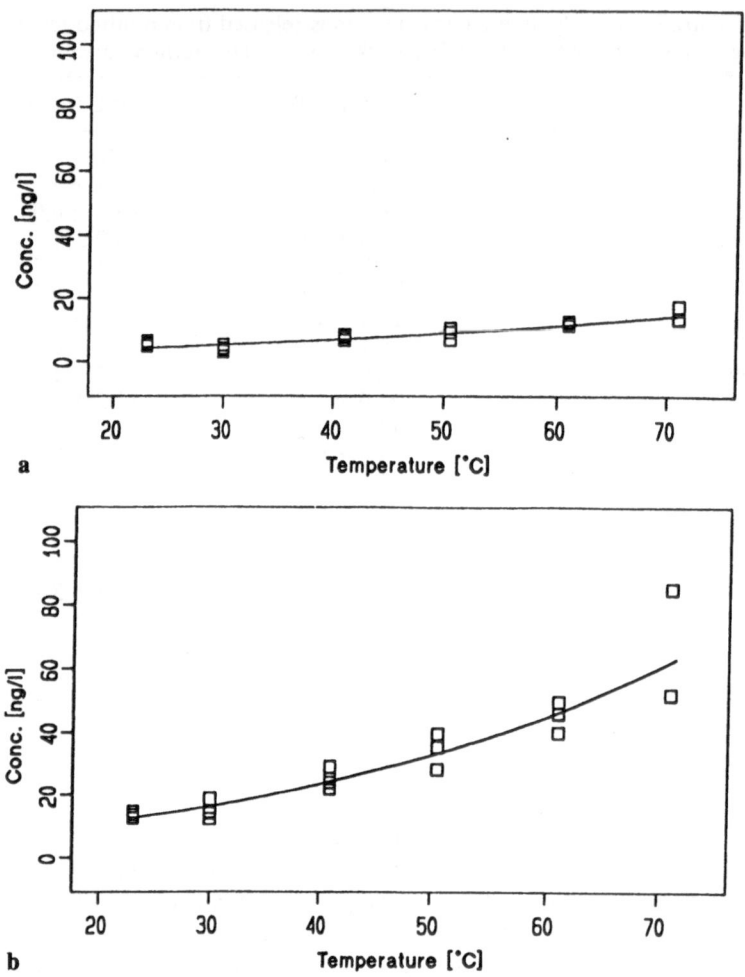

Fig. 4a–d. Temperature dependence of the emissions. **a** Styrene. **b** n-Hexanal

pound of low polar properties) shows little dependence on the temperature. The same behavior is observed for most alkylbenzenes. The temperature dependence is more pronounced for n-hexanal (Fig. 4b), a compound which is more polar, but still of low volatility. n-Tetradecane, a compound of low volatility and low polarity, shows a temperature dependence comparable to n-hexanal (Fig. 4c). Finally, a particularly strong dependence is found for benzothiazole (Fig. 4d). In a real indoor environment only temperatures between 20° and 30°C are expected, so that the high emissions found for polar compounds of low volatility and at high temperatures are of minor relevance for the actual indoor situation. However, it cannot be excluded that, under direct irradiation by sunlight, surface temperatures higher than 30°C are reached.

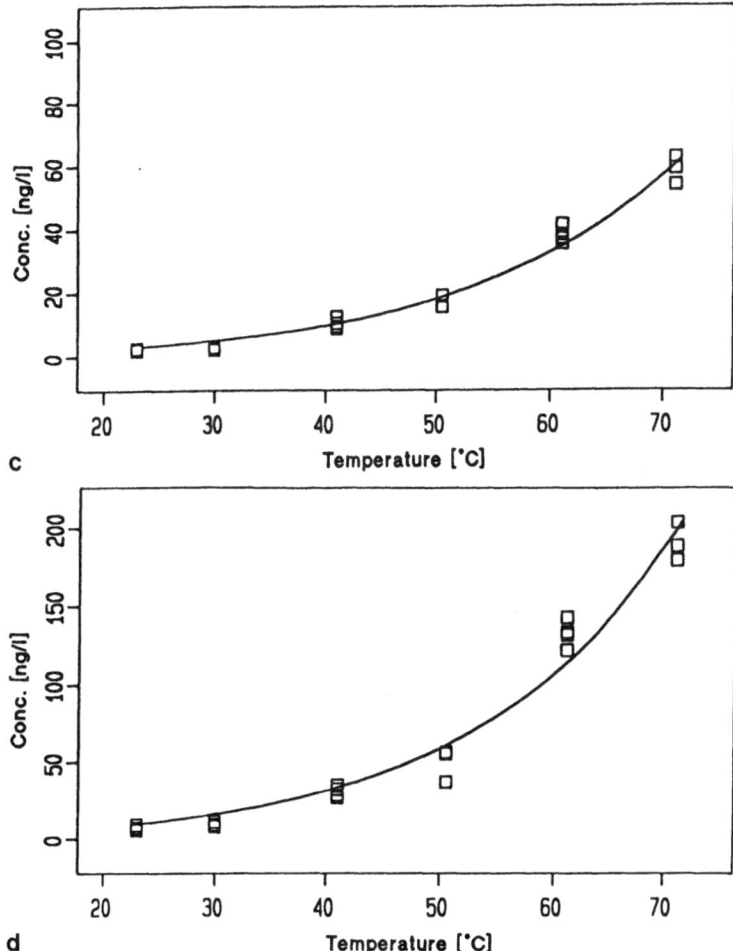

Fig. 4. c n-Tetradecane. **d** Benzothiazole

Dependence on Humidity

It has been observed that the emission of formaldehyde from particle-board depends strongly on the relative humidity, which must be taken into account when these materials are examined in climate chamber studies. The dependence of the concentration of 15 compounds emitted from the same textile floor covering at 0% and 45% relative humidity is shown in Table 3. Taking the standard deviation into account, the table demonstrates that the emissions from this textile floor covering do not depend on humidity, with the possible exception of aniline, the emission of which increases slightly with increasing humidity. Thus, for the testing of textile floor coverings in climate chambers it is not necessary to maintain a constant and well-defined humidity.

54   S. Sollinger and K. Levsen

Table 3. Comparison of the Concentration of Volatile Organic Compounds Released from Textile Floor Covering with Styrene-Butadiene backing at Different Relative Humidities

	0% r.h. 40°C (ng/l)	45% r.h. 40°C (ng/l)
Toluene	316 ± 18	330 ± 30
Hexanal	23.3 ± 2.6	25.1 + 2.9
Ethylbenzene	54.8 ± 5.8	44.2 ± 4.0
Nonane	11.3 ± 1.0	10.9 ± 1.1
m-Xylene	81.0 ± 9.0	85.1 ± 7.2
Styrene	7.8 ± 0.9	7.6 ± 0.6
Cumene	14.0 ± 1.6	13.6 ± 2.4
1,3,5-Trimethylbenzene	10.2 ± 0.9	9.9 ± 0.9
2-Ethyltoluene	22.4 ± 1.7	9.2 ± 1.2
1,2,4-Trimethylbenzene	27.1 ± 2.3	26.4 ± 2.5
Aniline	66.2 ± 4.6	88.3 ± 8.0
2-Ethylhexanol	161 ± 14	174 ± 15
p-Cymene	12.9 ± 1.3	13.7 ± 0.5
1,4-Dichlorobenzene	95 ± 8.6	85.7 ± 8.1
1,2-Diethylbenzene	5.4 ± 0.5	4.9 ± 0.5
1-Dodecene	–	5.4 ± 0.8
n-Dodecane	22.9 ± 5.9	22.3 ± 2.7
n-Tridecane	5.1 ± 0.5	6.4 ± 0.7
Benzothiazole	25.9 ± 3.7	31.7 ± 3.4
n-Tetradecane	10.5 ± 1.4	15.3 ± 2.3
2,6-Di-tert-butyl-4-methylphenol	8.9 ± 1.8	10.3 ± 0.3
1-Hexadecane	2.2 ± 0.4	2.8 ± 0.5

Mean of at least five determinations.

Chamber Loading

It is apparent that under dynamic conditions, i.e., with air exchange, the concentrations of the compounds emitted from a textile floor covering depend on the loading of the chamber. To test the dependence of the concentration in the climate chamber on the sample size, the emissions released from two different sample sizes ($0.44\,\mathrm{m}^{-1}$ and $0.88\,\mathrm{m}^{-1}$ chamber loading) were determined. Under static conditions, Fig. 5 demonstrates that the concentration of six organic compounds typically released from a textile floor covering with SBR backing is (within the reproducibility of the experiment) independent of the chamber loading. This demonstrates that under the experimental conditions described above equilibrium between the gas phase and the rubber foam backing (as well as between the gas phase and the adsorbed layers on the wall of the chambers and on the surface of the pile) is reached, and that the concentration within the rubber backing must be large as compared to the concentration in the gas phase (i.e., no

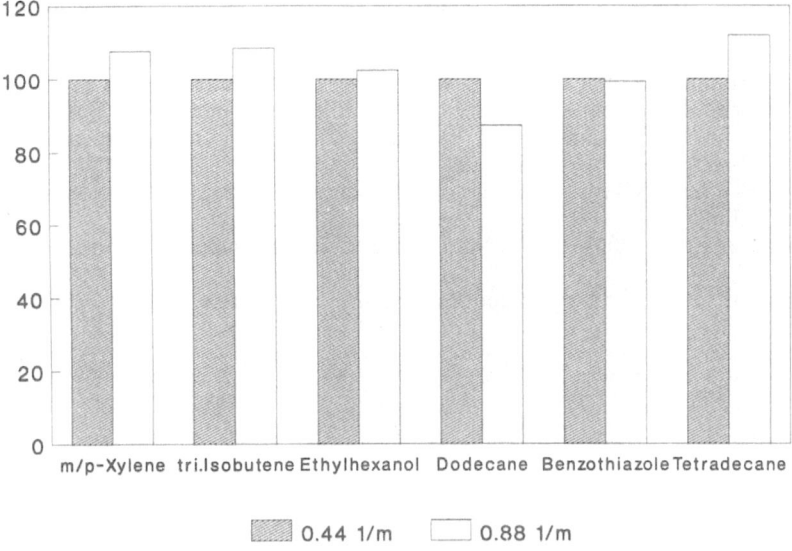

Fig. 5. Dependence of the concentrations of the emitted compounds on the chamber loading (relative to a loading of $0.44\,\text{m}^{-1} = 100\%$)

significant depletion of the organic compounds present in the rubber foam occurs).

References

Hawthorne AR, Gammage RB, Dudney CS (1986) An indoor air quality study of 40 east Tennessee homes. Environ Int 12:221–239

Krause C, Mailahn W, Nagel R, Schulz C, Seifert B, Ullrich D (1987) Pentachlorphenol containing wood preservatives: analyses and evaluation. Proceedings of the 4th international conference on indoor air quality and climate, vol 1. Berlin, 17–21 Aug 1987, p 201

Lebret E, van de Wiel HJ, Bos HP, Noij D, Boleig JSM (1986) Volatile organic compounds in Dutch homes. Environ Int 12:323–332

Matthews TG (1987) Environmental chamber test methodology for characterizing organic vapors from solid emission sources. Atmos Environ 21:321–329

Molhave L, Jensen JG, Larsen S (1991) Subjective reactions to volatile organic compounds as air pollutants. Atmos Environ 24A:1283–93

Repace JL (1982) Indoor air pollution. Environ Int 8:21–36

Schröder E, Klingenberger H (1988) Abhängigkeit der chemischen Zusammensetzung der Emissionen SBR-beschichteter textiler Bodenbeläge von der Compoundierung und von den Produktionsbedingungen. Deutsches Teppichforschungsinstitut, Aachen

Seifer B (1987) Luftverunreinigungen im Innenraum unter Berücksichtung der Situation bei Smogwetterlagen. Schriftenr Ver Wasser Boden Lufthyg Berlin Dahlem 69:143–149

Sexton K, Hayward SB (1987) Source apportionment of indoor air pollution. Atmos Environ 21:407–418

Sollinger S, Levsen K, Wünsch G (1991) Indoor air pollution by organic emission from textile floor coverings. Atmos Environ (submitted)

Sollinger S, Levsen K, Seidel P (1992) Eine Prüfkammer zur Bestimmung der Emissionen leichtflüchtiger Verbindungen (VOC's) aus Innenraum-materialien. Staub Reinhalt Luft 52:31–34

Wallace LA, Pellizari E, Leaderer B, Jelon H, Sheldon L (1987) Atmos Environ 21:385–393

Wanner HK, Kuhn M (1986) Indoor air pollution by building materials. Environ Int 12:311–315

Yocom JE (1982) Indoor-outdoor air quality relationships. JAPCA 32:500

Dust Measurements at Workplaces: State of the Art and Future Demands

W. Koch

Fraunhofer-Institut für Toxikologie und Aerosolforschung, Nikolai-Fuchs-Straße 1, W-3000 Hannover 61, FRG

Introduction

Special concern must be directed to hazardous airborne particles at workplaces. The concentrations may be one or two orders of magnitude higher than those at ambient sites. The particles may also have higher toxicity than particles usually found in outdoor air, posing an acute toxic risk to persons at work. Furthermore, workers may face life-long continuous exposure to noxious dusts. This can lead to serious chronic, even fatal diseases of the respiratory system. The pneumoconiosis of coal miners and the asbestosis, bronchogenic carcinoma, and mesothelioma of workers exposed to fibrous asbestos materials are examples where a direct relationship between exposure to dust and chronic occupational diseases has been confirmed on the basis of epidemiology.

Consequently, together with other measures, maximum concentrations of airborne hazardous substances have been established to protect the workers against adverse health effects (Senatskommission 1990). These include, in Germany, the *Maximale Arbeitsplatzkonzentration* (MAK) and the *Technische Richtkonzentration* (TAK). They are based on toxicological and epidemiological evidence. The MAK is a threshold value below which a health risk can normally be ruled out. For carcinogenic substances the assignment of a safe MAK value is not permitted, however; here, the TRK values are established, determined mainly by their technical feasibility and set standards according to the best technology available.

Historically, the MAK values are 8-h average values. To account for the actual concentration fluctuations at work places a more detailed classification scheme has been established to set limits also to the maximum tolerable deviation from the mean value. The overwhelming number of substances listed in the MAK list are classified into one of five categories determined by the tolerable height, duration, and frequency of concentration peaks. The categories reflect special mechanisms of short-term health effects of the substance under consideration. For example, peak concentrations of

U. Mohr et al. (Eds.)
Advances in Controlled Clinical
Inhalation Studies
© Springer-Verlag Berlin Heidelberg 1993

substances with locally irritating effects must always be lower than twice the MAK value. Concentration peaks should occur less than eight times per working shift. It is especially for the (reversible) short-term effects that controlled human inhalation experiments could be a helpful supplement or alternative to animal studies or other toxicological investigations in support-ing or revising the established limit values. The overall goal is always to minimize the health hazards at workplaces.

In order not only to comply with the legal regulations but also to obtain detailed information about the realistic exposure patterns to be simulated in controlled inhalation experiments, a reliable monitoring of the actual work-place situation is of utmost importance. It is essential to have measuring techniques available that are sufficiently sensitive to measure workplace con-centrations correctly and with a time resolution that is at least in accordance with the demands of the short-term classification scheme of the substance under consideration.

The purpose of this paper is briefly to review the workplace measuring techniques for airborne particulate materials and to compare the current situation with the future needs, especially with respect to the impending European standardization. Some examples of our own research activities in workplace aerosol monitoring are also mentioned.

Health-Related Sampling Criteria

The biological effects of airborne particulates such as dusts, fumes, mists, etc. depend on where the particles deposit in the human respiratory system (Lippmann et al. 1983). The probability that a particle will get into the respiratory system during breathing and the location and probability of deposition depends strongly on the particle size. Particles with different sizes may have quite different physiological relevance. For the purpose of health-related sampling, the most appropriate parameter to characterize the size of a particle is the so-called aerodynamic particle diameter. This deter-mines location and probability of particle deposition in the size range above $0.5\,\mu m$. Here, the mechanisms responsible for deposition are sedimentation and inertial impaction.

For health-related particle sampling in industrial hygiene two subfrac-tions of the total suspended particulate matter (TSP) have been defined, among others: the inhalable (inspirable) fraction and the respirable fraction, also called fine dust. The definition curves for the dust fractions are given for example in the International Standards Organization (ISO) convention TR/7708 (1983) (Fig. 1). The inspirable fraction is a subfraction of the TSP. The definition curve reflects the efficiency of dust intake through the nose and mouth. The ISO regulations are used in the United States. German regulations for health-related sampling do not specifically refer to this curve but define the total dust as the fraction of the TSP that is sucked in by a

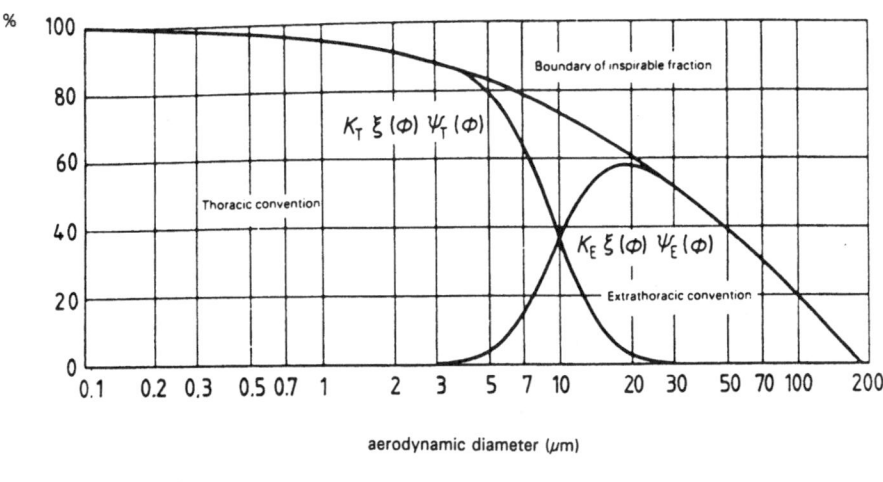

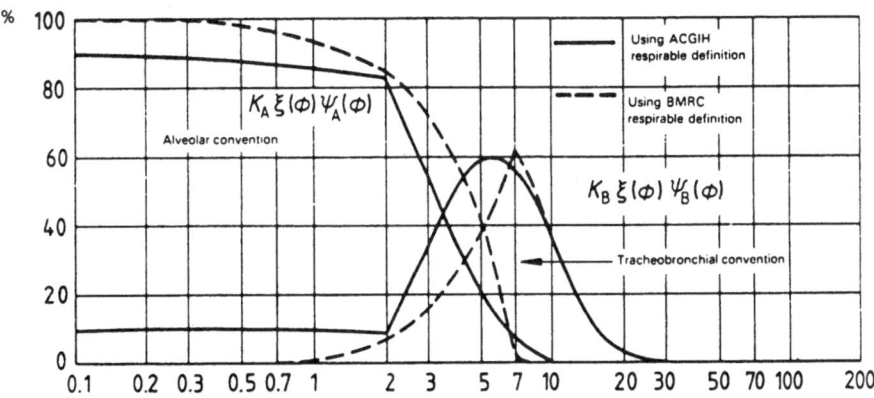

Fig. 1. Definitions for health-related sampling

sampling instrument operated at an intake velocity of 1.25 m/s. The two are highly correlated and in qualitative agreement for particles smaller than 50 μm but deviate for larger particles. The ISO definition for inspirability is based on data of Ogden and Birkett (1977). They were the first to use life-sized head and shoulders of a mannequin and to measure the aspiration efficiency of the human head. The Ogden data were later revised by Vincent and Armbruster (1981), who proposed a curve which was then adopted also by the American Conference of Governmental Industrial Hygienists (ACGIH). Particles are respirable, i.e., can penetrate into the alveolar region of the lung, if they are smaller than about 7 μm. There exist two (very similar) definitions for the fine dust following the ACGIH (ISO 1983) and the British Medical Research Council (BMRC; 1952) convention. Both curves are defined according to the penetration curves of size selective samplers. The ACGIH curve used in the United States resembles the efficiency curve of a cyclone whereas the BMRC curve used in Europe matches the separation curve of a horizontal elutriator. A third definition that is not yet in use as a sampling cirterion for sampling at workplaces but is the basis for taking ambient samples is the thoracic fraction, also called the PM 10. Current standardization activities within the European Community will take up the thoracic dust as a third fraction in addition to the total and the fine dust to be measured mandatorily at workplaces (Siekmann 1990).

The MAK list contains a total of 81 substances occurring as particulates or being adsorbed onto or incorporated into particles. The overwhelming majority must be measured as total dust; only 15 limit values refer to the fine dust concentration. With respect to short-term effects the 81 substances are classified according to Table 1. This table clearly shows that in order to comply with the legal regulations measuring techniques should be available that measure different dust fractions simultaneously and with sufficient time resolution.

Measuring Strategy and Instrumentation

Guidelines describing the measuring strategies and the instrumentation for workplace measurements are given in the "Technical Rules for Dangerous Substances" (TRGS 1986). The MAK list is a part of this system of regulations. These more general guidelines are eventually to be supplemented by

Table 1. Short-term dust classification (MAK list; number of substances classified)

Category	Peak			Size fraction	
	Concentration	Duration	Occurrence	Fine	Total
I Locally irritating	2 × MAK	5 min, peak[a]	8/shift	–	10
II Effects after resorption within 2 h					
II/1 Half time < 2 h	2 × MAK		4/shift		
II/2 Half time > 2 h	5 × MAK		3/shift		
		30 min, average[b]		5	46
III Effects after resorption after 2 h					
Half life > 8 h	10 × MAK		1/shift		
IV Weak effects	2 × MAK	60 min, peak	3/shift	3	
V Odorous substances	2 × MAK	10 min, peak	4/shift	–	–
No classification				10	17

[a] Instantaneous concentration value must not exceed limit value at any time.
[b] Average concentration value must not exceed limit value.

more specific ones which provide more detailed information on certain groups of dangereous substances. For aerosols, for example, the VDI guideline 2265 "Determination of Dust Concentrations at Workplaces for Industrial Hygiene Purposes" (VDI 1980) gives practical instructions on how the measurements should be conducted.

We do not provide a detailed description here but give a rough survey of the measuring techniques and the available instrumentation. It is shown that there is a gap between the demands of the regulations and the technical tools that are available to the authorities and the industry to meet these requirements.

In the MAK list all the limit values except those for fibrous materials are given in terms of mass concentrations. According to the TRGS 402 the following measurements must be made to fully characterize a working area:

- Concentration measurements to determine the current dust situation. This comprises 8-h average values, short-term measurements, measurements close to the emission source, and measurements of the spatial and the temporal concentration distribution.
- Control measurements, which must be performed to check the observance of the limiting values (8-h average value, peak value).
- Eventually a continuous monitoring of the concentration.

These rules apply to gaseous substances as well as to the airborne particulate material or specific subfractions to be measured.

A very elementary but reliable method to determine the dust concentration is the filter method. There exists a wide variety of different filter samplers, static as well as personal, that are able to sample the various dust fractions either separately or simultaneously. An excellent review of aerosol sampling at workplaces is given by Vincent (1989).

Instruments that measure the total dust suck in the air through special sampling heads designed to have aspiration efficiencies that match more or less accurately the definition curves for total dust. Widely used sampling instruments are the ORB sampler in the United Kingdom and the VC 25 Gravikon in Germany. These are static samplers located at a fixed position within the working area and therefore do not accurately assess the individual exposure of the workers. For this purpose so-called personal filter samplers have been developed that are worn by the workers during the entire work shift. A variety of different sampling heads exists on the market.

The fine fraction of the TSP is obtained by samplers using preseparators that remove the coarse particles. Instruments that closely follow the BMRC fine-dust definition use horizontal elutriators for the separation of the coarse dust. Air is drawn through an assembly of parallel plates designed so that particles larger than $7 \mu m$ are collected on the plates. The fine fraction passes the elutriator and is deposited on a filter. Commercially available instruments of this type are the British Cassella sampler MRE type 113a and

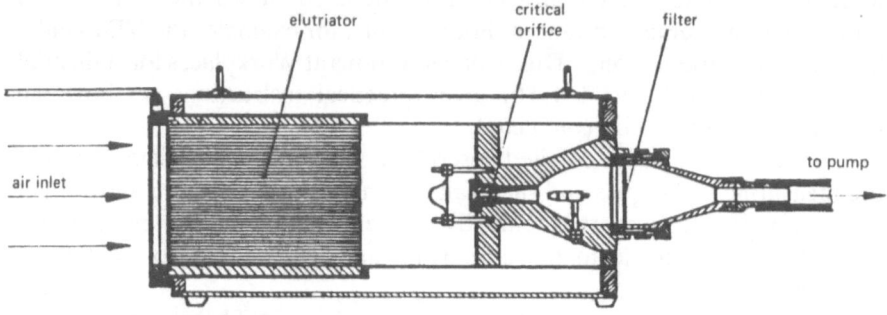

Fig. 2. Fine-dust sampler using horizontal elutriator

the German MPG II (Fig. 2) sampler. Cyclones are also widely used for particle size selective sampling. These are easily designed for a broad variety of flow rates to meet the suction capacity of numerous static as well as personal samplers. Other instruments, such as the German VC 25 F (Fig. 2), use impaction as a separation mechanism for coarse particles. All these separation mechanisms are tolerable for health-related sampling as long as the results correlate with the standard method of the horizontal elutriator. Conversion factors are allowed in the range between 0.7 and 1.3.

It is quite obvious that the classical filter method is of limited use for the characterization of fluctuating dust situations, for the localization of dust sources, and in most cases for measuring concentration peaks, especially if one does not know when these occur. Here, direct reading instruments with sufficient time resolution are highly desirable, particularly in view of future demands on workplace monitoring systems. Physical principles that can be used to measure mass concentrations more or less directly are the beta attenuation technique and the shift in resonance frequency of a mechanical oscillator (quartz crystal, glass tube) with increasing mass loading. Instruments that incorporate these principles are available on the market (Beta dust monitor, pieco balance). The Beta dust monitor can be operated with or without preseparator to measure the fine or the total dust, respectively. However, the instruments of this type are bulky, expensive, and often complicated to use. Therefore they are not suitable for widespread application for routine monitoring at workplaces under rough industrial conditions. Pieco balances usually measure fine dust because large particles do not sufficiently adhere to the oscillating surface.

Another group of instruments that have found application in workplace monitoring use the light-scattering properties of small particles; these instruments are called aerosol photometers. The aerosol moves through the measuring cell of the instrument; light is scattered by particles inside the sensing volume and is detected under a certain level by a photodetector. The signal is proportional to the mass concentration but also depends on the size distribution, and the optical constants of the aerosol material. The different size fractions composing the aerosol do not contribute equally to the overall scattering signal (Friedlander 1977). The sensitivity per aerosol mass is maximum for particles with sizes in the order of the wavelength of the light source used (usually around 500–800 mm). Thus large particles are strongly underrepresented. By properly choosing the scattering angle and the wavelength of the light it is possible to match the sensitivity curve approximately with the probability curve for particle deposition in the alveolar region of the human lung (Armbruster 1984). This makes aerosol photometry suitable for the measurement of the respirable dust fraction. Excellent time resolution is combined with a low detection limit and easy handling. However, it must be pointed out that by using light scattering one does not measure the mass concentration directly. A calibration, either internal or external, is always necessary. There are several aerosol photometers commercially available. The German TM Digital (Fig. 3) and the American Mini-Ram use an open measuring cell. The aerosol is sampled passively by the natural movement of the air. On the other hand, the British Simslin instrument samples actively. In this instrument coarse particles are removed by a horizontal elutriator before entering the optical cell. Interference with coarse particles is therefore excluded even if the coarse fraction is dominant. The Simslin instrument also offers the advantage of internal calibration whereas the passive samplers must be calibrated using separate filter samplers.

There is no direct reading instrument that is able to measure the three health-related fractions (fine, thoracic, total fraction) of the airborne

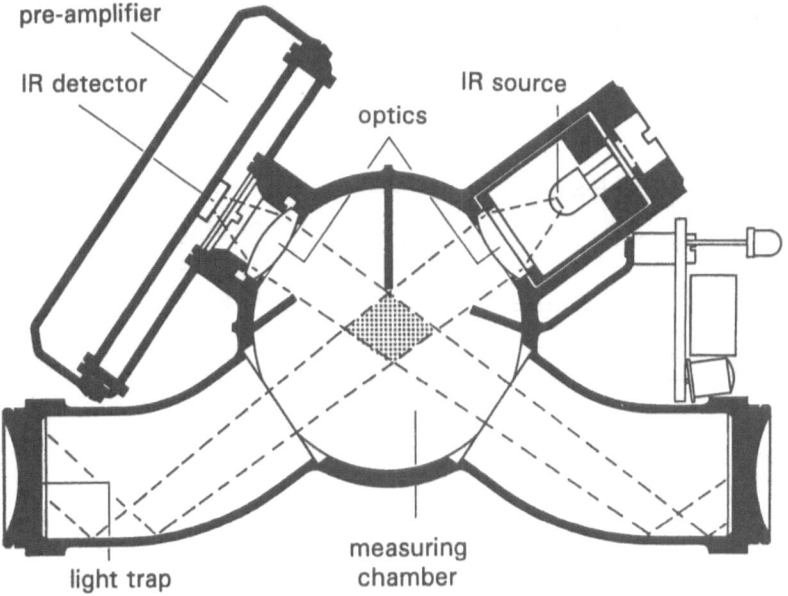

Fig. 3. Measuring cell for a fine-dust photometer that samples passively (TM digital)

dust simultaneously. There is a definite need of such instruments in view of an improved and more comprehensive short-term characterization of the working area, as will be recommended by the impending European standardization. In the draft of the standard "General Requirements for the Performance of Procedures of Workplace Measurements" the determination of spatial and temporal variation of the concentration is mentioned explicitly (Siekmann 1990). This can be achieved only using a direct-reading instrument. Furthermore, the measurement of the three above-mentioned dust fractions will be prescribed in the future European standards. Obviously, more research is needed into instrumentation. Although having superior dust characterization properties, the instruments to be developed must be simple and cheap enough to find broad application in routine monitoring, particularly in small companies.

A Direct Reading Instrument for the Fine and the Total Dust

Initiated by the health hazards related to wood dust, where fine and coarse particles seemed to be of importance, an instrument was developed at the Fraunhofer Institute that is a first step in the direction of on-line and simultaneous measurement of several dust fractions at workplaces. The use of aerosol photometry was extended to monitor simultaneously the fine and the total fraction of the airborne dust (Koch et al. 1988). Similar to the Simslin instrument, the modified instrument samples actively, and it uses both the aerodynamic and the light scattering properties of small particles. The instrument (Fig. 4) consists of a two-stage virtual impactor (the

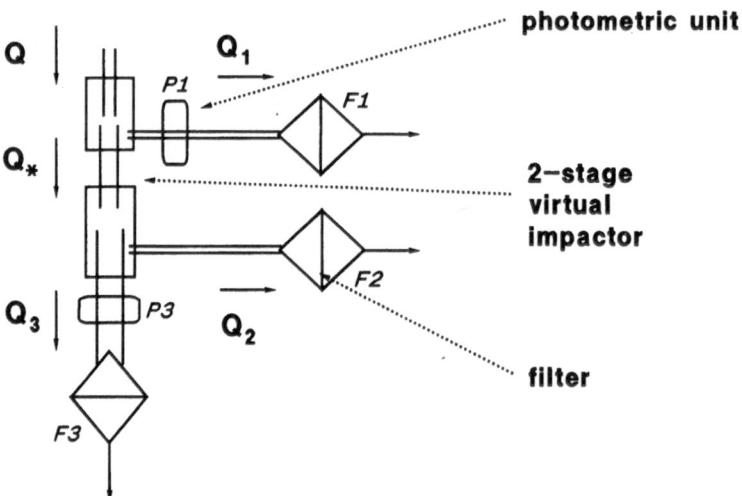

Fig. 4. Schematic description of an instrument using a combination of inertial enrichment/separation and optical aerosol detection

aerodynamic part) and two photometers (the optical part of the instrument). In each of the two stages of the virtual impactor the inlet flow is divided into two streams of 15% and 85%, respectively. Particles that are larger than a certain cutoff value (for example, 3 μm in the first stage and 10 μm in the second) are enriched in concentration in the channel with the minor flow whereas the complementary fraction is removed from the major flow channel. In total, the photometer placed in the minor flow rate channel of the second stage sees a 40-fold higher coarse dust concentration than a pure photometer. This compensates for the decreasing light-scattering efficiency of the large particles with respect to their mass. On the other hand, all particles that are larger than 3 μm are removed from the major flow of the first virtual impactor stage so that only fine particles are detected by a photometer placed in this channel (Fig. 5). Both photometers must be calibrated in situ using simultaneously taken filter samples. A microprocessor controls the instrument and stores the concentration data.

Measurements have been carried out various workplaces. Figure 6 shows a temporal concentration pattern that was taken very close to a drilling machine where fiber-reinforced plastics were proceesed. Samples were taken from a box covering the machine. Coarse dust is generated intermittently and settles out immediately after operation stops. Fine particles accumulate during the drilling process. They have a long residence time afterwards. Various samples were taken representing different process parameters and different materials. Calibration factors for the fine and the total dust were obtained by averaging the photometer voltage and dividing

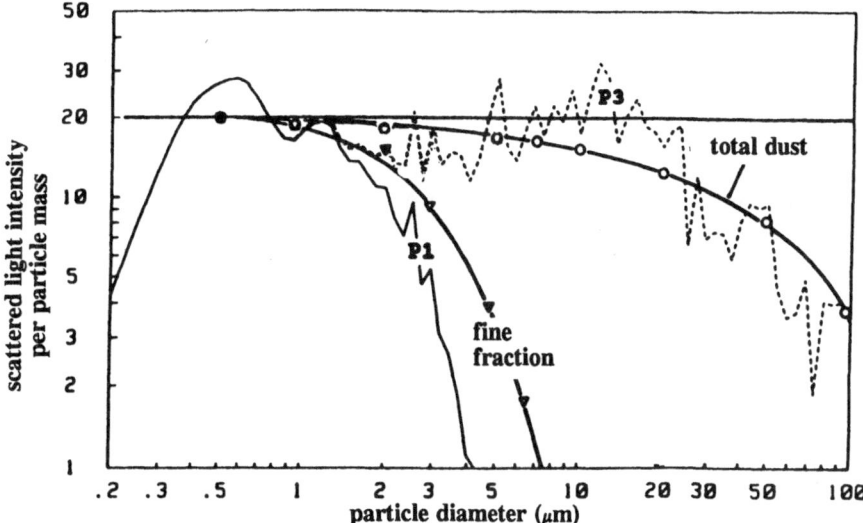

Fig. 5. Theoretical sensitivity curves obtained from the characteristics of the virtual impactor and Mie calculations for spherical particles ($\theta = 90$ xo, $\lambda = 800$ nm, $n = 1.55$)

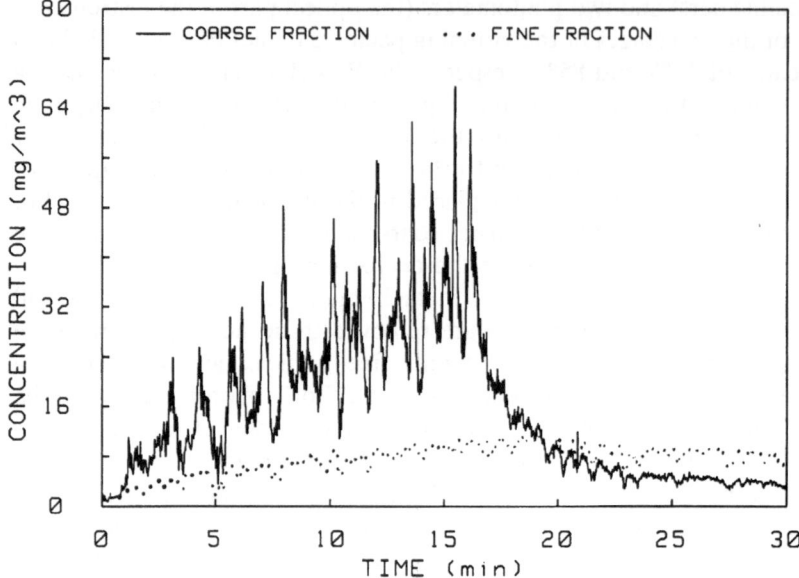

Fig. 6. Temporal concentration pattern for a highly polluted workplace. Note that the graph shows the concentration of the coarse fraction that was determined by substracting total and fine dust concentrations

by the mass concentration obtained from the in situ filter samples. The sensitivity was found to be constant irrespective of the dust composition.

The combination of aerodynamic separation and enrichment by a virtual impactor and aerosol detection by light-scattering offers a promising way for simultaneous, on line measurement of different health-related dust fractions. Future work in this direction must focus on also incorporating the thoracic fraction and miniaturizing the instrument to make it suitable for personal monitoring. This would allow one to characterize the actual exposure pattern of a worker much better than before and may thus help to take optimal measures to reduce the health risks at workplaces.

References

Armbruster L, Breuer H, Gebhart J, Neulinger S (1984) Photometric determination of respirable dust concentration without elutriation of coarse particles. Part Charact 1:96–101

British Medical Research Council (BMRC) (1952) Recommendations of the BMRC panels relating to selective sampling

Friedlander SK (1977) Smoke, dust and haze. Wiley, New York, p 133

International Standards Organization (ISO) (1983) Air-quality–particle size fraction definitions for health related sampling. Technical Report ISO/TR/7708-1983. ISO, Geneva

Koch W, Lödding H, Dunkhorst W, Scheffel H (1988) A measuring system with combined size and time reolution capability for the characterization of dust in the workplace environment. J Aerosol Sci 19:1453–1456

Lippmann M, Gurmann J, Schlesinger RB (1983) Role of particle deposition in occupational lung disease. In: Marple VA, Liu BYH (eds) Aerosols in the mining and work environment. Arbor, New York, pp 119–126

Ogden TL, Birkett JL (1977) The human head as a dust sampler. In: Walton WH (ed) Inhaled particles IV. Pergamon, Oxford, pp 93–105

Senatskommission zur Prüfung gesundheitsgefährlicher Arbeitsstoffe (1990) Maximale Arbeitsplatzkonzentrationen. Deutsche Forschungsgemeinschaft, Bonn

Siekmann H (1990) Messverfahren für Gefahrstoffe am Arbeitsphatz – Stand der Normung. Staub Reinhalt Luft 10:411–413

Technische Regeln für Gefahrstoffe (1986) Ermittlung und Beurteilung der Konzentrationen gefährlicher Stoffe in der Luft am Arbeitsbereich. TRGS 402. In: Markblätter für gefährliche Arbeitsstoffe. Ecomed, Landsberg

Verein Deutscher Ingenieure (VDI) (1980) VDI-Richtlinie 2265. Feststellen der Staubsituation am Arbeitsplatz zur gewerbehygienischen Beurteilung. In: VDI-Handbuch Reinhaltung der Luft. VDI, Düsseldorf

Vincent JH (1989) Aerosol sampling, science and practice. Wiley, New York

Vincent JH, Armbruster L (1981) On the quantitative definition of the inhalability of airborne dust. Ann Occup Hyg 24:245–248

Health Effects of Indoor Air Exposures

M. LIPPMANN

N.Y. University Medical Center, Nelson Inst. of Environmental Medicine, Long
Meadow Road, Tuxedo NY 10987, USA

Introduction

The pollutants inhaled in nonoccupational indoor settings can produce a
variety of health effects, with the impacts being dependent on the nature of
the pollutants, their concentrations, time spent indoors, respiratory rates,
interindividual susceptibility to the effects of the specific pollutants, and
the interactive effects of the multiple pollutant exposures. These basic considerations are well-known to those engaged in inhalation research. There
have been a series of learned monographs on the health effects of indoor
air, beginning with a National Research Council Report (NRC 1981), as
well as international symposia on this topic at 3-year intervals since 1978
(Copenhagen, Amherst, Stockholm, Berlin, and Toronto). The Environmental Protection Agency has compiled a reference bibliography on indoor
air containing 4367 citations (EPA 1989). This purpose of this presentation is to summarize current knowledge on the risks to passive building
occupants from exposures to some of the indoor pollutants that have been
the subject of major concern: radon (Rn) and daughters, environmental
tobacco smoke (ETS), asbestos fibers, and unvented combustion products. Another important class of indoor air pollutants, the volatile organic
chemicals, is addressed by Dr. Mølhave in another chapter.

Radon and Daughters

There is a widespread distribution of uranium-238 ($t_{1/2} = 4.5 \times 10^9$ years) in
soils, where it is usually present in secular equilibrium with the isotopes in
its decay chain through radium-226 ($t_{1/2} = 1.6 \times 10^3$ years). When ^{226}Ra
decays to the noble gas radon-222 ($t_{1/2} = 3.82$ days), there is an opportunity
for molecular diffusion, and radon migrates through interstices and gaps in
the soil and foundations into the basements of buildings. From there, it can
diffuse or be further transported to various occupied spaces by natural or
mechanical convection.

U. Mohr et al. (Eds.)
Advances in Controlled Clinical
Inhalation Studies
© Springer-Verlag Berlin Heidelberg 1993

The major variables thought to control ^{222}Rn entry into a building are: (a) indoor-outdoor temperature difference which, in turn, causes a differential pressure known as the stack effect, (b) the radium content of the soil under the building, (c) the radon release rate into the soil air, (d) the soil porosity, (e) the fraction of the air exchange or infiltration rate that comes through the soil pathway, and (f) the air exchange rate.

There are four radon daughters present in the particulate phase that have half-lives $(t_{1/2}) \leqslant 27$ min. This decay chain leads to the relatively long-term decay product, ^{210}Pb $(t_{1/2} = 22$ years). Three of the four are α-emitters. As the molecular-sized particles form, they rapidly coagulate and diffuse to available surfaces, such as other airborne particles and aggregates as well as the walls of the rooms and the airways of the lungs. Within the lungs, the particles are deposited preferentially at airway bifurcations in patterns closely matching the common sites of primary bronchial carcinoma (Schlesinger and Lippmann 1978).

The short-lived decay products are rarely in equilibrium or steady-state with the parent ^{222}Rn in practical situations. To circumvent this problem, exposures in mines were documented in terms of a unit called the working level (WL). The WL is the total decay energy of any combination of the short-lived daughters resulting in the release of 1.3×10^5 MeV of α energy and is equal to 3700 Bq $\cdot$ m^{-3} (100 pCi $\cdot$ l^{-1}) at equilibrium. Cumulative exposure was recorded for workers in units of the working level month (WLM). The relationship between radon concentrations and the short-lived daughters in WL depends mainly upon the ventilation rate and the atmospheric particle concentration in the space considered.

Radon released into an enclosed space, as in a mine or building, cannot disperse into the atmosphere and therefore gradually increases in concentration. The major source of radon in the air inside a building is the soil beneath and adjacent to the building, although release of dissolved radon from the water supply may also be significant in some locations. The observed values of indoor radon follow a log-normal distribution, the numbers of buildings with concentrations 10–100 times the average value being disproportionately large compared with the numbers expected from a normal distribution (NCRP 1984b). The highest indoor radon concentrations have been measured in the basements of single-family houses, with concentrations on higher floors decreasing somewhat. The concentrations in high-rise apartments and public buildings have generally been much lower, largely because of their greater ventilation and more substantial foundations, and the physical separation from basement air.

The average exposure of members of the American population has been estimated to range from 0.2 WLM per year (NCRP 1984b) to 0.25 WLM per year (Puskin and Nelson 1989), or possibly higher (NCRP 1987). The many radon measurements that have been made for exposure estimation were designed primarily to determine the maximum potential concentrations of radon in houses rather than the actual levels to which occupants are exposed. The commerical measurements are also biased by the fact that the customers requesting them usually have had reasons to suspect high concentrations of radon in their homes (Cohen 1988). Hence, there is a need for the statistically stratified program of radon sampling to estimate the average level of exposure in the USA, and such a survey has been initiated by the USEPA.

Toxicity and Health Effects

Human Epidemiology

Interpretation of the major studies of underground miners reported thus far is complicated by: (a) poorly documented exposures for many of the miners, (b) the uncertain contribution of smoking to the observed excess of lung cancer, and (c) the suitability of the control populations used.

Epidemiological studies are underway in the general population to estimate directly the risk of indoor radon. They are, however, subject to limitations from exposure misclassifications, inadequate sample size, and the possible confounding effects of extraneous risk factors. Because the general population has had lower levels of exposure than the miners, and, consequently, smaller effects are anticipated, the statistical power of the studies may prove to be inadequate. At this time estimates of the risks to the general population from exposure to radon have been based primarily on extrapolation from the experience of the miners.

From the lung cancer mortality reported in various cohorts of miners, the exposure-response relationship for lung cancer appears to be linear in the low-to-intermediate dose range. On the basis of this epidemiological evidence, supporting animal studies, and biological considerations, the frequency of lung cancer is assumed to increase linearly with exposure below 50 WLM. To assess the total magnitude of the radon risk, however, it is necessary to predict the lifetime lung cancer mortality in the various mining populations, many members of which still survive. For this purpose, the simple absolute risk model (which predicts a constant percentage increase in the annual age-dependent baseline risk following a given exposure) may not adequately describe the observed patterns of mortality. Instead, either a modified absolute risk model, in which the risk is reduced with time after exposure (NCRP 1984a), or a modified relative risk model in which the risk varies as a function of age and time after exposure (NAS/BEIR 1988), seems preferable. A model of the latter type has been adopted by the EPA for its radon risk assessment (Puskin and Nelson 1989).

It should be noted that the use of risk models for estimating risks to the general population from the data on miners involves additional uncertainties due to differences in age and sex distribution and potential differences between continuous exposure over a lifetime and short-term occupational exposure during working hours only. The apparent decrease in risk with time after cessation of radon exposure has not been precisely established. Since lung cancer is rare before the age of 40 years, exposure during childhood may possibly contribute little to the subsequent risk of the disease (NAS/BEIR 1989). On the other hand, the ICRP (1987) has considered risks to be greater for exposure during childhood. Other uncertainties complicating the assessment relate to estimation of the actual dose delivered to the lung, due to differences in breathing rate and aerosol particle size, the degree of radioactive equilibrium of the decay products in the atmosphere, and other variables (NCRP 1984a; Harley and Cohen 1987). The form of the interaction between the effects of smoking and those of radon is also uncertain, and assessment of this interaction is possible in only a few studies. The strongest evidence is available from the study of Colorado plateau uranium miners. It suggests a somewhat less than multiplicative interaction (NAS 1988). If the multiplicative interaction model is correct (e.g., NAS 1988), the absolute lifetime risk for a given level of radon exposure would be 6–10 times higher in smokers than in nonsmokers.

Animal Toxicology

Radon and radon decay products have been shown to increase the incidence of benign and malignant tumors of the respiratory tract in rats exposed to these radionuclides by chronic inhalation (Cross 1988); the magnitude of the increase varies, depending on the dose and the influence of other factors, such as inhalation of dust or cigarette smoke.

Risk Characterization

The average level of exposure to radon in members of the American population has not been characterized in a large nationwide survey. However, data from diverse sources suggest a mean concentration in US homes of about $1.5 \, pCi \cdot l^{-1}$. If annual exposure is assumed to approximate 0.25 WLM per year (Puskin and Nelson 1989), the lifetime risk of mortality from lung cancer can be calculated with the use of the risk models cited. With the use of such models, the lifetime risk of lung cancer from exposure to radon in the US population can be estimated to range from roughly 0.4%–1.8%. On this basis, exposure to radon can be estimated to account for some 5000–40 000 deaths from lung cancer each year in the USA or about 4%–30% of all lung cancer deaths in the US population (Puskin and Nelson 1989). The EPA's current estimate is that indoor radon and daughter exposures produce an annual increase in lung cancer deaths in the US of 16 000. All of these estimates may, however, overstate the actual impact, since most of the exposure estimates are based on measurements in basements.

In any case, these estimates strongly suggest that radon exposure presents a significant public health problem. Since the uncertainties in the exposure levels and in the risk estimates are large, vigorous efforts to refine the levels and the risk estimates are warranted.

Environmental Tobacco Smoke

ETS is a complex mixture of gases, vapors, droplets, and ash from burning cigarettes, and their admixtures with other components of ambient indoor air. Most of the ETS derives from sidestream smoke emitted from the burning end of the cigarette, with the rest being associated with the small fraction of the mainstream smoke that is exhaled. As the smoke ages, the submicrometer-sized condensation aerosols can grow by coagulation and/or shrink by evaporation. Further variation in the composition and particle size distribution of ETS results from variations in: (a) composition of the cigarettes (tobacco, packing density, humectants, filters, paper, etc.), (b) the rate and pattern of combustion; and (c) butt length. The concentrations achieved in an occupied space depend upon the size of the space, the ventilation rate, and the occupancy pattern and cigarette consumption by the occupants. As the smoke ages in the short term, the concentration ratios within the mixture increase for the relatively nonreactive, poorly adsorbed components such as carbon monoxide (CO). In the longer term, semivolatile organic compounds that deposit on internal surfaces by diffusion may cause tobacco odor in a room long after the CO has dissipated.

Extensive toxicologic, experimental, and epidemiologic data, largely collected since the 1950s, have established that active cigarette smoking is the major preventable cause of morbidity and mortality in the USA (USDHEW 1979; USDHHS 1989). More recently, involuntary exposure to tobacco smoke (passive smoke exposure) has been investigated as a risk factor for disease and also found to be a cause of preventable morbidity and mortality in nonsmokers. The 1986 Report of the Surgeon General on Smoking and Health (USDHHS 1986) and a report by the National Research Council (NRC 1986), also published in 1986, comprehensively reviewed the data on involuntary exposure to tobacco smoke and reached comparable conclusions with significant public health implications; both reports concluded that involuntary smoking was a cause of disease in nonsmokers. Authoritative reviews prepared more recently have reached essentially the same conclusions (Spitzer et al. 1990; Samet 1991; EPA 1990; SAB 1991).

The conclusions were based more on the cumulative weight of a large body of epidemiological evidence rather than on any single or small group of definitive population-based studies. Clinical studies and experimental animal studies have provided supporting information that added to the weight of evidence but have not been able to demonstrate independent evidence that ETS exposure, per se, produces diseases comparable with those implicated in the epidemiologic studies. Clinical studies are, by their very nature, limited to brief exposures that produce measurable, but transient physiological responses. The lack of documented disease in rodents chronically exposed to heavy concentrations of mainstream smoke has discouraged inhalation toxicologists from under-taking chronic exposure studies with ETS at lower concentrations.

The nature of the epidemiologic evidence is illustrated in Fig. 1 from the National Research Council Report (NRC 1986). It summarizes the results of 13 population studies of lung cancer among nonsmokers with spousal exposures to ETS, in relation to control groups of nonsmokers married to nonsmokers. It also shows the odds ratios determined from meta-analyses that combined the data from either all or selected subsets of the 13 studies. While most individual studies show odds ratios greater than unity, only a few were statistically significant. However, when the data were combined, the confidence intervals were greatly reduced, with the odds ratios of approximately 1.3 being significant. In general, studies of American populations show smaller odds ratios and less statistical significance than those conducted elsewhere. This may be due to a greater degree of misclassifica-

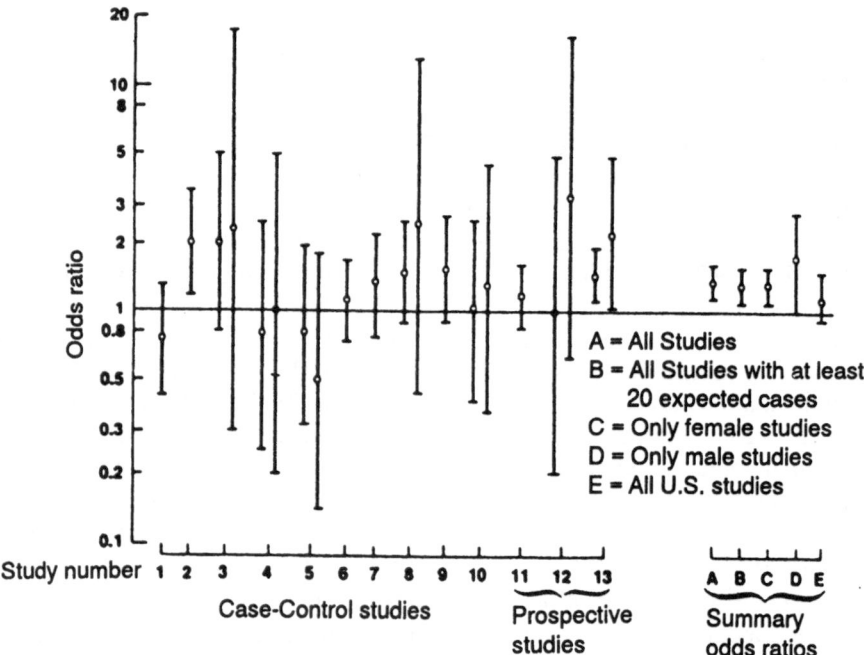

Fig. 1. Relative risk (point estimate and 95% confidence interval) of lung cancer in nonsmokers whose spouses smoke compared with nonsmokers whose spouses do not smoke for each of 13 studies and the summary estimate based on all the studies combined. The figures for females are shown first for studies based on male and female subjects (NRC 1986)

tion of exposure status for the nonsmoking women married to nonsmokers. It is likely that more of them are exposed to ETS at work and at leisure activities than are their counterparts in other countries, resulting in smaller differences in overall ETS exposure than in the spousal exposure surrogate used to define the groups.

It is rare for relative risks below about 1.5 to be considered as demonstrating causality, since the effects of misclassification and confounding by unanalyzed cofactors could account for the results. However, in this case, careful consideration of such factors has failed to demonstrate any systematic biases that could account for the elevated odds ratios. Furthermore, even if the odds ratio is low, very large numbers of people are exposed, and several thousands of additional lung cancers can result from such exposures. Thus, the estimates of the population impact are similar in magnitude to those for indoor exposures to radon and daughters.

While most attention has been focussed on the associations between ETS and lung cancer, there may be much greater human health impacts of ETS. In terms of other fatal outcomes associated with exposure, the greatest concern involves premature death from coronary heart disease or myocardial infarction. Fig. 2 shows that the meta-analysis by Glantz and Parmley (1991) of 10 epidemiological studies indicates a significant combined odds ratio of 1.3, similar to that for the several meta-analyses for lung cancer. Glantz and Parmley also reviewed data indicating that ETS adversely affects platelet

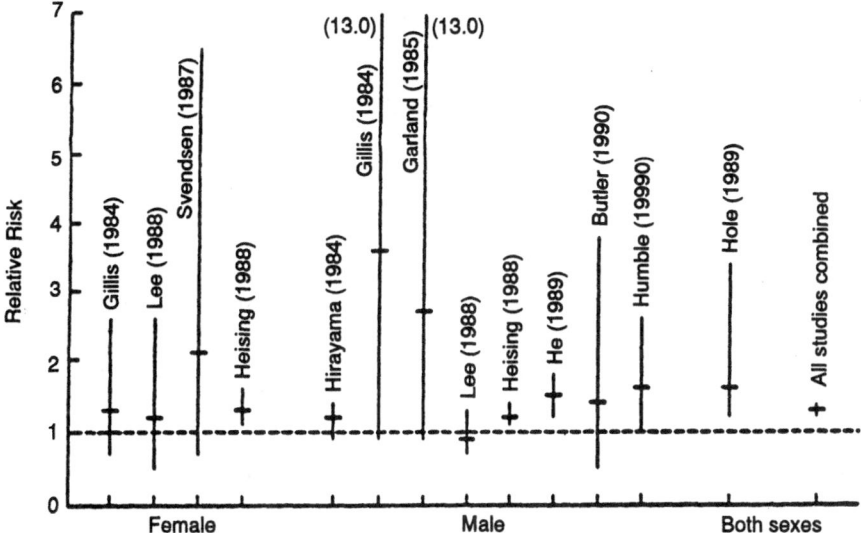

Fig. 2. Graph of relative risk in epidemiological studies of the risk of death from coronary heart disease or myocardial infarction among nonsmokers living with smokers compared with nonsmokers living with nonsmokers. Lines indicate 95% confidence intervals. (Note: two studies have upper bounds to the 95% confidence interval off the scale of the graph) (Glantz and Parmley 1991)

function, damages arterial endothelium, and reduces exercise capacity and argue that these responses are consistent with the augmented mortality rates. Their analysis has not been extensively reviewed in the manner that the Surgeon General (USDHHS 1986), the National Research Council (NRC 1986), the EPA (EPA 1990), and the EPA's Science Advisory Board (SAB 1991) have reviewed the ETS-lung cancer association, but the potential population impact may be much larger, i.e., they estimate about 37000 excess cardiovascular deaths per year attributable to ETS exposure, as compared with about one-tenth that many from lung cancer.

The public health impact of nonfatal outcome measures may also be considerable. For example, the NRC (1986) report concluded that:

- Children of parents who smoke compared with the children of parents who do not smoke show increased prevalence of respiratory symptoms, usually cough, sputum, and wheezing. The odds ratios from the larger studies, adjusted for the presence of parental symptoms, were 1.2–1.8, depending on the symptoms. These findings imply that ETS exposure causes respiratory symptoms in some children.
- Estimates of the magnitude of the effect of parental smoking on FEV_1 function of children range from zero to approximately 0.5% decrease per year. This small effect is unlikely by itself to be clinically significant. However, it may reflect pathophysiologic effects of exposure to ETS in the lungs of the growing child and, as such, may be a factor in the development of chronic airflow obstruction in later life.
- Bronchitis, pneumonia, and other lower-respiratory-tract illnesses occur up to twice as often during the first year of life in children who have one or more parents who smoke than in children of nonsmokers.
- Household exposure to ETS is linked with increased rates of chronic ear infections and middle-ear effusions in young children. For children with nasal allergies and recurrent otitis media, ETS exposure may synergistically increase their risk of persistent middle-ear effusions.
- Evidence has accumulated indicating that nonsmoking pregnant women exposed to ETS on a daily basis for several hours are at increased risk for producing low-birthweight babies through mechanisms which are, as yet, unknown. Recent studies show a dose-respone relationship between the number of cigarettes smoked by the father and birthweight of the children of nonsmoking pregnant women.

Additional evidence for these effects was summarized by the EPA in its Draft Risk Assessment (EPA 1990), and the Science Advisory Board (SAB 1991) concluded that this evidence warranted stronger concern in the overall risk assessment than that presented by the EPA.

Asbestos

Asbestos, a naturally occurring group of mineral silicates in fibrous crystalline forms, was hailed as a miracle fiber earlier in this century. Asbestos fibers have excellent mechanical and insulating properties and are highly resistant to heat and chemical corrosion under most conditions. Thus, they were widely used for insulation and fireproofing and were incorporated into composite materials such as asbestos-cement tiles and pipes, brake and clutch linings, vinyl-asbestos floor tiles, etc. for heat resistance and mechanical strength. Asbestos fibers also proved to have unique properties in terms of toxicity. Many workers who inhaled asbestos fibers at relatively high concentrations, generally over many years, developed asbestosis, a diffuse form of lung fibrosis; lung cancer; and/or cancer of the pleural or peritoneal membranes (mesothelioma). These chronic diseases, usually occurring decades after initial occupational exposure, are often progressive and fatal. In recent years, it has been found that maintenance and custodial workers in schools and other public buildings have been exposed to airborne fibers from friable asbestos and damaged asbestos-containing materials (ACMs) that they disturb during their work activities. Many of them develop pleural plaques, which are markers of exposure, may restrict lung function (HEI-AR 1991), and may be precursor lesions for mesothelioma.

Reviews of the worker experience and laboratory studies of animals have indicated that the cancer risks fits linear, nonthreshold dose-response models reasonably well. It is therefore prudent to consider that any exposure to airborne asbestos fibers produces some finite added risk of cancer. Worker exposure has long been defined in terms of the number of fibers that are longer than $5\,\mu m$ per milliliter of air (f/ml), as measured by phase-contrast optical microscopy (PCOM), and the risk models have been developed using this measure of exposure. It has long been known that fibers longer than $5\,\mu m$ are a minority of all fibers. On the other hand, it has also long been known that long fibers are much more toxic than shorter ones. Recent analyses of chronic animal inhalation study data, in vitro study data, and data from worker lung autopsy studies confirm the critical dependency of fiber toxicity and carcinogenicity on fiber length and justify retaining the $5\,\mu m$ length criterion for risk assessments for hazardous fibers (HEI-AR 1991).

Fiber concentrations in schools and public buildings are usually measured by transmission electron microscopy (TEM), which has a much better resolving power than PCOM. Since fibers as thin or thinner than $0.05\,\mu m$ are seen by TEM, while only fibers thicker than about $0.25\,\mu m$ are seen by PCOM, the TEM analyses generally show higher fiber concentrations, even when the counts are restricted to long fibers. Building concentrations are much lower than those that occurred in the industries where disease incidence was high. Historic occupational exposures were often in the range of 5–20 f/ml

(PCOM). The permissible exposure limit for workers in the USA was 2 f/ml between 1976 and 1986, when it was lowered to 0.2 f/ml. In 1990, the Occupational Safety and Health Administration (OSHA) proposed reducing it to 0.1 f/ml.

There are few published data on fiber concentrations in background air, schools, or other public buildings. In 1991, the Health Effects Institute – Asbestos Research (HEI-AR) Literature Review Panel gathered all available concentration data and reported that airborne concentrations of asbestos fibers of the dimensions most relevant to human health (i.e., fibers >5 μm long) show average concentrations on the order of 0.00001 f/ml for outdoor rural air (except near asbestos-containing rock outcroppings) and average concentrations up to about one order of magnitude higher in the outdoor air of urban environments. However, outdoor urban airborne concentrations above 0.0001 f/ml have been reported in certain circumstances as a result of local sources, e.g., downwind from, or close to, frequent vehicle braking or activities involving the demolition or spray application of asbestos products. Data on ambient indoor levels of asbestos from direct TEM measurements were averaged for a number of individual buildings. The following are based on some 1377 air samples obtained in 198 different buildings not involved in litigation. Excluding one outlier value (0.00243 f/ml), the overall means of the studies on these buildings range from 0.00004 to 0.00063 f/ml. Grouped by building category, the mean concentrations are 0.00051, 0.00019, and 0.00020 f/ml in schools, residences, and public and commercial buildings,

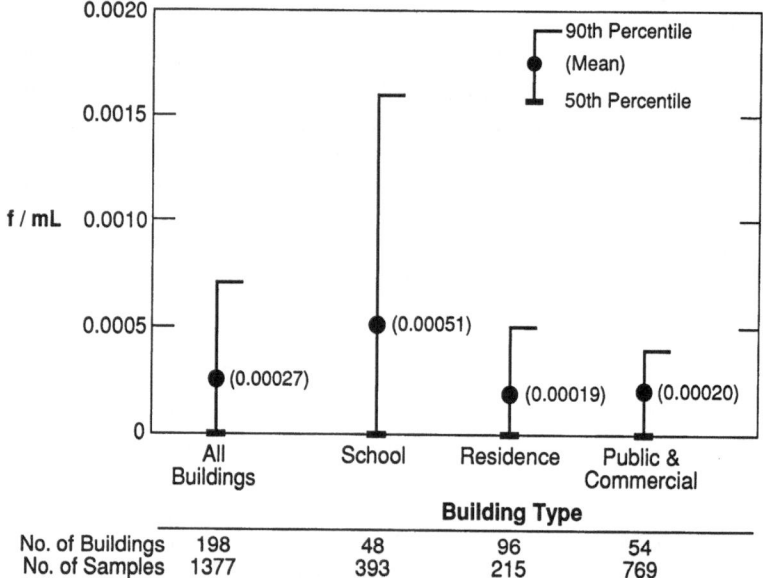

Fig. 3. Distribution of building average concentrations of airborne asbestos fibers (>5 μm in length) for nonlitigation samples (data extracted from HEI-AR 1991)

respectively, with upper 90th percentiles of 0.0016, 0.0005, and 0.004, respectively (Fig. 3). The outlier value was from the commercial and public building category. Without it, the mean value in this category was 0.00008 f/ml.

For each exposure increment of 0.0001 f/ml, the cancer risk models predict an increase in cancer risk of about 0.002%. About 10% of smokers develop lung cancer in the USA, as do about 0.5% of nonsmokers. For mesothelioma, which is not influenced by smoking, the incidence is about 0.02%.

In most situations, public concern over asbestos in buildings has focused primarily on potential risks to general building occupants. However, the potential risk to more highly exposed custodial and maintenance workers should be the primary consideration in determining whether to take remedial action. The averaged measured levels of airborne asbestos fibers in most asbestos-containing buildings are now so low that no increase over ambient background has been demonstrated directly. Asbestos removal activities sometimes cause a considerable and persistent increase in measured levels, and it is impossible to be certain, on the basis of available data, whether removal will, in practice, reduce or increase lifetime exposures of general building occupants. In most situations, the potential risks to occupationally exposed custodial and maintenance workers should constitute the primary consideration in determining appropriate remedial action, if any (HEI-AR 1991).

Unvented Combustion Products

Indoor combustion sources that are not vented to the outside release a wide variety of combustion products into the indoor air. One complex mixture of such pollutants, ETS, has already been discussed. This section covers the effluents from unvented cooking and heating appliances that use natural gas or kerosene as fuels. These include gas stoves, ovens, and water heaters, as well as gas and kerosene space heaters. All of them generate a variety of nitrogen oxides (NO_x) at varying rates and proportions, including nitric oxide (NO), nitrogen dioxide (NO_2), nitrous acid (HONO), and nitric acid (HNO_3). Commercial kerosenes often contain enough sulfur for the combustion effluent to contain sulfur dioxide (SO_2) and sulfuric acid (H_2SO_4) in appreciable concentrations. Other combustion products include water vapor (H_2O), carbon dioxide (CO_2), and carbon monoxide (CO). In some cases, the added water vapor can increase humidity to the point that the growth of mold and mildew is facilitated, creating a confounding factor affecting the interpretation of increased respiratory effects. When burner adjustments are improper, there can be enough generation of CO and products of incomplete combustion to cause serious consequences, but these will not be discussed here.

When gas is used for cooking and baking, there will be additional releases of water and organic vapors that add further complexity to the composition of the indoor air.

In the absence of malfunctioning combustion appliances, none of the combustion effluents are likely to be present in indoor air at concentrations and durations that have produced measurable responses in controlled exposure studies in humans or animals. On the other hand, a number of studies of populations of humans living in homes with unvented combustion appliances have reported abnormalities in respiratory function and/or symptoms that were greater than those found in control populations without such sources. In children from randomly selected areas of Great Britain, Melia et al. (1979) found a gradient of increased respiratory symptoms with increasing indoor levels of NO_2. In another study by Melia et al. (1982) of children aged 5–6 years from the same communities, there was no significant relationship between levels of NO_2 and the prevalence of respiratory illness. The levels of NO_2 in the bedrooms of homes with a gas stove were 0.005–0.029 ppm.

Results of the Harvard Six-Cities Study from 1974 to 1977 on over 8000 children aged 6–10 years indicated a significant increase in the rate of respiratory illness before age 2 years in homes with gas-fired vs. electric stoves (Speizer et al. 1980). Estimated levels of exposure were 0.004–0.026 ppm NO_2, based upon stove measures. However, examination of the same communities over a longer time period, namely 1974–1979 (Ware et al. 1984), did not show any statistically significant increase in respiratory illness in these young children. In a later analysis from this study, Dockery et al. (1989) reported results from a sample of over 5000 children aged 7–11 years during the period 1983–1986. Marginal significance was noted for physician diagnosed respiratory illness prior to age 2 years in homes using gas-fired stoves compared with those using electric stoves; estimated exposures to NO_2 were similar to those above.

Ware et al. (1984) examined various pulmonary mechanical indices in the above children. The use of gas stoves was associated with significant reductions in parameters of expiratory flow (FEV_1, FVC) in a first examination, but not in a second. In another study, which examined a sample of over 100 children in Tucson (Lebowitz et al. 1985), a borderline significant effect between peak flow reduction in healthy children in homes with gas stoves was found, while for asthmatic subjects, peak flow was highly significantly associated with the use of such stoves. In Connecticut, respiratory symptoms were measured in adult women and children (aged 13 years and younger) (Berwick et al. 1984). Children under the age of 7 years exposed to ≥0.016 ppm were found to be at an increased risk of lower respiratory tract symptoms than those who were not so exposed; there was also an increased, but lesser, risk of upper respiratory symptoms. No increased risk was found in older children or adults. Comstock et al. (1981) noted a relationship between the use of gas stoves and increased prevalence of respiratory symptoms (cough) and reduction in some pulmonary function indices in adults in Maryland. Other studies have found various results, such as no association between gas stove use and symptoms or lung function changes in children (Schenker et al. 1983; Dodge 1982), or an association between such use and hospitalization for acute respiratory illness in children under 2 years of age (Ekwo et al. 1983).

The effect of NO_2 on respiratory health in 6 to 9-year-old Dutch children was examined by Houthuijs et al. (1987). Personal exposures to NO_2 were measured as indoor levels in the home. The prevalence of lung disease was found to be associated with the presence of unvented gas water heaters, with weekly (average) exposures estimated at 0.021 ppm. Koo et al. (1990) used personal samplers to monitor NO_2 exposure in children aged 7–13 years in Hong Kong. No association was noted between exposure levels (means ranged from 0.013 to 0.023 ppm for a 1-week period) and respiratory symptoms, such as wheeze, running nose, or cough.

Berwick et al. (1989) presented results of an epidemiologic study of reported upper and lower respiratory tract symptoms in 121 children (59 with kerosene heaters and 62 without) conducted during the 1982–1983 heating season in New Haven, Connecticut. Using measured values of NO_2 in the homes ($n = 113$), children (under 7 years old) with NO_2 levels greater than $30\,\mu g/m^3$ showed an odds ratio of 1.33 (1.19–1.49) for upper and 2.17 (1.69–2.79) for lower respiratory tract symptoms. The effects in this study were greater than expected on the basis of the NO_2 exposures and could have been due to the elevations in concentration of SO_2, H_2SO_4, and HONO condensed on ultrafine carbon particles that are also elevated by unvented kerosene heaters. Leaderer et al. (1990) reported the results of chamber studies of particle acid, sulfate, and respirable mass emissions from kerosene heaters, showing that the heaters are an important source of fine carbon particles, sulfate aerosol, and acid aerosol indoors. The projected levels in homes of acid particles was from less than 1–$4\,\mu g/m^3$, sulfate aerosol from 7 to $15\,\mu g/m^3$, and for respirable mass $20\,\mu g/m^3$ or more. Maltuned heaters could produce much higher levels.

It is not possible on the basis of the available data to draw any definitive conclusions regarding adverse health effects of NO_2 or the other effluents. There have been both positive and negative findings at various levels of NO_2 exposure, with various degrees of precision in measuring actual outdoor exposure levels, and generally with gas stove use as a surrogate measure of indoor exposure. Some results suggest that an increase in acute respiratory illness, especially in young children, may be associated with chronic ambient exposure to NO_2 at concentrations generally found in the home or outdoors. Although the extent of any such effect is small, this result is consistent with the increased bacterial infectivity found in toxicological studies at much higher concentrations.

Conclusions

Chronic exposures to indoor air pollutants at elevated levels can produce a variety of fatal outcomes and/or debilitating chronic diseases, thereby elevating the incidence of these diseases above background rates. The risks to any given individual are generally small, but when large proportions of the public receive elevated exposure, the overall public health impact can be appreciable.

The four kinds of indoor air pollution discussed in this paper, i.e., radon and daughters, ETS, asbestos, and the products of unvented combustion, have been the subjects of the greatest concern. They differ considerably in the nature of the sources, the factors influencing exposures to building occupants, and the kinds of health effects of primary concern.

Lung cancer is involved with three of the pollutants reviewed here, i.e., radon daughters, ETS, and asbestos. While effects other than cancer have not been associated with indoor air exposures to radon daughters and asbestos, the elevation in lung cancer incidence associated with ETS may represent only a small part of its overall adverse effects on general population health. Its effects on cardiovascular mortality may be 10 times as high, and its effects on respiratory morbidity in children, while difficult to interpret in terms of disease incidence or severity, may represent its greatest public health impact. Some of the same respiratory disease morbidity effects have been associated with the unvented products of combustion. It is still not clear what contributions the individual products, e.g., NO_2, HONO, increased humidity, make to the overall effects. In any case, the net effects are less well established than those of ETS exposure, and they almost certainly have lesser overall impacts on public health.

Acknowledgements. This work was supported, in part, by Cooperative Agreement CR 818325 from the U.S. Environmental Protective Agency, and is part of a Center Program supported by Grant ES 00260 from the National Institute of Environmental Health Sciences.

References

Berwick M, Zagraniski RT, Leaderer BP, Stolwijk JA (1984) Respiratory illness in children exposed to unvented combustion sources, vol 2. In: Berglund B, Lindvall T, Sundell J (eds) Indoor air. Swedish Council for Building Research, Stockholm, pp 225–260

Berwick M, Leaderer BP, Stolwijk JAJ, Zagranski RT (1989) Association between nitrogen dioxide levels and lower respiratory symptoms in children exposed to unvented combustion sources. Environmental International 15:225–232

Cohen BL (1988) Radon Levels by States and Counties. Report of the Radon Project Data through February 1988. Radon Project, Pittsburgh, 1988

Comstock GW, Meger MB, Helsing KJ, Tockman MJ (1981) Respiratory effects of household exposures to tobacco smoke and gas cooking. Am Rev Respir Dis 124:143–148

Cross FT (1988) Evidence of lung cancer from animal studies. In: Nazaroff WW, Nero AV Jr (eds) Radon and its decay products in indoor air. Wiley, New York, pp 373–406

Dockery DW, Speizer FE, Stram DO, Ware JH, Spengler JD, Ferris BG Jr (1989) Effects of inhalable particles on respiratory health of children. Am Rev Respir Dis 139:587–594

Dodge R (1982) The effects of indoor pollution on Arizona children. Arch Environ Health 37:151–155

Ekwo EE, Weinberger MW, Lachenbruch PA, Huntley WH (1983) Relationship of parental smoking and gas cooking to respiratory disease in children. Chest 84:662–668

EPA (Environmental Protection Agency) (1989) Indoor air-reference bibliography. EPA/600/8-89/067F, USEPA, ECAO, Research Triangle Park, NC

EPA (Environmental Protection Agency) (1990) Health effects of passive smoking: assessment of lung cancer in adults and respiratory disorders in children. EPA/600/6-90/006A, USEPA, Washington, DC

Glantz SA, Parmley WW (1991) Passive smoking and heart disease – epidemiology, physiology, and biochemistry. Circulation 83:1–12

Harley NH, Cohen BS (1987) Updating radon daughter dosimetry. In: Hopke PK (ed) Radon and its duaghter products. American Chemical Society, Washington, p 419

HEI-AR (Health Effects Institute – Asbestos Research) (1991) Report of the literature review panel on asbestos in public and commercial buildings. HEI-AR, Cambridge, MA

Houthuijs D, Remijn B, Brunekreef B, de Koning R (1987) Exposure to nitrogen dioxide and tobacco smoke and respiratory health of children, vol 1. In: Seifert B, Esdom H, Fischer M, Rueden H, Wegner J (eds) Indoor air '87. Institute for Water, Soil and Air Hygiene, Berlin, pp 463–467

ICRP (International Commission on Radiological Protection) (1987) Lung cancer risk from indoor exposures to radon daughters. International Commission on Radiological Protection Publication No. 50. Pergamon, New York

Koo LC, Ho JHC, Ho C-Y, Matsuki H, Shimizu H, Mori T, Tominaga S (1990) Personal exposure to nitrogen dioxide and its association with respiratory illness in Hong Kong. Am Rev Respir Dis 141:1119–1126

Leaderer BP, Boone PM, White JB, Hammond KS (1990) Total particle sulfate and acidic aerosol emissions from kerosene space heaters. Environ Sci Technol 24:908–912

Lebowitz MD, Holberg CJ, Boyer B, Hayes C (1985) Respiratory symptoms and peak flow associated with indoor and outdoor air pollutants in the southwest. J Air Pollut Control Assoc 35:1154–1158

Melia RJW, Florey CDV, Chinn S (1979) The relation between respiratory illness in primary schoolchildren and the use of gas for cooking: I. Results from a national survey. Int J Epidemiol 8:333–339

Melia RJW, Florey CDV, Morris RW, Goldstein BD, John HH, Clark D, Craighead IB, Mackinlay JC (1982) Childhood respiratory illness and the home environment: II. Association between respiratory illness and nitrogen dioxide, temperature and relative humidity. Int J Epidemiol 11:164–169

NAS/BEIR (National Academy of Sciences – National Research Council) (1988) Health risks of radon and other internally deposited alpha-emitters (BEIR IV). National Academy, Washington

NAS/BEIR (National Academy of Sciences – National Research Council) (1989) Health effects of exposure to low levels of ionizing radiation (BEIR V). National Academy, Washington

NCRP (National Council on Radiation Protection and Measurements) (1984a) Evaluation of occupational and environmental exposures to radon and radon daughters in the United States. National Council on Radiation Protection and Measurements Report No. 78. National Council on Radiation Protection and Measurements, Bethesda

NCRP (National Council on Radiation Protection and Measurements) (1984b) Exposures from the uranium series with emphasis on radon and its daughters. National Council on Radiation Protection and Measurements Report No. 77. National Council on Radiation Protection and Measurements, Bethesda

NCRP (National Council on Radiation Protection and Measurements) (1987) Ionizing radiation exposure of the population of the United States. National Council on Radiation Protection and Measurements Report No. 93. National Council on Radiation Protection and Measurements, Bethesda

NRC (National Research Council) (1981) Indoor pollutants. National Academy, Washington

NRC (National Research Council, Committee on Passive Smoking) (1986) Environmental tobacco smoke: measuring exposures and assessing health effects. National Academy, Washington

Puskin JS, Nelson CB (1989) EPA's perspective on risks from residential radon exposure. J Air Pollut Control Assoc 39:915–920

SAB (Science Advisory Board, USEPA) (1991) Health effects of passive smoking: assessment of lung cancer in adults and respiratory disorders in children. Report of the Indoor Air Quality and Total Human Exposure Committee – Review of the ORD Draft Report (EPA/600/6-90/00GA), EPA-SAB-IAQTHE-91-007 USEPA, Washington, DC

Samet JM (1991) The health effects of environmental tobacco smoke. In: Lippmann M (ed) Environmental toxicants – human exposures and their health effects. Van Nostrand Reinhold, New York

Schenker MB, Samet JM, Speizer FE (1983) Risk factors for childhood respiratory disease: the effect of host factors and home environmental exposures. Am Rev Respir Dis 28:1038–1043

Schlesinger RB, Lippmann M (1978) Selective particle deposition and bronchogenic carcinoma. Environ Res 15:424–431

Speizer FE, Ferris B Jr, Bishop YMM, Spengler J (1980) Respiratory disease rates and pulmonary function in children associated with NO_2 exposure. Am Rev Respir Dis 121:3–10

Spitzer WO, Lawrence V, Dales R, Hill G, Archer MC, Clark P, Abenhaim L, Hardy J, Sampolis J, Pinfold SP, Morgan PP (1990) Links between passive smoking and disease: a best-evidence synthesis. Clin Invest Med 13:17–42

USDHEW (US Department of Health, Education, and Welfare) (1979) Smoking and health. A report of the Surgeon General. DHEW Publication No. (PHS) 79-50066. US Government Printing Office, Washington

USDHHS (US Department of Health and Human Services) (1986) The health consequences of involuntary smoking. DHHS, PHS Publication No. (CDC) 87-8398. U.S. Government Printing Office, Washington

USDHHS (US Department of Health and Human Services) (1989) Reducing the health consequences of smoking. 25 years of progress. A report of the Surgeon General 1989. DHHS Publication No. (CDC) 89-8411. US Government Printing Office, Washington

Ware JH, Dockery DW, Spiro III A, Speizer FE, Ferris BG Jr (1984) Passive smoking, gas cooking, and respiratory health of children living in six cities. Am Rev Respir Dis 129:366–374

Inhalation Studies in Investigation of the Sick Building Syndrome

L. MØLHAVE

Institut of Occupational and Environmental Medicine, University of Aarhus, Ole Worms Allé, Bdg. 180, 8000 Aarhus C, Denmark

Introduction

Volatile organic compounds (VOC) are frequent air pollutants in non-industrial environments. Organic compounds have been categorized into four groups, of which the VOC category is defined by a boiling point range with an lower limit between 50° and 100°C and an upper limit between 240° and 260°C. The higher values refer to polar compounds (WHO 1989).

In indoor air, 307 VOCs have been identified. The World Health Organization report (WHO 1989) summarizes concentrations found in four recent studies. Each compound seldom exceeds $50\,\mu g/m^3$, which is 100 to 1000 times lower than the concentrations found in industrial environments. The total concentrations of VOC (TVOC) are normally below $1\,mg/m^3$, which is only about 0.2% of the occupational threshold limit value (TLV) of toluene.

The toxic effects of VOCs may be classified into those common to most compounds and those specific for individual compounds. Lists of the former known from high level exposures to VOCs and of the latter, like genotoxic effects or effects involving the immune system, are found in textbooks on toxicology together with lists of commonly used toxicological tests.

The effects associated with the sick building syndrome (SBS) are similar to those known from low levels of exposures to VOC. They and their causality are mostly unexplained in textbooks. Therefore, this paper focusses on these VOC as an example of exposures which may contribute to the occurrence of the SBS. No investigations of the SBS have been reported in which a complete and well-defined spectrum of symptoms have been given. In general, the descriptions of the symptoms in the literature are anecdotic and unsystematic. Criteria for causality like those used in epidemiology are not yet fulfilled, and the SBS is therefore still hypothetical.

U. Mohr et al. (Eds.)
Advances in Controlled Clinical
Inhalation Studies
© Springer-Verlag Berlin Heidelberg 1993

Health Effects and VOC Exposures at Low Levels

A Biological Model of Human Reactions to VOC Exposure

The most frequent effects of VOC exposure at low levels fall into three classes: (a) changed perception of the environment caused by acute stimulation of the senses, (b) perceptions or observations of weak acute or subacute, inflammatory-like reactions in the exposed tissues, and (c) a number of subacute effects which may be described as environmental stress reactions. The three types of effects expected to follow from low level exposure are summarized in Mølhave (1990a).

Perceived Air Quality. VOC are perceived by the odorous sense at the top of the nasal cavity, the gustatory senses on the tongue, or by the set of senses often called the general chemical sense. The chemical sense includes both the trigeminal sense in the facial skin, sensors in mucosal membranes of eyes, nose, and mouth, and other similar non-myelinated nerves in other skin areas.

The three sensory systems (olfactory, gustatory, and chemical sense) respond to airborne chemicals but to different qualities of the exposure. Stimulation of one, two, or all three seems to result in a combined perception which may be called the perceived indoor air quality (PIAQ).

Inflammation. In medicine, inflammatory reactions are related to microbiologic, metabolic, or immune system reactions and are generally considered to be protective. Only acute reversible reactions seem to be relevant to the low level VOC exposures in nonindustrial environments. Generally, the first sign of acute inflammation is peripheral dilatation of vessels, causing color and temperature changes of tissue. Subsequently, granulocytes and other cell types are activated.

If the exposure increases in intensity or duration beyond the point of comfort, the body may react by initiating protective reflexes or mechanisms. These reflexes are activated either by chemical mediators or through sensory perception and other nervous signals. Examples include running eyes or nose, cough, changes in respiratory pattern, increased nucosal secretion, increased blood flow to exposed skin areas, etc.

Environmental Stress. The constant effort to identify the wanted and to override the unwanted sensory information as well as to maintain protective reflexes is a strain to humans and may by itself cause effects. If such stress situations continue for extended periods of time, subacute stress like complaints will be heard, of which headache seems to be most important.

Symptoms of weak environmental stress are well-known from both the indoor and the outdoor environment. Many different physical or chemical exposures have been shown to cause the typical stress symptoms which have been reviewed by Evans et al. (1989).

The intensity of each of the symptoms may be modified by such factors as age, smoking habits, and gender. Furthermore, the number of symptoms observed and their intensity may affect the individual's behavior, leading them, for example, to modify their environment or to focus on certain symptoms and suppress others. As a consequence of individual differences in these modifying factors, each subject may react differently to the mixed exposure and exhibit only a few of the symptoms observed in the whole population.

This model of the mechanisms associated with VOC exposure describes the effects as unspecific. They may be caused by other environmental conditions than chemical explosure. For example, physical exposure to temperature extremes or inert dust may cause a similar spectrum of symptoms. A discussion of the causality between VOCs and the symptoms, therefore, must consider not only the exposure levels but also the extent of other contributing factors.

Measuring the Exposure

At present, few acceptable methods are available for objective measurements of low VOC exposures and the relevant cofactors. Two reasons for this are that the relevant exposure variables have not yet been identified and that the sensitivity of the available measuring techniques is insufficient.

Measuring methods exist for the concentrations of most VOC, but often two problems prevent their use at low exposure levels. The first is the extreme sensitivity of humans to, e.g., odorants. This sensitivity is difficult to match with existing measuring techniques. Second, many compounds are present at the same time, which makes any detailed measuring program time-consuming and expensive.

Three shortcuts are employed to overcome these difficulties. Human subjects may be used as detectors, e.g., by using panels to assess the Olf/Decipol levels (Fanger et al. 1988). Tracer compounds are taken as indicators for the level of pollution (like CO_2 or H_2O), or compounds which themselves are potent air pollutants (like CH_2O) may be used as an estimate of the general potential of the indoor air to cause in effect. These shortcuts are described in most textbooks on indoor climate.

Another one focuses on indicator or index measures of the total measurable level of air pollution. One of these is called total volatile organic compounds (TVOC). No procedure has been established for the calculation of the combined effects of the many different compounds found in most indoor atmospheres. Summation in mg/m^3 of masses of polluting molecules is, therefore, suggested and is called the TVOC indicator. Details about the limitations and use of this indicator are found in Mølhave (1990a).

Some Investigations of Health Effects Caused by Low Level VOC Exposure

The limitations of low level clinical experiments and field investigations are reviewed in Mølhave (1992). They reduce the usefulness of conclusions about the causality of most experiments at low exposure levels. In addition, experiments at higher exposure levels, e.g., around occupational threshold limit values, often focus on health effects which have adverse consequences for the subjects and pay little attention to the relative harmless but frequently appearing comfort reduction caused by, e.g., odors or sensory irritation. Also, these high level exposure experiments may involve only an adult and healthy population, excluding more sensitive groups like children or old people. The high level exposure experiments may further use exposure times different from normal nonindustrial occupancy.

Therefore, few occupational experiments are relevant for extrapolation to the low concentrations found in most nonindustrial environments. Some experiments have been done in which humans were exposed to low levels of VOC as reviewed in Mølhave (1990b, 1991).

Discussion

Henle-Koch Criteria

In epidemiology, the Henle-Koch criteria (Evans 1976) were developed for the causality of diseases described by a spectrum of responses and caused by specific agents. These criteria have been revised for use with VOC (Mølhave 1991). In short, they are:

1. A measurable response following exposure to VOC should regularly appear among occupants lacking this before exposure or should increase in magnitude if present before exposure.
2. Exposure to VOC should be present more commonly among occupants showing the effect than in controls without the effects when all risk factors are held constant.
3. A spectrum of responses should follow exposure to VOC along a predicted biological gradient from mild to severe.
4. Temporally, the effects should follow the exposure to VOCs (possibly with a delay time).
5. Experimental reproduction of the effects should produce a higher incidence in animals or men appropriately exposed to VOC than in those not so exposed.
6. Elimination or modification of the VOC exposure or modification of the occupants' sensitivity to exposure should decrease or eliminate the effect.
7. An etiology which makes biological sense must have been suggested. This implies that:

- Reasonable and documented biological mechanisms must be used for the explanation of the observed symptoms or effects.
- The effects or symptoms and expected mechanisms should preferably be known from similar or higher exposure levels to VOC.
- The etiology must explain any delay (latency) in response following exposure to VOC.
- The variables (effects, exposures, and cofactors) involved in the suggested etiology must be measurable. Alternatively, acceptable indicators must be available.

A proposed causality between exposure to VOC and health effects must fulfill criteria like these Henle-Koch criteria in order to be accepted. However, although fulfillment of these criteria is strong evidence for the proposed causality, it may not be a sufficient or final proof. In the following, the present knowledge about VOC and health is discussed in the light of the criteria described above.

Does a Causality Exist between Exposure to VOC and Health Effects?

Experiments indicate that during controlled exposures effects follow exposures to VOC as required according to criteria 1 and 5.

In most cases, the concentrations reported from field investigations are improperly documented, and the selection of the sampling locations may have been biased. Furthermore, the symptoms are unsystematically reported, which makes comparison of the reports difficult. Published field investigations do, however, indicate that the concentrations of VOC are generally higher in problem buildings than in buildings without problems (Mølhave 1986). It was found that complaints seem to arise when concentrations exceed $1.7\,mg/m^3$. Below $1.7\,mg/m^3$ complaints may occur if other types of simultaneous exposure are present (Mølhave 1986).

From the field experiments, it appears that symptoms are more frequent among exposed than nonexposed subjects. This conclusion has been confirmed in controlled experiments. The second criterion may therefore also be fulfilled, although only future research can finally settle this.

The effects follow a gradient as required in the third criterion, starting with perceptive effects, followed by weak inflammatory-like reactions and environmental stress reactions at higher exposure levels.

In the Danish Town Hall Study, the lower threshold of no effect was in the exposure range of $0.19-0.66\,mg/m^3$ (Zweeers et al. 1990). This range corresponds to the lowest concentrations found in other studies of complaints buildings (Mølhave 1986), and at present the best estimate of the lower limit of no effect of VOCs, therefore, seems to be about $0.2\,mg/m^3$.

Few inflammatory reactions have been reported, although some of the irritative effects may be of inflammatory origin or may be caused by chemical mediators. Changed tear film stability and cell counts have been seen at 25 mg/m^3. Subjects also reported changed temperature sensation in exposed skin areas at 25 mg/m^3. These effects may be weak inflammatory reactions.

The concentration 25 mg/m^3 also seems to cause weak environmental stress symptoms like headache and drowsiness. Associated psychological effects like changed performance, confusion, and fatigue are also found at 25 mg/m^3. These effects are known from higher exposure levels but have not been consistently seen in controlled experiments with low level exposures. At present, 25 mg/m^3 appears to be the lowest controlled exposure which has caused such effects.

Measurable responses, therefore, are found in controlled exposure experiments. They follow a gradient from sensory effects (odor 3 mg/m^3) to indications of subacute inflammatory reactions (changed leukocytes in liquids, perceived skin temperature at 25 mg/m^3) and of subacute stress reactions at 25 mg/m^3. The third criterion of progression of effects also seems to be fulfilled.

Laboratory experiments indicate that the effects which are expected according to the biological model can be experimentally reproduced and are acute following exposure. Criteria 4 and 5, therefore, are also fulfilled. No field investigations have reported the effects of elimination or modification of the exposure or sensitivity of the occupants. Postexposure measurements during controlled experiments, however, indicate that the effects are reversible and disappear shortly after exposure. The sixth criterion, therefore, also may be fulfilled.

Has an Acceptable Biological Explanation Been Given for the Causality?

Previously, a set of four criteria was outlined for the acceptance of a suggested biological model for causality. The first is that the model must explain the observed effects. The effects expected after low level exposure to VOC coincide very well with those observed both in epidemiological field investigations and in controlled clinical experiments. The model explains why sensory irritation, olfaction, and weak inflammatory or neurological effects seem to dominate during low level exposures. The first criterion for an acceptable biological model, therefore, seems to be fulfilled. The list of effects may include other effects, for example, those related to productivity or performance. Such influences have not yet been positively identified.

The effects are all known from similar or higher exposure levels. The second criterion, therefore, is fulfilled. Any delay in the effects caused by the exposure has yet to be identified. Some indications of a subacute latency exists. According to the model, such a latency is explained by the subacute skin or stress reactions. Therefore, the fourth criterion also may be fulfilled, although this will have to be investigated in more detail.

The model does not include acceptable objective measures of the subjective comfort effects which are the dominating results caused by these exposures. Also, estimates of the combined exposure to the many compounds found in most indoor environments are lacking. Some indicator measures have been developed, but they have not yet been investigated in detail. The fourth criterion for the model, which demands acceptable measures of effects and exposures, is thus not yet fulfilled.

In conclusion, no evidence is known to contradict the proposed causality between the effects tentatively related to low level exposures to VOC. On the contrary, evidence from both field investigations and controlled clinical experiments support it. However, existing evidence is too little to allow a final conclusion.

Tentative Guidelines for Nonindustrial Indoor Environments

Exposures in most field investigations are multifactorial, and other factors than VOC exposure may exceed their threshold for effects. Most of the effects reported in field investigations, therefore, may have more than one cause. It is, consequently, not surprising that effects of exposure to VOC in field investigations seem to occur at lower exposure levels than in controlled experiments. In these clinical tests, other influences than VOC normally are held below their no-effect level, and due to ethical reasons the VOC exposure may consist of less reactive compounds than those found in the field. Furthermore, in the clinical experiments the exposure times are normally less than 3 h, which from field experience seems too short to cause severe subacute effects at low exposure levels.

Under these multifactorial exposure conditions, three exposure ranges are of interest. They are defined by the relative contribution of the VOC exposure to the prevalence of effects or symptoms. Below a lower threshold (the no-effect level), no effects are expected to follow from the exposures to VOC. At present, the best estimate of this is 0.2 mg/m^3.

Above an upper threshold (the effect level), an effect of exposure to VOC is always expected, even when all other factors are controlled and acceptable. Between the two thresholds, a correlation may or may not occur between exposure to VOC and prevalence of effects, depending on the interactions from other elements. This range is called the multifactorial exposure range and is often associated with the postulated and yet unexplained SBS (Mølhave 1990a).

The tentative conclusion of the available field and laboratory studies (Mølhave 1986, 1990b) is that at concentrations higher than about 3 mg/m^3 complaints seem to arise in all investigated buildings with occupants having symptoms. In controlled experiments, odors are significant at 3 mg/m^3. At present, the concentration $3 \, mg/m^3$ seems to be the best estimate of the effect level of VOC.

At $5 \, mg/m^3$, objective effects were indicated in addition to the subjective feeling of irritation. Exposures for 50 min to $8 \, mg/m^3$ led to significant irritation of mucous membranes in the eyes, nose, and throat.

In the literature, few acceptable indicators of exposure levels are given which would allow an estimate of the threshold of headache. Concentrations below $3 \, mg/m^3$ in field investigations produced a significant difference in the frequency of headache between problem buildings and control buildings. On the other hand, headache was found in only one of the exposure experiments and then at $25 \, mg/m^3$.

The reason for the lower thresholds found in field investigations may be either the interaction of other factors or the effect of the longer exposure duration found in the field. Therefore, based on the present information, the threshold for headache and other weak neurotoxic effects caused by exposure of less than a few hours' duration is expected to lie between 3 and $25 \, mg/m^3$.

These conclusions refer to the most prevalent effects of VOC exposure on the normal population. Risk groups may exist which will respond more strongly than the normal population. Furthermore, future investigations dealing with larger groups of subjects may reveal special effects like allergy or genotoxicity from low level exposure to VOC. These special effects have not been demonstrated to follow from exposures to VOC at the concentrations found in the nonindustrial indoor environments.

References

Evans AS (1976) Causation and diseases. The Henle-Koch postulates revisited. Yale J Biol Med 49:175–195

Evans GW, Carrere S, Hohansson G (1989) A multivariate perspective on environmental stress. Arch Complex Environ Studies 8(1):1–5

Fanger PO, Lauridsen J, Bluyssen P, Clausen G (1988) Air pollution sources in offices and assembly halls, quantified by the Olf unit. Energy Building 12:7–19

Mølhave L (1986) Indoor air quality in relation to sensory irritation due to volatile organic compounds. Paper 2954, ASHRAE (American Society of Heating, Refrigerating and Air-Conditioning Engineers) Transactions 92(1)

Mølhave L (1990a) Volatile organic compounds, indoor air quality and health. 5: 15–33 In: Walkinshaw D (ed) Indoor Air 90'. Canadian Mortgage and Housing Corp., Ottawa

Mølhave L (1990b) The sick building syndrome (SBS) caused by exposures to volatile organic compounds (VOCs). In: Weekes DM, Gammages RB (eds) The practitioner's approach to indoor air quality investigations. Am Ind Hyg Ass, Akron Ohio, USA, chap. 1

Mølhave L (1991) Indoor climate, air poleution and human comfort. J Expos Anal Environ Epidemiol 1:63–81

Mølhave L (1992) Design considerations for exposure experiments at Exposure levels below TLV. Eur J Appl Psychol 41(3):229–238

WHO (1989) Indoor air quality: organic pollutants. Report on a WHO-meeting. EURO Rep Stud 111 WHO regional Office for Europe, Copenhagen

Zweers T, Skov P, Valjørn O, Mølhave (1990) The effect of ventilation and air pollution on perceived indoor air quality. Energy Building 14:175–181

Section 3. Assessing Personal Exposure

Personal Exposure Assessment: Implications for Clinical Studies of Inhaled Pollutants*

J.M. SAMET and W.E. LAMBERT

The University of New Mexico, Medical Center, New Mexico Tumor Registry, 900 Camino de Salud NE, Albuquerque, NM 87131, USA

Introduction

In clinical studies of inhaled pollutants, the investigator controls the concentration of the pollutants and the temporal profile of exposure; by varying the degree of exertion during exposure, the investigator can further affect the dose delivered to the respiratory tract. Of necessity, the protocols for clinical studies limit exposures to brief periods, typically from 1 h or less to no more than 5 or 6 h. In most protocols, subjects are exposed at only a single concentration, although a recent study imposed "peaks" of NO_2 exposure on a lower background (Utell et al. 1990). In selecting concentrations of inhaled pollutants for a clinical study, some relevant considerations include expectations of producing effects on outcome measures based on the results of previous studies, evidence from animal studies, the need to describe "safe" levels of exposure for regulatory purposes, and ethical constraints.

By contrast to the controlled circumstances of exposure in clinical studies, many exposures in the community setting have widely varying temporal profiles reflecting the multiple microenvironments, i.e., locations having homogeneous concentrations over a specified time interval in which exposure occurs (Duan 1982). Varying levels of exertion throughout the day further modify pollutant doses. These variations in concentration and temporal profile should be further considerations in developing clinical studies of inhaled pollutants. To the extent that exposures in clinical studies reflect exposures in the community, results of clinical studies can be extended with more certainty to the population setting. Optimally, exposures to

---

*Supported in part by a contract from the Health Effects Institute (HEI), an organization jointly funded by the United States Environmental Protection Agency (EPA) (Assistance Agreement X-812059), automotive manufacturers, and the Gas Research Institute. The contents of this article do not necessarily reflect the views of the HEI, nor do they necessarily reflect the policies of the EPA, automotive manufacturers, or Gas Research Institute.

U. Mohr et al. (Eds.)
Advances in Controlled Clinical
Inhalation Studies
© Springer-Verlag Berlin Heidelberg 1993

inhaled pollutants in clinical studies should be based on population patterns of exposures, perhaps paralleling average or more extreme conditions of the population's distribution of exposures.

Clinical studies of inhaled pollutants are brief and directed at acute effects on the lung or other organs. Thus, if clinical studies are to be linked to exposures of the general population, data on personal exposures are needed that afford sufficient temporal resolution, i.e., measurement of concentrations over periods of hours. Continuous rather than integrated exposure data are preferable if the exposure profiles of the clinical studies are to be closely comparable with those of the microenvironments of interest.

Personal Exposure to Inhaled Pollutants

Patterns of time use and activity place children and adults in diverse indoor and outdoor environments throughout the day, each environment having its own unique set of air contaminants. Personal exposure represents the time-weighted average of pollutant concentrations in each microenvironment (Duan 1982; Sexton and Ryan 1988). Total integrated exposure (E) can be represented as the linear combination of concentrations in various micro-environments (c_i, in the ith microenvironment) weighted by the time spent (t_i) in each microenvironment: $E = \sum_{\tau} c_i t_i$. Thus, approaches for capturing total personal exposures need to provide either integrated measurements across microenvironments or the c_i and t_i for each microenvironment. As a basis for designing clinical studies, these data should be available with sufficient temporal resolution to serve as a template for controlled exposures; biologically relevant temporal variation in exposure profile must also be captured.

Assessment of Personal Exposure

Personal exposure can be estimated by collecting information on time spent in relevant microenvironments and on their pollutant concentrations. Using this approach, an investigator places area monitors in the microenvironments where exposure occurs. This microenvironmental approach may be limited by the type of microenvironments and the availability of suitable equipment, particularly for capturing continuous data.

Alternatively, personal exposures can be directly measured. The measurement instrumentation to support direct personal monitoring on continuous or short time scales is limited (Table 1). Two classes of personal monitoring instrumentation are available: (1) passive samplers which bind the pollutant to a reactive surface or matrix provide integrated measure-ments over relatively short periods of time, e.g., hours, and (2) continuous

Table 1. Personal exposure monitoring instrumentation capable of quantitative measurements at ambient concentrations (adapted from Sexton and Ryan 1988)

Pollutant	Monitor type	Collection method	Analytical method
Particles			
Mass	Integrated, active	Pump/impactor	Gravimetric
Sulfates, nitrates, metals	Integrated, active	Pump/impactor	Gravimetric, chemical analysis, PIXE
Gases			
Carbon monoxide	Continuous, active, integrated, passive	Pump or diffusion Diffusion	Electrochemical sensor Electrochemical
Formaldehyde	Integrated, diffusion	Diffusion tube	Chromotropic acid
Nicotine	Active, integrated	Pump, treated filter	Gas chromatograph
	Passive	Badge	Gas chromatograph
NO_2	Integrated, active	Pump/impingers	Colorimetric
	Integrated, passive	Diffusion tube	Colorimetric
	Continuous, active	Pump	Electrochemical sensor
O_3 (under development)	Integrated, passive	Badge	Electrochemical
Volatile organic compounds	Integrated, active	TENAX cartridge	GC/MS

PIXE, proton-induced X-ray emission; GC/MS, gas chromatography – mass spectroscopy.

monitors which measure pollutant concentrations in real time and process and store the measurement in electronic memory. Both approaches require intensive laboratory support of field measurements.

While passive samplers are simple in design, construction and quantitative analyses require strict quality control to maximize sensitivity for use in the community. Similarly, accurate measurements by continuous monitoring instrumentation require careful and regular calibration against gas standards and, at times, extensive maintenance. The paucity of continuous data on personal exposures may be attributed to the high cost of electronic instrumentation and the labor required to maintain the monitors. For this reason, epidemiologic studies have tended to incorporate passive samplers to obtain exposure measurements. Continuous monitoring has been limited to smaller numbers of subjects and has been used to validate integrated measurements from passive devices. The development of personal monitoring instrumentation has been constrained by the design requirements of portability, independent powering, sensitivity and accuracy in a low concentration range, and expense (Wallace and Ott 1982).

Biological monitoring of chemical contaminants or metabolites is another possibility for estimating personal exposures. However, this usually provides measures of integrated exposures over longer averaging times than are relevant for typical clinical studies. Markers indicative of exposures over periods of several hours include carboxyhemoglobin or carbon monoxide in exhaled air, nicotine levels in body fluids, and levels of some volatile organic compounds in exhaled air.

An Example: Clinical Studies of NO_2

Clinical studies have been conducted to assess the effects of NO_2 on people with asthma and on healthy people without respiratory disease (Samet and Utell 1990) (Table 2). Exposure to NO_2 takes place both outdoors, where the principal sources are vehicles, power plants, and industry, and indoors, where the principal sources are combustion appliances, gas ranges and ovens and unvented space heaters. Scant data are available on short-term variation in NO_2 concentrations outdoors; excursions of concentration would be anticipated in relation to vehicle traffic, meteorology, and other factors. Hourly data at monitoring sites are available, but data from continuous personal monitoring are extremely limited.

Indoors, the burning of natural gas in pilot lights of stoves maintains a relatively steady elevation of NO_2. Cooking further elevates concentrations. The elevation persists during cooking and decays quickly when the burners or oven are turned off (Harlos 1988). NO_2 is also released during the operation of unvented kerosene and propane space heaters (Leaderer 1982; Samet et al. 1987). Thus, consideration of sources of NO_2 indicates several microenvironments relevant to human exposure: outdoors, homes with gas stoves at times when the range or oven is not in use, homes with gas stoves at times when the range or oven is in use, homes with electric stoves, and homes with operating, unvented space heaters.

Some data are now available on NO_2 concentrations in these microenvironments. Residences with gas stoves have integrated NO_2 concentrations in the range of 20–40 ppb average over 1- to 2-week monitoring periods (Spengler et al. 1983; Samet et al. 1987); concentrations tend to be highest in the kitchen. Homes have been monitored either continuously or

Table 2. Exposure scenarios in selected clinical studies of NO_2 and asthma sufferers

Investigation	NO_2 concentration/duration	Circumstances
Orehek et al. 1976	0.1 ppm/1 h	Rest
Hazucha et al. 1983	0.1 ppm/1 h	Rest
Kleinman et al. 1983	0.2 ppm/2 h	Rest, exercise
Bylin et al. 1985	0.1–0.5 ppm/20 min	Rest
Bauer et al. 1986	0.3 ppm/30 min	Rest, exercise
Linn et al. 1986	0.3–3.0 ppm/1 h	Moderate exercise

over short averaging times during the use of gas stoves (see Harlos 1988 for a review).

In the most extensive study, Harlos (1988) used a portable, electro-chemical cell monitor to measure concentrations in the kitchen and at the breathing zone of the person cooking during meal preparation. Mean personal exposures and concentrations in the kitchen were about 100 ppb, but substantial variation in the continuously recorded concentrations was documented with occasional spikes of NO_2 near 1 ppm in the cook's breathing zone. Similarly, Goldstein (1988) showed that exposures to NO_2 during stove use in small urban apartments averaged 0.3–0.4 ppm with brief peaks up to 1.5 ppm. Harlos and colleagues (1987) assessed personal exposures of infants to NO_2; concentrations in the kitchen during cooking averaged about 100 ppb, whereas the 1-day averaged value was 66 ppb and the 1-week averaged value, 37. Lebret (1985) monitored kitchens, bedrooms, and living rooms in 12 Dutch homes; sources of NO_2 included gas stoves and unvented gas water heaters. One-minute values as high as 1.5 ppm were observed, and the highest 1-h average was 1 ppm. We have been making continuous measurements of NO_2 in the kitchen, family room, and bedroom in homes of infants enrolled in a study of respiratory illness. Our results confirm that spikes of exposure occur during cooking with frequent 5-min peaks of 200 ppb or more. These peaks are transmitted to other rooms but are damped to a variable extent among the homes.

Harlos (1988) reported a small number of continuous NO_2 samples taken during transit. Spikes were observed during times of close contact with sources, e.g., trucks or other sources of combustion emissions. The maximum values were only about one-fifth of those measured indoors using the same instrumentation.

Although the data on the microenvironments of interest in regard to NO_2 exposure are limited, temporal patterns are evident. Spikes of exposure occur indoors in relation to source use and outdoors in relation to proximity to sources. However, only one clinical study (Utell et al. 1990) has included spikes in the exposure protocol.

Conclusions

Clinical studies have proven informative for studying the acute effects of inhaled pollutants. The investigative method permits control of the level and pattern of exposure and detailed assessment of health effects. The extent to which the results can be generalized may be limited, however, by uncertainty concerning the relation between exposures used in clinical studies and those experienced in the population setting. New techniques for personal monitoring can provide information on concentrations for some pollutants on time scales relevant for clinical studies.

In designing clinical studies of particular inhaled pollutants, considera-tion should be given to the microenvironments in which exposure occurs and the concentrations in these microenvironments. The expanding population-based data on personal exposure need to be examined. The choice of concentration and temporal profile of exposure for a clinical study should be made in reference to these data, thereby assuring that results can be extended to the population setting.

References

Bauer MA, Utell MJ, Morrow PE, Speers DM, Gibb FR (1986) Inhalation of 0.30 ppm nitrogen dioxide potentiates exercise-induced bronchospasm in asthmatics. Am Rev Respir Dis 134:1203–1208

Bylin G, Lindvall T, Rehn T, Sundin B (1985) Effects of short-term exposure to ambient nitrogen dioxide concentrations on human bronchial reactivity and lung function. Eur J Respir Dis 66:205–217

Duan N (1982) Models for human exposure to air pollution. Environ Int 8:305–309

Goldstein IF (1988) Effects of peak exposure to nitrogen dioxide on pulmonary function. In: Harper JP (ed) Combustion processes and the quality of the indoor environment. Air and Waste Management Association, Pittsburg, pp 294–295

Harlos DP (1988) Acute exposures to nitrogen dioxide during cooking or commuting. Thesis, Harvard School of Public Health, Boston

Harlos, DP, Marbury M, Samet J, Spengler JD (1987) Relating indoor NO_2 levels to infant personal exposures. Atmos Environ 21:369–376

Hazucha MJ, Ginsberg JF, McDonnell WF, Haak ED Jr, Pimmel RL, Salaam SA, House DE, Bromberg PA (1983) Effects of 0.1 ppm nitrogen dioxide on airways of normal and asthmatic subjects. J Appl Physiol 54:730–739

Kleinman MT, Bailey RM, Linn WS, Anderson KR, Whynot JD, Shamoo DA, Hackney JD (1983) Effects of 0.2 ppm nitrogen dioxide on pulmonary function and response to bronchoprovocation in asthmatics. J Toxicol Environ Health 12:815–826.

Leaderer BP (1982) air pollutant emissions from kerosene space heaters. Science 218:1113–1115

Lebret E (1985) Air pollution in Dutch homes: an exploratory study in environmental epidemiology. Thesis, Department of Air Pollution, Department of Environmental and Tropical Health, Wageningen Agricultural University

Linn WS, Shamoo DA, Avol EL, Whynot JD, Anderson KR, Venet TG, Hackney JD (1986) Dose-response study of asthmatic volunteers exposed to nitrogen dioxide during intermittent exercise. Arch Environ Health 41:292–296

Orehek J, Massari JP, Gayrard P, Grimaud C, Charpin J (1976) Effect of short-term, low-level nitrogen dioxide exposure on bronchial sensitivity of asthmatic patients. J Clin Invest 57:301–307

Samet JM, Utell MJ (1990) The risk of nitrogen dioxide: what have we learned from epidemiological and clinical studies? Toxicol Ind Health 6:247–262

Samet JM, Marbury MC, Spengler JD (1987) Health effects and sources of indoor air pollution, part 1. Am Rev Respir Dis 136:1486–1508

Sexton K, Ryan PB (1988) Assessment of human exposure to air pollution: methods, measurements, and models. In: Watson AY, Bates RR, Kennedy D (eds) Air pollution, the automobile, and public health. National Academy Press, Washington, DC, pp 207–238

Spengler JD, Duffy CP, Letz R, Tibbitts TW, Ferris BG Jr (1983) Nitrogen dioxide inside and outside 137 homes and implications for ambient air quality standards and health effects research. Environ Sci Technol 17:164–168

Utell MJ, Morrow PE, Bauer MA (1990) Effects of inhaled nitrogen dioxide on respiratory function: controlled clinical studies. Presented at the 83rd Annual Meeting and Exhibition, Pittsburg: Air and Waste Management Association (Paper no. 90-147.3)

Wallace LA, Ott WR (1982) Personal monitors: a state-of-the-art survey. J Air Pollut Control Assoc 32:601–610

Regional Deposition of Inhaled Particles in the Human Respiratory Tract

J. Heyder

GSF Forschungszentrum für Umwelt und Gesundheit, Projekt Inhalation,
W-8042 Neuherberg, FRG

Introduction

Clinical inhalation studies with surrogates of ambient aerosols are useful tools for estimating health hazards associated with air pollutants. These studies are usually performed with aerosols of known composition and concentration over known periods of time so that dose-effect relationships can be established. However, the estimation of the dose received by an individual further requires the knowledge of particle deposition and particle deposition rate in the respiratory tract of this individual. This report covers strategies in lung dosimetry for controlled clinical inhalation studies.

Particle Deposition

Total deposition is the mean probability of an inspired particle being deposited in the respiratory tract. Regional deposition is the mean probability of an inspired particle being deposited in a region of the respiratory tract.

Regions of the Respiratory Tract

To estimate local effects of inhaled particulate pollutants in the respiratory tract it would be desirable to know the spatial distribution of deposited particles in anatomical structures of the entire respiratory tract. However, very little information on particle deposition in anatomical regions is available to date so that "regions" other than anatomical regions must be considered.

A way of looking upon particle deposition in various regions of the respiratory tract is by making use of the aerosol bolus technique and by studying particle losses from inspired boluses penetrating to different depths into the respiratory tract upon inspiration (Heyder et al. 1988). In this case the respiratory tract is considered as a one-dimensional structure composed

U. Mohr et al. (Eds.)
Advances in Controlled Clinical
Inhalation Studies
© Springer-Verlag Berlin Heidelberg 1993

of *regions of equal volume*. The approach which has most often been used to study regional deposition utilizes the distinctive removal rates of two *functional regions* in the respiratory tract by studying removal of labeled particles from the thorax after short-term aerosol exposure (Albert and Arnett 1955). This approach partitions the lungs into a proximal region composed of airways covered with ciliated epithelium (bronchial region) and a distal region without this epithelium (alveolar region).

Deposition in Functional Lung Regions

The assessment of particle deposition in functional lung regions is based upon measuring total deposition while steadily breathing radio- or magnetolabeled monodisperse aerosol for a short period of time, partitioning total deposition into an extrathoracic and a thoracic component by external detection of deposited label in head and thorax immediately after aerosol administration, and partitioning thoracic deposition into a bronchial and a alveolar component by external detection of label removal from the thorax. Mean deposition of unit density spheres in the respiratory tract of a standard person for oral breathing at rest from experiments summarized by Heyder et al. (1986) is illustrated in Fig. 1.

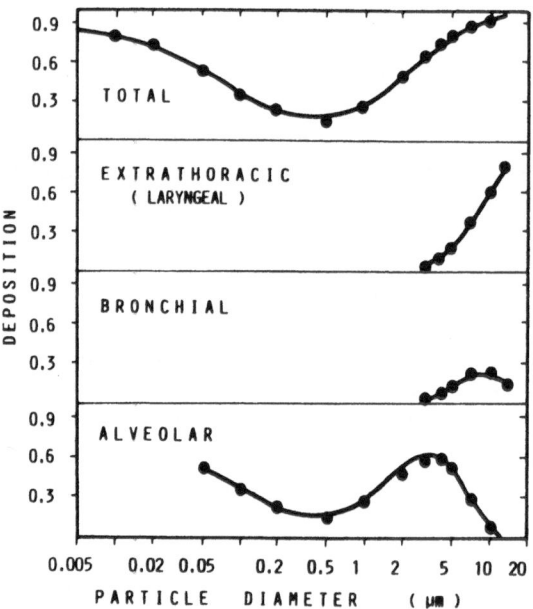

Fig. 1. Deposition of unit density spheres in the respiratory tract of a standard person for steady oral breathing at a mean flow rate of $250 \, \text{cm}^3 \text{s}^{-1}$ and a breathing cycle period of $8 \, \text{s}$. The curves represent experimental values, the point values calculated with a compartmental algebraic deposition model. (From Heyder et al. 1986)

The concept of studying particle deposition in these functional regions is based on the assumption that the fast phase of particle removal from the thorax reflects removal from ciliated thoracic airways, and that all particles deposited in these airways are removed from the lungs within about 1 day after aerosol administration. These assumptions were recently challanged by experiments in which aerosol boluses containing monodisperse radiolabeled particles with an aerodynamic diameter of 3 μm were delivered to either the ciliated or the nonciliated portion of the lungs (Stahlhofen 1989). The results indicate the possibility that not all particles deposited in ciliated airways are cleared within 1 day, but that a fraction of deposited particles is retained for a much longer period of time. The suggestion was therefore made to partition the lungs into a fast-cleared and a slow-cleared thoracic region. However, deposition in these regions is very similar to deposition in the bronchial and alveolar region. Maximum deposition in the slow-cleared region is 0.55 as compared to 0.62 in the alveolar region. Maximum deposition in the fast-cleared region is 0.26 and 0.22 in the bronchial region (Stahlhofen et al. 1990).

Modeling Particle Deposition in Functional Lung Regions

Since the transport of inspired particles toward airway surfaces is ruled by physical mechanisms, it is possible to express regional deposition in terms of algebraic functions. The compartimental algebraic model developed by Rudolf (1985) considers the respiratory tract as a series of three regions which collect aerosol particles: extrathoracic region, bronchial region (ciliated intrapulmonary airways), and alveolar region. It formulates the relationship between particle collection efficiencies, depositions, and volumes of these regions. It has been shown that extrathoracic deposition is ruled by inertial impaction, bronchial deposition by diffusion, gravitational sedimentation, and inertial impaction, and alveolar deposition by diffusion and gravitational sedimentation. This semiempirical model enables regional deposition to be calculated for a standard healthy person as a function of particle characteristics and breathing pattern. There is a very good agreement between experimentally determined and empirically calculated deposition values for oral breathing (Fig. 1). Figure 2 shows empirically calculated deposition values for nasal breathing at rest.

Assessment of Individual Regional Dose

To estimate the dose received by an individual participating in a clinical inhalation study, first of all the particle number concentration and the particle size distribution of the aerosol available for inspiration must be determined as well as the breathing pattern of the individual. The compart-

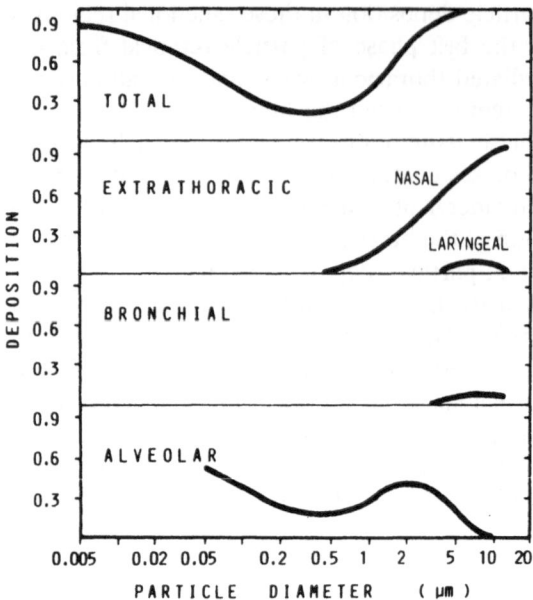

Fig. 2. Deposition of unit density spheres in the respiratory tract of a standard person for steady nasal breathing at a mean flow rate of $250\,\mathrm{cm^3\,s^{-1}}$ and a breathing cycle period of $8\,\mathrm{s}$ calculated with a compartmental algebraic deposition model. (From Heyder et al. 1986)

mental algebraic model can then be used to calculate the mass of particles deposited in various regions of a standard person breathing at the pattern of this individual.

Since particle deposition in healthy individuals exhibits a large inter-individual variability (Stahlhofen et al. 1981; Heyder et al. 1982), estimation of the lung dose received by the individual requires the knowledge of particle deposition in the individual. When total deposition in the individual is measured for quiet, controlled, steady oral breathing of unit density spheres of 3 and $8\,\mu m$ diameter, deposition of 3-μm particles simulates gravitational deposition in the alveolar and bronchial region and deposition of 8-μm particles inertial deposition in the extrathoracic and bronchial region. The comparison of these deposition values with regional deposition values of 3- and 8-μm particles calculated for a standard person breathing at the pattern of the considered individual results in correction factors which can be used to estimate regional deposition and thus deposited mass accumulated during the exposure time in the various regions of the respiratory tract of the individual.

Future Directions

The concept of lung dosimetry in clinical inhalation studies proposed in the previous section can be applied to short-term studies with healthy individuals at rest exposed to hydrophobic, uncharged particles larger than 0.1 μm in diameter. To expand the applicability of this concept to studies with other individuals and other aerosols the major issue to be addressed in the future is to determine regional deposition of ultrafine particles, hygroscopic particles, and electrically charged particles in the normal and diseased and/ or susceptible lung at rest and during exercise. In long-term studies the clearance of deposited particles from the respiratory tract must be taken into account for calculating accumulated dose in lung regions.

References

Albert RE, Arnett CL (1955) Clearance of radioactive dust from the human lung. A MAA Arch Ind Health 12:99–106

Heyder J, Gebhart J, Stahlhofen W, Stuck B (1982) Biological variability of particle deposition in the human respiratory tract during controlled and spontaneous mouth–breathing. Ann Occup Hyg 26:137–147

Heyder J, Gebhart J, Rudolf G, Schiller CF, Stahlhofen W (1986) Deposition of particles in the human respiratory tract in the size range 0.005–15 μm. J Aerosol Sci 17:811–825

Heyder J, Blanchard JD, Brain JD (1988) Particle deposition in volumetric regions of the human respiratory tract. Ann Occup Hyg 32:71–79

Rudolf G (1985) Ein mathematisches Modell zur Deposition von Aerosolteilchen im Atemtrakt des Menschen. Ph D thesis, University of Frankfurt am Main

Stahlhofen W (1989) Human lung clearance following bolus inhalation of radioaerosols. In: Crapo JD et al. (eds) Extrapolation of dosimetric relationships for inhaled particles and gases. Academic, San Diego, pp 153–166

Stahlhofen W, Gebhart J, Heyder J (1981) Biological variability of regional deposition of aerosol particles in the human respiratory tract. Am Ind Hyg Assoc J 42:348–398

Stahlhofen W, Köbrich R, Rudolf G, Scheuch G (1990) Short–term and long-term clearance of particles from the upper human respiratory tract as a function of particle size. J Aerosol Sci 21 [Suppl 1]:S407–S410

Calculation of Acid Aerosol Dose

T.V. LARSON, Q.S. HANLEY, J.Q. KOENIG, and O. BERNSTEIN

Dept. of Civil Engineering, University of Washington, Wilcox Hall Mail Stop FX-10, Seattle, WA 98105, USA

Introduction

Polluted air at times contains a number of acidic compounds, most notably particulate acid in the form of partially neutralized sulfuric acid (H_2SO_4) and acidic vapor in the form of nitric acid (HNO_3). This chapter discusses model estimates of the respiratory fate of acidic particles and gases with emphasis on the neutralization that occurs in the airways due to respiratory ammonia (NH_3). Such models seek to estimate the actual exposure of the lung, rather than using the values measured at the airway entrance. This is useful in calculating conditions under which acid exposures of the lung actually occur in laboratory experiments and in integrating the results of laboratory studies with field measurements of acidic air pollution.

We first discuss the sensitivity of these estimates to various clinical parameters and then use the models to evaluate the acidic exposure of 22 asthmatic subjects who showed changes in pulmonary function when exposed to H_2SO_4, but no observed changes when exposed to similarly low levels of HNO_3. The details of the laboratory exposures, the subjects' medical characteristics, and subsequent pulmonary function measurements have been reported previously (Hanley et al. 1991; Koenig et al. 1989).

Modeling the Fate of Inhaled, Acidic Particles

In order to consider the fate of inhaled acidic particles, we have used the neutralization model for H_2SO_4 from Larson (1989) and Larson et al. (1982). The extent of neutralization depends upon the residence time of acidic aerosol in the airway, the airway NH_3 concentration, the airway relative humidity profiles, and the H_2SO_4 particle size. For modeling purposes, the polydisperse aerosol entering the airways is subdivided into i size fractions. The estimated fraction of acid remaining in the ith particle size interval relative to the amount present prior to inhalation, P_i, is given by:

U. Mohr et al. (Eds.)
Advances in Controlled Clinical
Inhalation Studies
© Springer-Verlag Berlin Heidelberg 1993

$$P_i = \frac{2\pi D_{NH3} t_{airway} d_i [NH_3] f(Kn) \alpha}{\text{initial moles of acid in } i\text{th size class}} \qquad (1)$$

where:

D_{NH3} = diffusivity of gaseous NH_3 in cm^2/s (a value of 0.24 is assumed for all calculations based on a temperature of 36°C)

t_{airway} = particle residence time in the airway prior to deposition (s)

d_i = average particle diameter of the ith size fraction in cm (the value of d_i is based on respiratory RH)

$[NH_3]$ = respiratory NH_3 concentration (moles/cm^3)

$f(Kn)$ = noncontinuum mass transfer diffusion factor
= $[1 + Kn]/[1 + 1.71\,Kn + 1.33\,Kn^2]$

Kn = particle Knudsen number

α = ratio of reaction rate to diffusion rate
= $\{1 + [1.33\,Kn\,f(Kn)/[\alpha_r - 1]]\}^{-1}$

α_r = NH_3-H_2SO_4 reaction coefficient

An estimate is then made of the extent of chemical neutralization of each H_2SO_4 particle by respiratory NH_3 after passage of the inspired particle through the airways. This neutralization model is then coupled with the empirical deposition model of Rudolf et al. (1986) in order to estimate the total deposition of acidic particles at various regions of the airways. If the model is used to evaluate clinical experiments involving various periods of rest and exercise, we estimate the average value of P over all particle sizes for the jth exposure peirod, P_j, as follows:

$$P_j = \sum_i P_{i,j} F_i \qquad (2)$$

where F_i is the fraction of particle volume measured in the ith size interval and the subscript j refers to an exposure period of either rest or exercise.

As just mentioned, the traditional exposure measure reported in the literature is airborne mass concentration of acid measured at the exposure mouthpiece, C_{mp}. The average mass concentration of acid in air entering the trachea during the jth exposure period, $(C_{tr})_j$ can also be estimated from the above neutralization model as a function of C_{mp} and an appropriate value of P_j for that period:

$$(C_{tr})_j = C_{mp} P_j \qquad (3)$$

The average value of C_{tr} over all exposure periods is then a time-weighted average summed over j as shown:

$$C_{tr} = \frac{\sum_j (C_{tr})_j (\text{time})_j}{\sum_j \text{time}_j} \qquad (4)$$

We have also computed the number concentration of acid particles, N, as another possible index of exposure. An acid particle can be practically defined as any particle containing more than some threshold amount of acid per particle. Several definitions of an acid particle appear reasonable within the context of our H_2SO_4 exposure system: (a) any particle that has not been completely neutralized by NH_3, i.e., any particle with an ammonium to sulfate ion ratio less than 2.0; (b) any particle containing some amount of the fully dissociated first proton of H_2SO_4, i.e., any particle with an ammonium to sulfate ion ratio less than 1.0; or (c) any particle containing a sufficient amount of acid per particle temporarily to acidify a fixed amount of biologically buffered material.

The first definition postulates that any amount of acidity in the particle is important to its ultimate irritant potential. The relatively weak acidity of ammonium bisulfate particles compared with sulfuric acid particles does not matter in this view because the lung surface would act as a base relative to either solution, that is, the protons would be delivered to the biological solution no matter what the chemical state of the droplet prior to its landing on the lung surface.

The second definition considers only the strongest, fully dissociated proton as being important and ignores the weaker second proton that is not fully dissociated in the acid droplets. If the lung is ultimately a highly buffered organ and if the small amounts of acid particles inhaled are not altering the gross acidity of the lung, then it would appear that some local, transient "hot spots" of acid are produced. Therefore, the dynamics of this interaction is the important factor, not the final equilibrium pH after deposition which would be the buffered pH value of the lung. To the extent that this local pH transient is a "trigger" of some additional irritant mechanism, then a sulfuric acid particle could produce a local, transient pH decrease that is larger than that produced by an ammonium bisulfate particle, because it has a lower pH.

The third definition gives an acid threshold per particle that is determined by the localized buffering capacity of the lung surface. One version of this concept is the so-called irritation signaling hypothesis of Hattis et al. (1987). In this hypothesis, acidic particles below a certain size threshold would be neutralized by mucus droplets in the lung. To incorporate this concept into our models, we have to consider the amount of acid per particle, rather than the size of the particle. The advantage of acid quantity, as opposed to size, is that it allows consideration of particles partially or completely neutralized prior to deposition on the surface of the lung. According to Hattis's hypothesis, these particles require between 30 and 300 attomoles of acid per particle in order to neutralize the mucus membrane upon impact. Any amount of acid per particle greater than this could produce an irritant signal. The applicability of this concept is less clear for particles that deposit deep in the lung, beyond the mucus layer.

To estimate the relevant number concentration, we note that the density of sulfuric-acid-containing droplets is constant at a given humidity, and hence the number of particles that can be made from a given mass of sulfuric acid at a given humidity is constant for each size fraction. Let n_i be the number of particles per cubic meter of air in the ith size fraction, A_i the amount of acid per particle in the ith size fraction, and $T(i)$ a function that selects for irritating particles on the basis of the quantity of acid exceeding a threshold value. The actual threshold value can be computed for a given particle size based upon one of the three definitions of an acid particle described above. Then the number concentration entering the trachea of irritating acid particles remaining in all size fractions is:

$$N_{tr} = \Sigma n_i T(i) \tag{5}$$

where $T(i) = 0$ if $A_i <$ the threshold value and $T(i) = 1$ if $A_i >$ the threshold value.

With this approach, we can define N_{tr} as the number concentration of all particles that have not been completely neutralized; $N300_{tr}$ as the number concentration of all particles that have more than 300 attomoles of acid per particle; and $NK1_{tr}$ as the number concentration of all particles that contain some amount of the fully dissociated first proton of H_2SO_4. By analogy, we can also define two other measures of acid mass concentration, $C300_{tr}$ and $CK1_{tr}$.

Modeling Inhaled Acid Vapors

We have also considered the fate of an inhaled acid vapor, nitric acid (HNO_3). To date, no model for the neutralization of HNO_3 in the airways has been proposed. In the literature the rate constant of the reaction between HNO_3 and NH_3 has been estimated to be as high as $10^{-13}\,cm^3/$ molecule $\cdot$ s. Farrow and Richton (1981), using a photoacoustic technique, found the rate to be much lower, $2 \times 10^{-18}\,cm^3$/molecule-s. Assuming this latter value as well as a constant oral NH_3 concentration, the neutralization of HNO_3 follows pseudo-first order kinetics of the form:

$$[HNO_3]_{airway} = [HNO_3]_{initial} \exp\{-89\{NH_3\}t_{airway}\} \tag{6}$$

where $[HNO_3]_{initial}$ is the nitric acid vapor concentration prior to inhalation, and $\{NH_3\}$ is the concentration in ppb rather than mol/cm^3. The nitric acid reacts to form ammonium nitrate particles. The assumption of a constant oral NH_3 concentration is based on the view that these are steady state concentrations and on the observation that they are in excess of the inhaled acid vapor concentrations in our experiments. The equilibrium concentration of nitric acid vapor passing through the airways in the presence of these particles is then determined by its equilibrium value with oral ammonia as specified by the vapor pressure product at 36°C (Tang 1980):

$$K_p = [HNO_3][NH_3] = 51.1\,ppb^2 \tag{7}$$

Model Sensitivities

Tables 1 and 2 summarizes a systematic examination of the sensitivity of the predicted total airway deposition of acid particles to changes in the important clinical variables. In this analysis, we have computed the acid in three different ways: (1) all acid contained in particles at the point of impact in the airways, the obvious definition; (2) only the "strong" acid fraction (the first proton of H_2SO_4) in these particles; and (3) the deposition of all the acid only in those particles containing more than 300 attomoles of acid each at the point of impact. As shown in Table 1, the model predictions are relatively sensitive to all of the clinical variables considered. The sensitivity of the model predictions depends in part on which of the definitions of acid we adopt. For instance, if we adopt the third definition above, we see that the total airway deposition of acid is very sensitive to the average particle size prior to inhalation as well as to the SD of the size distribution. Figs. 1 and 2 demonstrates this latter point. In general, the most important clinical variables are the ventilation rate (rest versus exercise), the oral ammonia level, and the particle size.

The sensitivity of the HNO_3 neutralization model to the input parameters, NH_3 and residence time, is more obvious. For this reason, we have not done such an analysis. Rather, we will use this model later in briefly discussing its application to clinical observations.

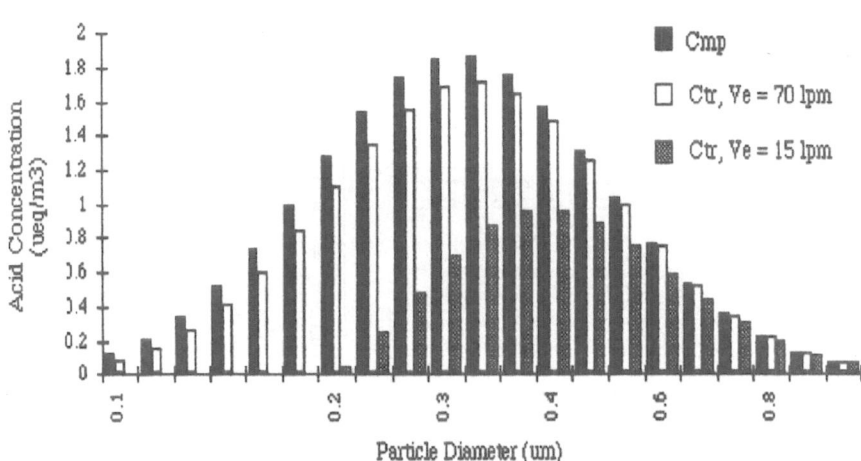

Fig. 1. Extent of neutralization of inhaled acid particles after passage through the mouth as a function of particle size. The particle diameter is reported at 50% RH, a typical value in exposure atmospheres prior to inhalation. As shown, the amount of acid remaining after oral passage is greater in the larger particles and with shorter passage times (high ventilation rates)

Table 1. Summary of model sensitivity analyses

When the variable below	Is changed		All other variables held constant[a], the predicted acid deposition in the airways changes by a factor of			Remarks
	From	To	Total	"Strong"	>300 attomol	
Oral NH$_3$	0.2	0.8 ppm	-4[b]	-30	-4	MMD = 0.3 μm
			-2	-3	-2	MMD = 0.6 μm
Reaction coefficient	0.1	0.9	-0.6	-0.5	-0.3	0.3 < MMD < 0.9 μm
Ventilation rate	15	70 lpm	5	10	10	0.3 < MMD < 0.9 μm
MMD and σ$_g$	0.3	0.5 μm	2	4	10 000	σ$_g$ = 1.2
	0.5	1.2 μm	2	5	30	σ$_g$ = 1.2
	0.3	0.5 μm	2	3	25	σ$_g$ = 1.4
	0.5	1.2 μm	2	3	<10	σ$_g$ = 1.4
	0.3	0.5 μm	2	3	10	σ$_g$ = 1.6
	0.5	1.2 μm	2	5	5	σ$_g$ = 1.6
Route of entry (total deposition)	Mouth	Nose	2	5	5	V$_e$ = 15 lpm
			2	3	4	V$_e$ = 70 lpm

[a] Base case: MMD = 0.3 μm, σ$_g$ = 1.4, C$_{mp}$ = 70 μg/m^3, [NH$_3$] = 0.3 ppm, reaction coefficient = 0.3, V$_e$ = 15 lpm at a breathing frequency of 7.5 breaths per minute.
[b] Negative sign indicates a decrease.
MMD, Mass median diameter; σ$_g$, geometric standard deviation; V$_e$, minute ventilation.

Table 2. Summary of model sensitivity analyses

When the variable below	Is changed		All other variables held constant[a], the predicted acid deposition in the airways changes by a factor of			Remarks
	From	To	Total	"Strong"	>300 attomol	
Oral NH$_3$	0.2	0.8 ppm	−1.2[b]	−2	−1.5	MMD = 0.8 μm
			−1.1	−1.1	−1.1	MMD = 1.5 μm
Reaction coefficient	0.1	0.9	<−1.1	<−1.1	<−1.1	0.8 < MMD < 2.5 μm
Ventilation rate	15	70 lpm	4	4	5	0.8 < MMD < 2.5 μm
MMD and σ$_g$	0.8	2.5 μm	2.5	3	3	σ$_g$ = 1.2
			2	3	3	σ$_g$ = 1.4
			2	2.5	2.5	σ$_g$ = 1.6
Route of entry (total deposition)	Mouth	Nose	1.5	2	2	V$_e$ = 15 lpm
			2.5	2.5	2.5	V$_e$ = 70 lpm

[a] Base case: MMD = 0.8 μm, σ$_g$ = 1.4, C$_{mp}$ = 70 μg/m^3, [NH$_3$] = 0.3 ppm, reaction coefficient = 0.3, Ve = 15 lpm at a breathing frequency of 7.5 breaths per minute.
[b] Negative sign indicates a decrease.
MMD, Mass median diameter; σ$_g$, geometric standard deviation; V$_e$, minute ventilation.

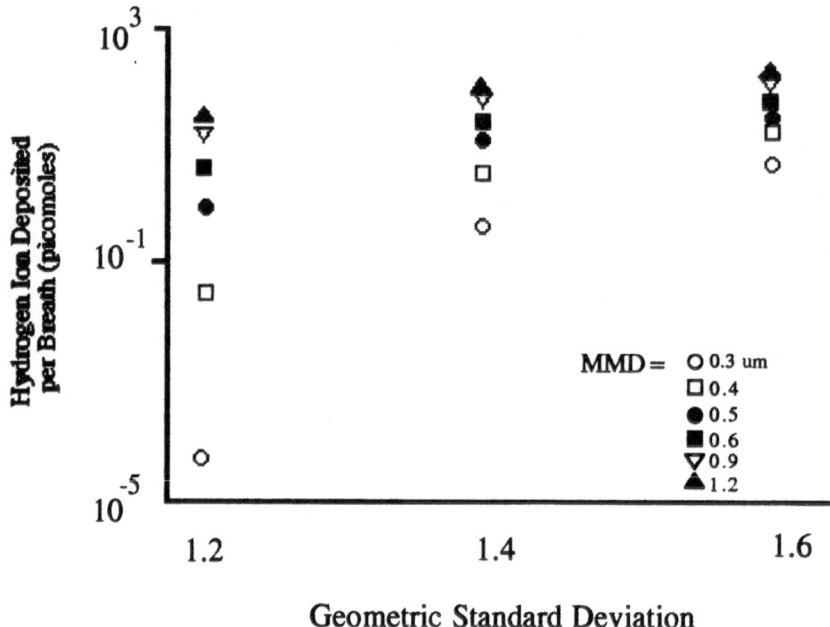

Fig. 2. Predicted changes in deposition of acid as a function of the width of the particle size distribution for various mass median diameters (MMD). The acid deposited is that contained in particles with >300 attomoles per particle. The MMD values are those at 50% RH prior to inhalation. C_{mp} = 70 μg/m^3, [NH$_3$] = 0.3 ppm, reaction coefficient = 0.3, Ve = 15 lpm at a breathing frequency of 7.5 breaths per minute

Application to a Human Clinical Experiment

We have used this model to estimate the exposure to inhaled acids in 22 allergic adolescent subjects studied clinically. We measured the concentration of H$_2$SO$_4$ particles or nitric acid vapor in the exposure chamber prior to their inhalation. However, we wanted to estimate the concentrations to which their lungs actually were exposed during their mouth breathing protocol. All subjects inhaled the test atmospheres through a mouthpiece with nose clips in place. The test atmospheres were clean air, H$_2$SO$_4$, or HNO$_3$. Oral NH$_3$ was measured before and after each exposure; during exposure, the subject's minute ventilation was also monitored as was either the concentration of HNO$_3$ or the particle concentration and size distribution of the H$_2$SO$_4$ aerosol. In the calculation of P$_j$ for the H$_2$SO$_4$ exposures, the pre- and post-exposure values of oral NH$_3$ were used to represent the first and last half of the exposure period, respectively. Fig. 3 summarizes the observations of oral ammonia level and minute ventilation in each subject for periods of both rest and exercise. As shown earlier, the combinations of high ammonia and low ventilation rate or low ammonia and high ventilation

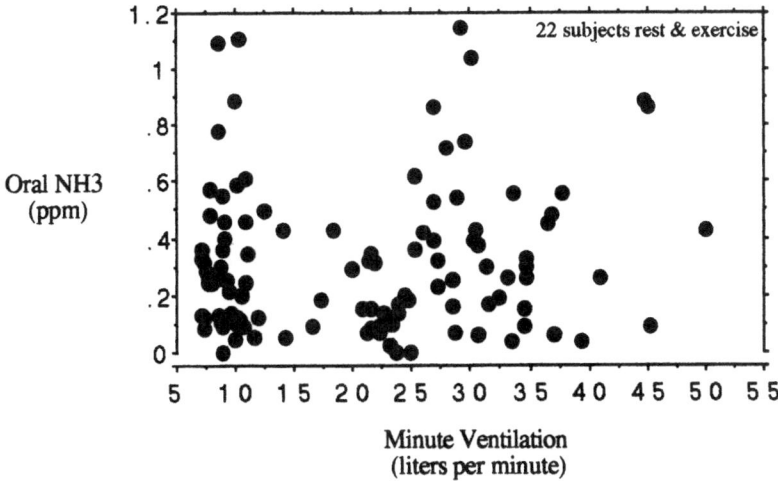

Fig. 3. Observed values of oral ammonia and ventilation rate in 22 subjects exposed to acid particles in the laboratory. A combination of high ammonia and low ventilation rate or low ammonia and high ventilation rate produce smaller or larger amounts of acid deposition, respectively

rate produce smaller or larger amounts of acid deposition, respectively, even if the acid concentration at the mouthpiece remains constant.

We estimate that HNO_3 was completely neutralized even at the lowest concentrations of oral NH_3 and the shortest oral residence times observed. From Eqn. (6), the mean lifetime of HNO_3 in the mouth of a person with 1 ppb of oral NH_3 is 11 ms. The lowest residence time in any of these subjects was >100 ms. According to our calculation, only 1 subject experienced a HNO_3 concentration entering the trachea greater than 2 ppb. This one instance of a higher concentration resulted from a very low observed oral NH_3 level (below the detection limit for the method used).

In contrast, all subjects inhaled substantial amounts of acid in particle form. The estimates of both the number and mass concentrations of particulate acid after passage through the mouth are summarized as frequency distributions in Figs. 4 and 5. As shown, there is a lower concentration of acid entering the trachea than inhaled at the mouthpiece. Most exposure indices are within one order of magnitude of that measured at the mouthpiece. One exposure index, $NK1_{tr}$, is as much as one order of magnitude less at the entrance to the trachea than at the mouthpiece. We have refrained from estimating the regional acid deposition because the modified model of Rudolf et al. (1986) is based on adult males, and these 22 subjects are adolescents of both sexes. However, the various concentrations estimated at the entrance to the trachea are useful indices of total deposition, as the full deposition/neutralization model does not predict much neutralization beyond this point.

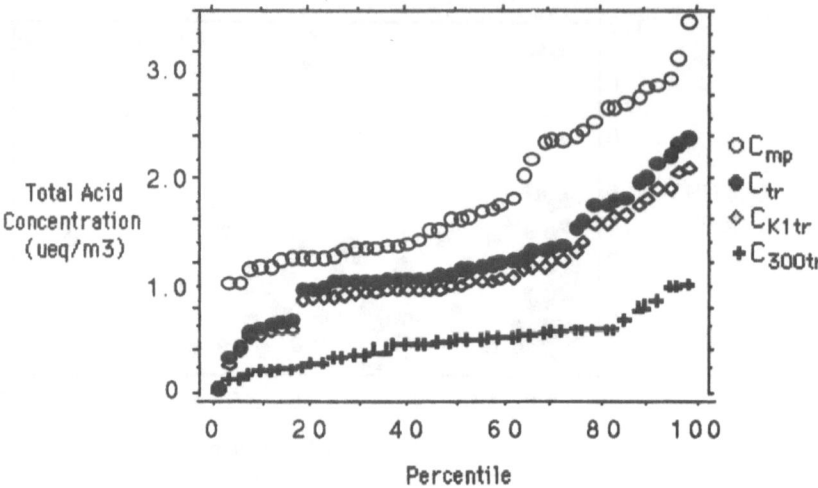

Fig. 4. Frequency distribution of the estimated mass concentration of acid particles at the entrance to the trachea for the 22 subjects exposed to H_2SO_4 particles at the mouthpiece. Each point represents the value during a given exposure averaged over periods of both rest and exercise. The variation is due to the variation in both oral ammonia levels and ventilation rates in these subjects (see Fig. 3). The various mass concentrations are defined in the text

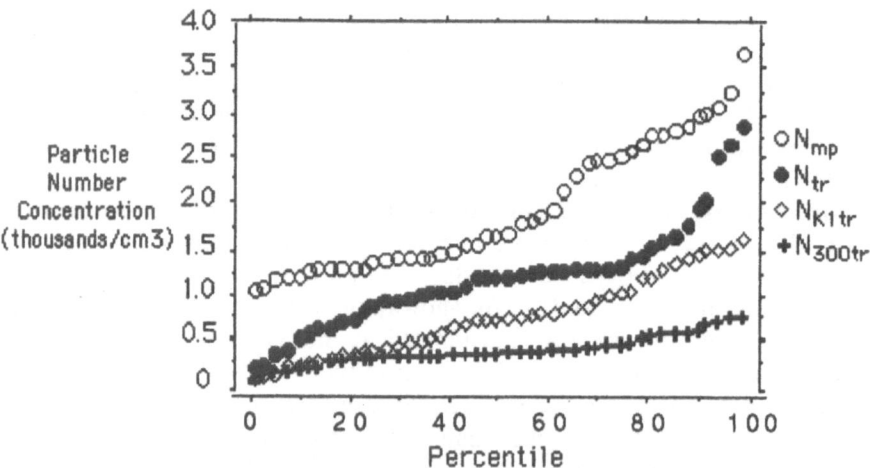

Fig. 5. Frequency distribution of the estimated number concentration of acid particles at the entrance to the trachea for the 22 subjects exposed to H_2SO_4 particles at the mouthpiece. Each point represents the value during a given exposure averaged over periods of both rest and exercise. The variation is due to the variation in both oral ammonia levels and ventilation rates in these subjects (see Fig. 3). The various number concentrations are defined in the text

Table 3. Correlations between C_{mp} and other exposure indices

Index	Overall correlation coefficient[a]	Within subject coefficient[b]
C_{tr}	0.73	0.98
$C300_{tr}$	0.74	0.94
$CK1_{tr}$	0.39	0.93
N_{tr}	0.46	0.85
$N300_{tr}$	0.70	0.94
$NK1_{tr}$	0.16	0.85

[a] Includes between and within subject variability for 22 asthmatic adolescents with varying oral NH_3 levels and ventilation rates (see also Fig. 3).
[b] Multiple R with C_{mp} as the dependent variable, index as a continuous independent variable, and subject as a category variable. In this analysis, all index and all subject-index interaction terms were significant ($P < 0.05$).

It is instructive to consider the correlations between these various exposure indices within and between this group of 22 subjects. For a fixed concentration of H_2SO_4 at the mouthpiece, there is a lot of subject to subject variability in the other exposure indices. The overall pairwise correlation coefficient between C_{mp} and other exposure indices is summarized in Table 3. In addition, the within subject correlations are also given.

General Considerations

From these results, we can make several general conclusions. First, it is instructive to consider the respiratory fate of inhaled acidic species in terms of the degree of neutralization in the airways. We predict that substantially more H_2SO_4 can be delivered to the lungs via inhalation than can HNO_3. This is consistent with our measurements of functional change (or the lack of it) in asthmatic subjects.

Second, our model of the fate of H_2SO_4 can provide insight into the design of clinical studies. A classic study design seeks to hold the inhaled concentrations constant for a group of subjects and examines differences in group response as a function of exposure concentration. We can see that in the case of inhaled acidic compounds, we will never achieve the first requirement of a constant exposure of the lung for all members of the group. If one of the exposure indices discussed here is related to the response of interest but is uncorrelated with the concentration at the entrance to the airways, the study may not be interpreted optimally. If the study design controls for subject, then high correlations between these same exposure indices make it difficult to decide which exposure metrics are valid. For instance, testing some version of the "irritation signaling" hypothesis (chronic or acute) is difficult due to the very high correlations between $N300_{tr}$ and $NK1_{tr}$.

One approach used in aerosol studies is to examine the differences between exposures to particles with different mean size and equal mass concentration. As an example, particles with 0.03 versus 0.3 μm mass median diameters (MMD) at the same mass concentration and geometric SD differ in particle number concentration by three orders of magnitude, a fact that may have biological consequences. It would appear plausible to make such particles and test the hypothesis clinically. The complication arises when the neutralization of these particles is considered. Our models predict that inhaling 0.03 μm MMD H_2SO_4 particles (geometric standard deviation less than 1.8) through either the nose or mouth will result in complete neutralization of these particles prior to their entering the lung in all 22 of the subjects we studied. In contrast, inhaling 0.3 μm MMD H_2SO_4 particles (geometric standard deviation less than 1.8) will result in significant quantities of acid being delivered to the lung. At these sizes this complication is not easily avoided.

Interestingly, Amdur and Chen (1989) have documented a number of convincing effects of 0.05-μm acid particles in guinea pigs. How can this be? On first glance, it contradicts our model results. However, if we consider the short residence times and potentially low NH_3 levels in these animals compared with humans (20–50 ms in the nose at 15 ppb NH_3), we can estimate from our models that substantial amounts of acid enters the lungs of these animals. The longer residence times and higher NH_3 levels in humans implies that these small particles will not deposit as acidic particles in the human lungs. This explanation is only speculative, in that the ammonia level in guinea pigs has not been reported. A value of 15 ppb was chosen because it represents the levels in the nose of humans. If this is the correct order of magnitude, then our hypothesis is plausible.

Finally, we must emphasize that these model estimates make one very fundamental and important assumption: the acid particles represented by H_2SO_4 aerosol behave both physically and chemically like the acidic particles actually found in the atmosphere. Most notably, we are assuming that these particles grow upon exposure to increasing RH and are readily neutralized upon exposure to respiratory NH_3 just as their laboratory counterparts are. Examining this question appears relatively straight-forward, sampling atmospheric acidity in the conventional manner and, in addition, passing the particles through a simulated upper airway, NH_3 and all.

Acknowledgements. This research was supported by grant no. RO 1 ES 02366 from the National Institute of Environmental Health Sciences.

References

Amdur MO, Chen LC (1989) Furnace-generated acid aerosols: speciation and pulmonary effects. Environ Health Perspect 79:147–150

Farrow LA, Richton RE (1981) Photoacoustic applications to chemical kinetics. SPIE J 286:18–23

Hanley QS, Koenig JQ, Larson TV, Anderson TL, van Belle G, Rebolledo V, Covert DS, Pierson W (1991) Response of young asthmatics to inhaled sulfuric acid. Am Rev Respir Dis (in press)

Hattis D, Wasson JM, Page GS, Stern B, Franklin CA (1987) Acid particles and the tracheobronchial region of the respiratory system – an "irritation signaling" model for possible health effects. J Air Pollut Control Assoc 37:1060

Koenig JQ (1989) An assessment of pulmonary function changes and oral ammonia levels after exposure of adolescent asthmatic subjects to sulfuric or nitric acid. Presentation at the 82nd annual meeting of the Air and Waste Management Association, Anaheim, California, 25–30 June

Larson TV (1989) The influence of chemical and physical forms of ambient air acids on airway doses. Environ Health Perspect 79:7–13

Larson TV, Frank R, Covert DS, Holub D, Morgan MS (1982) Measurement of respiratory ammonia and the chemical neutralization of inhaled sulfuric acid aerosol in anesthetized dogs. Am Rev Respir Dis 125:502–506

Rudolf G, Gebhardt J, Heyder J, Schiller CF, Stahlhofen W (1986) An empirical formula describing aerosol deposition in man for any particle size. J Aerosol Sci 17/3:350–355

Tang IN (1980) On the equilibrium partial pressures of nitric acid and ammonia in the atmosphere. Atmos Environ 14:819

Section 4. Clinical Inhalation Methodology

Generation of Complex Aerosols

W. Holländer

Fraunhofer Institut für Toxikologie und Aerosolforschung, Nikolai Fuchs Straße 1, W-3000 Hannover 61, FRG

Introduction

Airborne particulates may have acute and/or long-term adverse effects on human health. In order to study the underlying mechanisms and to set up guidelines for policy makers there is a need for aerosol inhalation studies. Since many of the epidemiologically relevant aerosols originate from complex natural and/or technological processes, and the exposure aerosols have to mimic them as closely as possible, it can not be expected either that the aerosol is simple itself in terms of, e.g., chemical composition, physical stability, and biological activity or that the aerosol generation and handling procedures are straightforward. The purpose of this chapter is therefore to outline the most important processes leading to suitable aerosols for inhalation toxicology experiments.

Parameters for Aerosol Characterization

Due to the fact that establishing unequivocal dose-response relationships is a very important goal for inhalation studies, the aerosol mass concentration is probably the single most important parameter. Since at least one of the study groups should be exposed to concentrations above the no-effect level, one typically deals with concentrations in the range of several mg/m^3 for nontoxic or moderately toxic substances. The full range of concentrations can therefore cover from a few $\mu g/m^3$ up to approximately $100\,mg/m^3$, at which point even nontoxic dust overloads the lung clearance capacity. As far as the particle size is concerned, one has to discriminate between the inhalable dust which extends up to approximately $100\,\mu m$ in diameter and the fine dust below approximately $10\,\mu m$ which is called thoracic because it enters the lungs. However, due to the different nose anatomy of the experimental animals as compared with man, in many cases the aerosol has to be smaller than $3\,\mu m$ in diameter. Due to the fact that different particle sizes are deposited in different places in the lung, it is sometimes necessary to have relatively monodispersed particles, i.e., the particles are of more or

U. Mohr et al. (Eds.)
Advances in Controlled Clinical
Inhalation Studies
© Springer-Verlag Berlin Heidelberg 1993

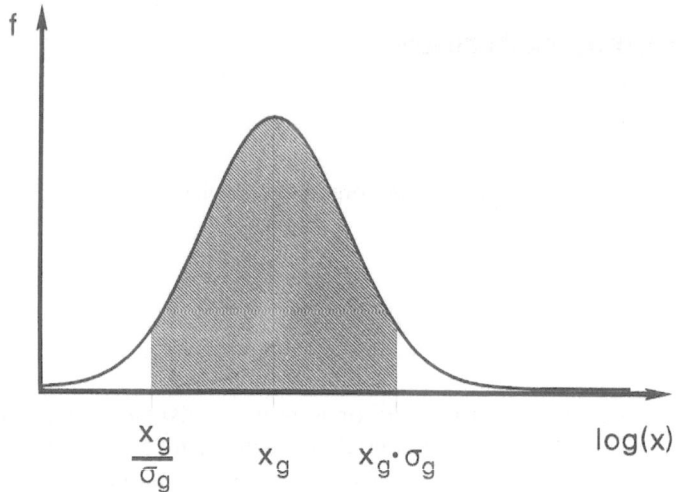

Fig. 1. Example of a log normal distribution, in which 86% of the population are within the diameter range x_g/σ_g and $x_g \cdot \sigma_g$.

less uniform size. Since under real conditions the particles do not have strictly the same size, the population must be described by a so-called particle size distribution which is characterized by an average particle size and a measure of the distribution width. For practical purposes, in most cases a so-called log normal distribution is applied, the width of which is called the geometric standard deviation, σ_g. If the particle population follows this distribution, 86% of all particles are located in the diameter range x_g/σ_g and $x_g \cdot \sigma_g$ (see Fig. 1), where x_g is the geometric average diameter. An aerosol is called monodisperse for $\sigma_g < 1.15$, quasimono-disperse for $1.15 < \sigma_g < 1.5$, and polydisperse for $\sigma_g > 1.5$. Of course, this description can be applied not only to number distributions but also to mass distributions, activity distributions, etc. One essential requirement for an aerosol to be "simple" is that its particle size distribution can be closely described by this log normal distribution. In reality, however, one very often encounters skew distributions or even a superposition of several log normal modes which may be produced by different generation processes. A very important question is the definition of particle size, because particles of the same volume but of different shape and from different material will behave differently. Since the settling velocity of a particle in the air is responsible to a large extent for its behaviour in the lung, the so-called aerodynamic diameter is defined in the following way: If an irregular particle of arbitrary density settles with a certain velocity, its aerodynamic diameter is the diameter of a sphere with density $1\,g/cm^3$ with the same settling speed (see Fig. 2). The aerodynamic diameter varies with the square root of the particle density. The effect of shape on the settling velocity can

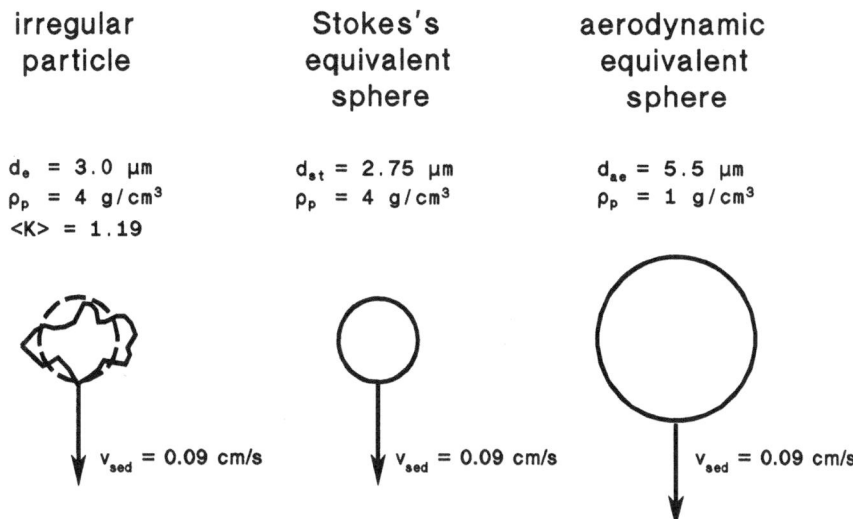

irregular particle	Stokes's equivalent sphere	aerodynamic equivalent sphere

d_e = 3.0 μm
ρ_p = 4 g/cm³
$\langle K \rangle$ = 1.19

d_{st} = 2.75 μm
ρ_p = 4 g/cm³

d_{ae} = 5.5 μm
ρ_p = 1 g/cm³

V_{sed} = 0.09 cm/s V_{sed} = 0.09 cm/s V_{sed} = 0.09 cm/s

Fig. 2. The aerodynamic diameter concept

be taken into account by a so-called dynamic shape factor which can be calculated for simple geometries for the different directions of motion so that in practice a certain average of these shape factors has to be used.

Basic Processes for the Generation of "Simple" Aerosols

There are essentially two basic mechanisms which lead to the production of aerosol particles. The first consists in dispersing solids or liquids. The second starts out with individual atoms and/or molecules and causes them to form clusters which may eventually grow to aerosol particles.

Cutting, grinding, and milling typically produce particles larger than 1 μm with a broad particle size distribution and irregular shape. However, these primary processes are rarely used for inhalation purposes because they are dangerous and costly. Very often, therefore, the powders produced by these processes are collected so that the secondary generation of the aerosol consists in dispersing these powders. Several instruments are commercially available and are described in VDI guidelines 3491 parts 8, 9, and 10 (VDI 1989a,b; 1990a). If a fluidized powder bed is shaken with a suitable frequency and amplitude the air permeating this fluidized bed will entrain particles (Fig. 3) (VDI 1990a). This technique has been widely used for dispersing fibrous powders. Another method uses a rotating brush for scraping off compacted powder fed by a piston from a cylindrical reservoir (Fig. 4) (VDI 1989a). A jet of carrier gas blows the particles away from the brush. The concentration is determined by the powder feed rate and the carrier gas

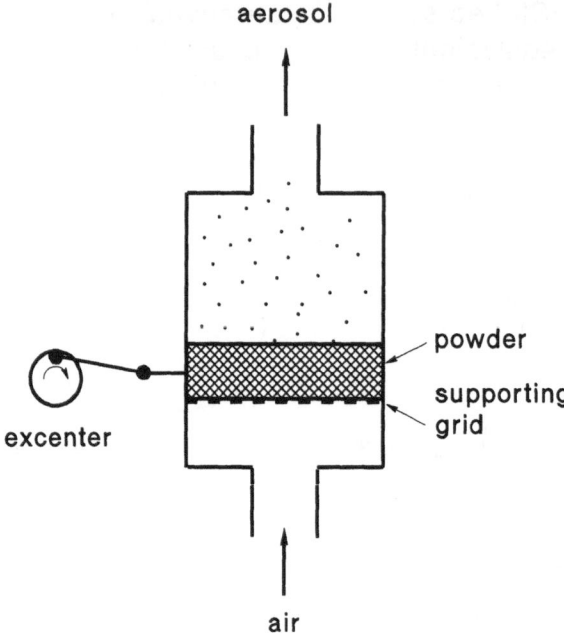

Fig. 3. Principle of a vibrating bed generator

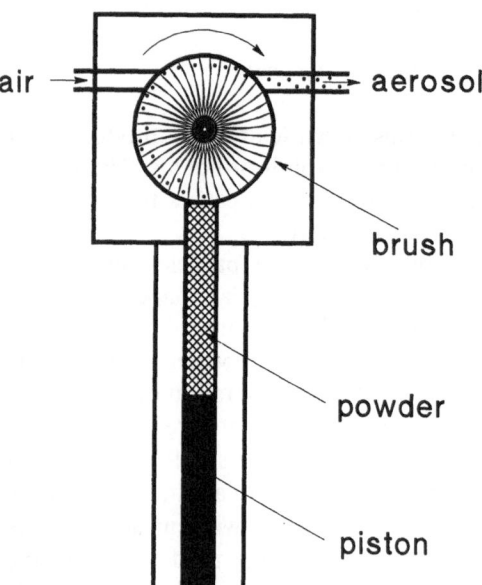

Fig. 4. Schematic of a rotating brush generator

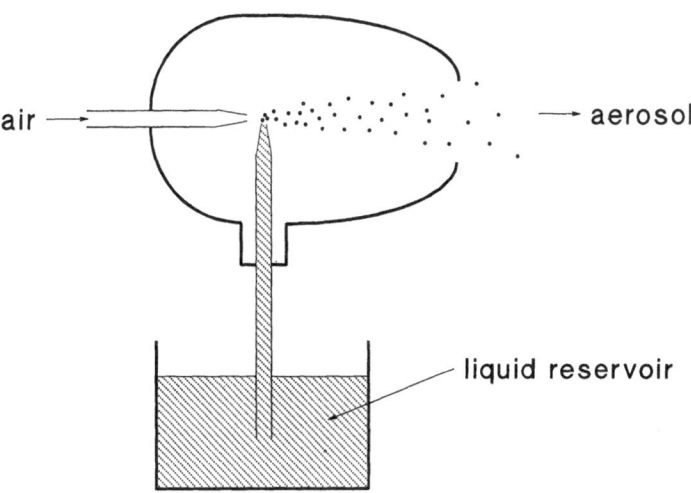

Fig. 5. Principle of air-jet liquid atomizer

volumetric flow rate. A very effective method is to use the suction produced by a fast air jet which disperses agglomerates by shear forces. Feeding can be done either by a screw feeder or by a belt feed unit as described in VDI (1989b). The advantage of the above-described methods is their simplicity; their disadvantage consists in the poor control over particle size distribution. Also, these techniques do not work with sticky powders. Application purpose permitting, additives like aerosil (amorphous silicon dioxide) may help to improve the dispersion characteristics. The same ejector principle can be used to disperse liquids provided they are not too viscous (Fig. 5) (VDI 1980a). Typical primary droplet size for water is in the range of several microns with a geometric standard deviation around 1.4–1.5. If a solution is atomized instead of a pure liquid, under suitable conditions the solvent may be evaporated and the solid or liquid residual particle will remain. Its size will depend on the third root of the solute concentration. For practical analytical reasons this technique is very often applied with fluorescein and methylene blue dyes, but salts like NaCl are popular, too. A convenient modification of this technique suitable for generating monodisperse aerosols consists in adding monodisperse Latex particles and thus forming suspensions. If the suspension concentration is low enough, most of the primary droplets will contain no particle, some of them will contain one particle, and the probability for multiple particles within one primary droplet will be negligible so that the resulting aerosol particle size distribution will be monodisperse to a very large degree. In addition to the above atomizers which are based on gas shear forces acting on liquid columns or sheets, liquid disintegration occurs solely through liquid film instability in the methods described below. The simplest atomizer is a jet issuing from an

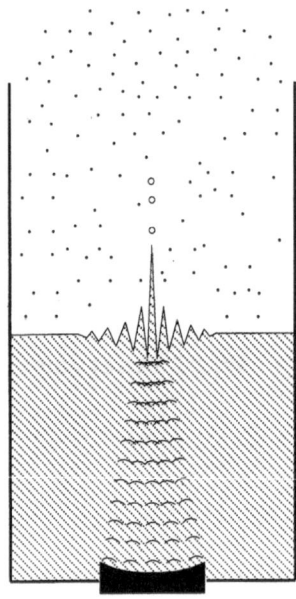

Fig. 6. Schematic of an ultrasonic generator

orifice; this principle is used in every diesel fuel injection pump and produces droplets of an approximate diameter of 100 μm. If a disturbance
of 4.5 jet diameters is superimposed onto the liquid jet it breaks up into
monodisperse droplets. Since the liquid flow rate drastically drops with
decreasing jet orifice diameter, resulting particle production rates are
generally too low for inhalation purposes, but this technique is very suitable
for calibration aerosols. Liquid films can also be produced by spinning discs
with very high rotational speeds (up to 100 000 rpm); with proper design
fairly monodisperse particles at comparatively high production rates in
the size range 0.5–100 μm can be produced (VDI 1990b). Application of
ultrasonic waves for liquid disintegration offer the advantage of high particle
production rates without the necessity of applying high volumetirc flow rates
so that high aerosol concentrations can be achieved (VDI 1990c). The
geometric standard deviation is in the range 1.4–1.5, and depending on the
applied frequency primary droplet sizes down to 2 μm can be obtained.
Standard ultrasonic nebulizers use a concave oscillator crystal immersed in
the liquid to be dispersed (Fig. 6). Under normal operating conditions, the
liquid level is at the focus of the crystal in order to achieve maximum energy
density for dispersion. A modification of this technique is the so-called
capillary wave generator (VDI 1988) which produces resonant capillary
waves on the surface of a disc (Fig. 7). With increasing oscillator amplitude
the capillary waves grow exponentially and therefore disintegrate from the
surface film. The resulting droplet size distributions are slightly skew but can
be approximated by a log normal distribution.

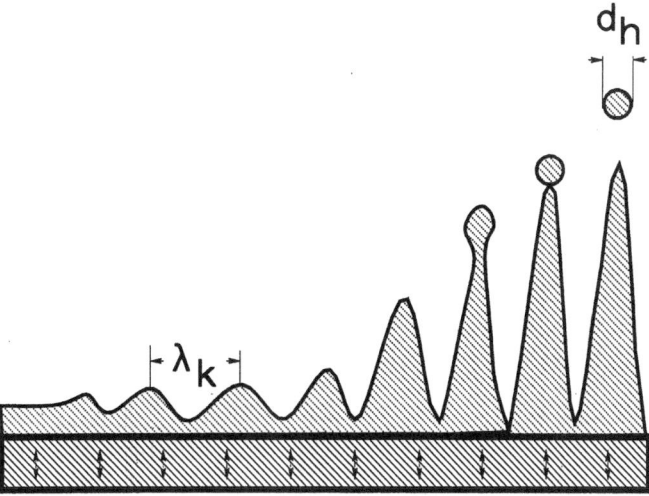

Fig. 7. Schematic of a capillary wave generator

If submicron particles at comparatively high concentrations are required, one has to resort to condensation methods. If a chemically stable liquid or solid can be evaporated thermally, by an electric arc, plasma torch, electron beam or any other means, subsequent temperature reduction in this volume leads to a supersaturation with condensation resulting. Even if there is convective or turbulent dilution of the vapor, supersaturation normally occurs because saturation vapor pressure is an exponential function of the temperature, and therefore actual vapor pressure may be considerably higher than saturation pressure. A typical example is the plume of a steam locomotive. If great care is taken and the supersaturation conditions are uniform within the generator, by these means a monodisperse aerosol can be obtained in the size range $0.1–10\,\mu m$. Depending on the required particle size and concentration, these techniques may be used with and without seed nuclei. In the presence of seed nuclei the supersaturation required for droplet growth is significantly reduced because no energetically unfavorable build-up of critical molecular clusters is required, and the vapor molecules can immediately condense onto preexisting surfaces. There is no big difference between the two popular generators after Rapaport-Weinstock (VDI 1987) and Sinclair and LaMer (VDI 1980b). The only difference is that the former uses natural impurities in the condensable liquid as condensation nuclei, whereas in the latter, foreign seed nuclei are used (Fig. 8). A very important pathway for the formation of relevant natural and anthropogenic aerosols is condensation after chemical reaction, which occurs if the saturation vapor pressures of the resulting compounds are considerably lower than those of the primary compounds. Examples include the production of carbon black by the combustion of acetylene, of very fine

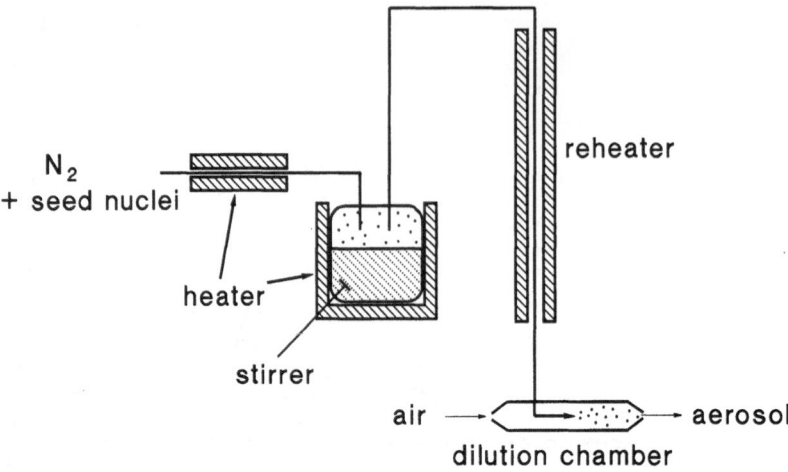

Fig. 8. Principle of a Sinclair-LaMer generator

ultraclean iron particles from the oxidation of iron pentacarbonyl, $Fe(CO)_5$, and of electronic grade silicon from silane reactions, as mentioned in a review by Flagan et al. (1990). The literature on photochemical aerosol production in the atmosphere fills whole libraries. The problem with natural and technical systems is that the chemistry of the resulting aerosol particles is usually very complex, which makes it very difficult to produce a nearly identical aerosol in a different or hopefully simpler process. Under some circumstances, aerosol generation can be hardly simplified, and the only way to economize consists in downscaling the technical process.

Generation and Handling of Moderately Complex Aerosols

Any aerosol produced by the above-described methods is called simple if no special means have been taken for controlling the constancy of output concentration, mean diameter, and geometric standard deviation. However, very often the inhalation toxicologist requires parameter combinations which are difficult to meet for fundamental or technical reasons. For instance, the requirement of a very high concentration is incompatible with a simultaneous excellent monodispersity because of particle coagulation. This can be easily seen from the following qualitative considerations (Fig. 9). If an aerosol consists of strictly monodisperse particles at high concentrations, they collide with each other, and the series of singulets, doublets, triplets, etc. forms an increasingly polydisperse aerosol. On the other hand, the width of a very broad distribution will shrink because very small particles will have a very high collision probability with very large particles. This means that over long times arbitrary initial distributions reach an asymptotic distribution

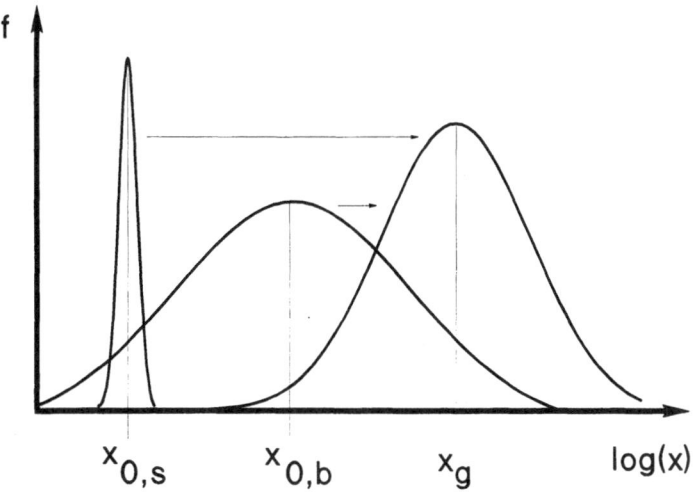

Fig. 9. The coagulation process of aerosols with wide and narrow size distributions leads to the same asymptotic distribution

with a σ_g in the range 1.35–1.45 depending on the particle size. Another change of size spectrum of droplets or volatile solid particles may occur due to the fact that because of the Kelvin effect the vapor pressure over small particles is greater than that over large particles. That means that large particles will grow at the expense of small particles, which will eventually evaporate completely. Depending on the vapor pressure of the substance under consideration, the time scale for this so-called Ostwald ripening is in the 0.1 to 10-min range. A similar, even more pronounced effect occurs if the total substance concentration is only slightly larger than the saturation concentration, because only the fraction in excess of the saturation concentration will remain in particulate form. Since the saturation concentration is a nearly exponential function of the temperature, even temperature fluctuations considerably smaller than 1 Kelvin will affect the aerosol concentration dramatically. Different size distributions at different locations in the exposure chamber will also result due to sedimentation losses of large particles if the geometric standard deviation is very large. Similar losses which affect different sizes of the particle spectrum in different ways may be due to electrical charges acquired during the generation process. Generally, dispersion techniques produce large particle charges, which lead to image force deposition if the charges are not removed by bipolar ion sources. In addition to these fundamental problems which can be taken into account comparatively easily during the planning stage, technical problems may turn out to be very difficult to deal with sometimes. Since a chronic inhalation study requires very good long-term constancy of the aerosol parameters concentration, mass median aerodynamic diameter, and geometric standard deviation even for highly toxic, sticky, and polymerizing material for which no aerosol literature data are available, there is no general a priori way available to avoid technical difficulties. Very often, strong deposition occurs in the tubing, especially at bends or at orifices for the determination of flow rates. The latter is particularly detrimental, because due to the automatic control there will be a gradual shift in dilution ratios and so on. In most cases, heating of critical components reduces particle deposition due to thermophoretic repulsion to a noncritical level, but care has to be taken that the temperature is not too high, thus thermally degrading the material which may lead to the build-up of very annoying crusts.

Examples of "Complex" Aerosols

The complexity of the aerosol generation procedure generally increases with number and stringency of requirements, which may even be incompatible with each other. In general, all multielement and all multicompound particles will be termed complex. Even generation of one-component aerosol particles may require complex equipment, e.g., if a special particle shape is needed. For example, in a technique recently proposed for preparing monosized carbon fibers, a high power CO_2-laser is necessary for cutting fiber bundles (Loo et al. 1982). An even more flexible technique as far as shapes is concerned was described by Hoover et al. (1990), who used integrated circuit fabrication techniques, but because of the high price of approximately 1 cent per 10^8 particles, this method is out of the range of inhalation experiments while certainly very useful for calibration and other specialized purposes. The simplest conceivable way of producing a two-component aerosol is by coating a simple aerosol with the required second component, which may be sulfuric acid, or polycyclic aromatic hydrocarbons (which are of epidemiological interest), or by tagging them with radioactive labels (^{51}Cr, ^{95}Zr) (Newton et al. 1980; Walters et al. 1988). Inhalation of metallic vapors (Zn, Ni, Mn, Cd, etc.) may cause vomiting, headache, and cramps, which are therefore of occupational relevance, as well as the corresponding metal oxide fumes, which can adsorb and react with industrial flue gases such as SO_2, NO_x, H_2S, and hydrocarbons. Probably this group of complex aerosols is the most important one in terms of epidemiology. A variety of slightly modified condensation techniques can be applied to produce such aerosols, like evaporation of metal organic compounds with subsequent thermal degradation using the exploding wire technique or burning of the metal in oxygen or electrical heating of a wire, if only low particle fluxes are required. The techniques are described in much more detail in the original papers (Conte et al. 1989; McCarthy et al. 1982; Amdur et al. 1988). Another aspect which enhances the technical complexity of aerosol generation appreciably is low aerosol stability. Water droplets of a size of 10 µm for instance will evaporate within 500 ms in a dry atmosphere, and even in 99% relative humidity they need only 2 s for evaporation. Fortunately, clean water is not very interesting for inhalation purposes, so one has the option to stabilize the droplets by adding some electrolytes such as salt, sulfuric acid, etc. which may compensate for the Kelvin effect sufficiently so that stable droplets can result. Nevertheless, retrofitting of an existing inhalation facility for use with fog aerosol would be hardly feasible because of the limited stability and the large droplet size, which lead to enormous losses in all tubings.

Even with the best technology, however, there are some highly complex natural or technical aerosol processes which cannot be simulated in a reasonable way, for instance, formation of photochemical smog, diesel soot, coal oven aerosol, cigarette aerosol, and so on. In these cases, there is no other way than to use the original process scaled down to a minimum size as required by the laboratory conditions.

Additional information on aerosol generation can be found in (Willeke et al. 1980; Dennis 1976).

References

Amdur MO, Sarofim AF, Neville M, Quann RJ, McCarthy JF, Elliott JF, Lam HF, Rogers AE, Conner MW (1988) Coal combustion aerosols and SO_2: an interdisciplinary analysis. Environ Sci Technol 20:138–145

Conte C, Devitorfrancesco G, Di Castro V (1989) Surface reactions of SO_2 on metallic particles. Atmos Environ 23:1939–1943

Dennis R (1976) Handbook on aerosols. National Technical Information Service, Center Energy Research and Development Administration, Springfield

Flagan RC (1990) Aerosol processes for material synthesis. In: Masuda S, Takahashi K (eds) Aerosols. Pergamon, New York, pp 50–54

Hoover MD, Casalnuovo SA, Lipowicz, PJ, Yeh HC, Hanson RW, Hurd AJ (1990) A method for producing non-spherical monodisperse particles using integrated circuit fabrication techniques. J Aerosol Sci 21:569–575

Loo BW, Cork CP, Madden NW (1982) A laser-based monodisperse carbon fiber generator. J Aerosol Sci 13:241–248

McCarthy JF, Yurek GJ, Elliott JF, Amdur MO (1982) Generation and characterization of submicron aerosols of zinc oxide. Am Ind Hyg Assoc J 43:880–886

Newton GJ, Kanapilly GM, Boecker BB, Raabe OG (1980) Radioactive labeling of aerosols; generation methods and characteristics. In: Wilke K (ed) Generation of aerosols and facilities for exposure experiments. Ann Arbour Science, Ann Arbor

VDI (1980a) Messen von Partikeln; Herstellen von Prüfaerosolen aus Farbstofflösungen mit Düsenzerstäubern. VDI, Düsseldorf (VDI Handbuch Reinhaltung der Luft, vol 4, guideline 3491, part 3)

VDI (1980b) Messen von Partikeln; Herstellungsverfahren für Prüfaerosole; Aerosolgenerator nach Sinclair und La Mer. VDI, Düsseldorf (VDI-Handbuch Reinhaltung der Luft, vol 4, guideline 3491, part 4)

VDI (1987) Particulate matter measurement; generation of test aerosols; Rapaport-Weinstock generator. VDI, Düsseldorf (VDI Handbuch Reinhaltung der Luft, vol 4, guideline 3491, part 7)

VDI (1988) Messen von Partikeln; Herstellen von Prüfaerosolen unter Verwendung eines Kapillarwellengenerators. VDI, Düsseldorf (VDI Handbuch Reinhaltung der Luft, vol 4, guideline 3491, part 14)

VDI (1989a) Particulate matter measurement; generation of test aerosols with a rotating brush generator. VDI, Düsseldorf (VDI Handbuch Reinhaltung der Luft, vol 4, guideline 3491, part 9)

VDI (1989b) Particulate matter measurement; generation of test aerosols from powders using a belt feed unit. VDI, Düsseldorf (VDI Handbuch Reinhaltung der Luft, vol 4, guideline 3491, part 8)

VDI (1990a) Particulate matter measurement; generation of test aerosols from fibrous powders using a vibrating bed aerosol generator. VDI, Düsseldorf (VDI Handbuch Reinhaltung der Luft, vol 4, guideline 3491, part 10)

VDI (1990b) Particulate matter measurement; generation of test aerosols with centrifugal atomizers. VDI, Düsseldorf (VDI Handbuch Reinhaltung der Luft, vol 4, guideline 3491, part 12)

VDI (1990c) Particulate matter measurement; generation of test aerosols using ultrasonic atomizers. VDI, Düsseldorf (VDI Handbuch Reinhaltung der Luft, vol 4, guideline 3491, part 11)

Walters RB, Nordenstam BJ, Phalen RF (1988) A generator for the production of sulfuric acid-coated diesel soot aerosols. Atmos Environ 22:17–23

Willeke K (1980) Generation of aerosols and facilities for exposure experiments. Ann Arbor Science, Ann Arbor

Assessment of Ambient Exposures and Their Effects on Health in Chambers*

J.D. HACKNEY and W.S. LINN

University of Southern California, Rancho Los Amigos Med. Center, 51 Medical Science Building, 7601 East Imperial Highway, Downey, CA 90424, USA

Introduction

Clinical inhalation studies typically take place in whole-body exposure chambers with tightly controlled atmospheric conditions and with exposure protocols intended to be representative of actual community or occupational exposure conditions, with respect to pollutant concentration, exposure duration, and activity patterns (Hackney et al. 1985). Chamber studies usually employ free-living volunteers drawn from segments of the population which are considered to be especially at risk from exposure to the pollutant(s) in question. The special risk may relate to increased responsiveness or decreased functional reserve, as in patients with chronic cardiopulmonary disease. Alternatively, the special risk may relate to unusually high inhaled doses of pollutants, as in healthy manual laborers and athletes who experience high ventilation rates for long periods of time.

In health risk assessment, conventional laboratory-based exposure-chamber studies of human volunteers have many obvious strengths, but they address certain important questions inadequately, if at all (Table 1). To help answer these questions, scientists need to adapt their laboratory measurement methods for use in the field. They can then measure volunteers' activities and health changes before and after chamber exposure and make direct comparisons of the voluteers' experience between the chamber and their usual environments.

In this paper we examine several methodologies which may be useful to integrate chamber and field investigations and present preliminary results from our initial applications of them.

---

*The work discussed here has been supported by Southern California Edison Company, the Electric Power Research Institute, and the Health Effects Institute.

U. Mohr et al. (Eds.)
Advances in Controlled Clinical
Inhalation Studies
© Springer-Verlag Berlin Heidelberg 1993

Table 1. Some important questions raised by chamber exposure studies

1. How would responses compare between the volunteer groups actually studied and random samples of the populations whose health risks are being assessed? (Are the most responsive individuals underrepresented or overrepresented in volunteer groups?)
2. How do volunteers' physiologic or clinical responses in a chamber compare with their typical hourly, daily, or seasonal variability in health status? (Are the responses to pollutants in chambers medically important in comparison with other typical short-term health changes?)
3. How representative of usual physical activities are the exercise protocols used in chambers? (Do chamber protocols provide realistic inhaled doses of pollutants and realistic levels of other accompanying stresses?)
4. Are volunteers in their typical state of health at the beginning of an exposure study? (Do undocumented variations in preexposure health status cause misleading experimental results?)
5. Are there persistent or delayed effects of chamber exposures not documented in conventional experimental protocols?

Methodology to Integrate Field and Chamber Investigations

Volunteer Recruitment by Random Sampling

Chamber studies usually can employ only 10–100 volunteers, although they intend to document health risks in populations thousands or millions of times larger. Such small-scale studies are inherently likely to underestimate the "worst case" health effect, because they are unlikely to include the most exposed/most responsive individuals in a large population. For that reason, investigators commonly focus on suspected high-risk volunteers, as mentioned before. That approach has been successful in confirming that certain high-risk groups respond unfavourably to ambient exposures which seem not to bother most people, in particular, exercising asthmatics exposed to sulfur dioxide (Sheppard et al. 1981) and athletes/heavy laborers exposed to ozone (Folinsbee et al. 1988). Even so, typical studies of self-selected volunteers probably underestimate worst-case responses, because individuals who are (or think they are) very sensitive to pollution probably are reluctant to volunteer. On the other hand, such individuals might be overrepresented in volunteer groups, if they expect to receive medical help by volunteering. In any case, it seems unlikely that a typical volunteer group's data can accurately predict the distribution of responses in an entire exposed population, the information most important to health risk assessors.

In theory, one could select chamber subjects by randomly sampling the exposed population and thereby predict the entire population's response accurately. In practice, not all individuals contacted in a random survey would volunteer for chamber studies. But if a substantial percentage volunteered and if both volunteers and nonvolunteers answered questions concerning their health and exposure status, then one could elucidate the relationship between health and volunteering behavior. This would not necessarily allow an accurate prediction of responses in the entire exposed population but would at least identify potential sources of bias in data from self-selected volunteers.

We are attempting to apply the strategy described above to estimate the range of responses to ozone in 18-to-55-year-old nonsmoking adult residents of a socioeconomically diverse Los Angeles suburb (Hackney et al. 1991a). Results of the initial effort have not been entirely encouraging. Only about half the individuals in a randomly selected sample provided usable questionnaire data, fewer than 4% of the original sample volunteered for an ozone exposure study when offered the same payment typically given to self-selected volunteers, and fewer than 2% actually participated in the exposure. Thus, the self-selection process operating on chamber volunteers seems very strong. On the other hand, volunteers and nonvolunteers showed similar patterns of questionnaire responses (although the statistical power to detect differences was low because there were so few volunteers). The two groups' age and gender distributions were similar. About 30% of each group considered themselves unusually sensitive to air pollution, and a similar number said they limited their activity during pollution episodes. About 10%–15% of each group gave a history of asthma, 30%–35% gave a history of respiratory allergy, and 70% reported living in the Los Angeles area for 10 years or longer. Additional random-sampling subject recruitment efforts seem worthwhile, but to have a chance of success, they must be designed very carefully to make participation in exposure studies convenient and to provide strong positive motivations for volunteering.

Adaptation of Laboratory Measurements for Field Use: Self-Monitoring of Activity Patterns and Health Status

In a typical chamber study of a respiratory irritant air pollutant, the investigator estimates inhaled doses on the basis of pollutant concentration, duration of exposure, and subjects' ventilation rates and then relates inhaled doses to health responses (e.g., changes in lung function or symptoms during exposure). Ideally, one would like to measure these same exposure and health variables in the field as precisely as in the laboratory. Then, by monitoring a number of subjects for several days while they go about their normal activities, one could determine whether the responses found in chamber studies also occur in "real life," and if so, how they compare with other short-term health changes experienced in the normal course of life, independent of pollution exposure.

In practice, of course, neither exposure nor health status can be measured as precisely in the field as in the laboratory, and many extra complicating factors are encountered in the field: pathogens, allergens, respiratory medications, exposures to occupational and household pollutants, etc. Even so, field monitoring technology has advanced such that it is now practical to measure physical activity and health status with time resolution in the minute or hour range. Exposures to nitrogen dioxide can be measured with 24-h time resolution using convenient, commercially available, passive dosimeters (see, for example, Yanagisawa and Nishimura 1982), and analogous devices to measure ozone exposure are under development (see, for example, Koutrakis et al. 1990). We have developed techniques to allow panels of volunteer subjects to monitor their own lung function, clinical status, and activities over periods of 1–2 weeks (Linn et al. 1990). The lung function measurement system, employing a conventional survey spirometer interfaced to a comparatively inexpensive personal computer, can be placed in the subject's home. It displays instructions to the subject and records all the test data, along with the dates and times of testing. Subjects are asked to test themselves three times a day. Concurrently, they record ventilation rates (self-estimated in terms of "slow," "medium," or "fast" physical activity), symptoms, and medication usage every waking hour on a diary form. More objective estimates of ventilation are obtained by recording heart rates every minute with inexpensive athletic training instruments. Graded exercise tests are performed to determine each individual's relationship between heart rate and ventilation rate. Raizenne and Spengler (1989) first demonstrated the usefulness of this technique in a summer camp study involving supervised exercise. We have found that most volunteers can record their heart rates successfully without supervision, although some data are lost due to operating mistakes or unfavorable recording conditions.

To test the capabilities of these techniques, we studied a panel of Los Angeles area asthmatic volunteers for 1 week each in summer and winter (Shamoo et al. 1991; Stram et al. 1991). No personal exposure monitoring or chamber exposures were performed. In all 45 persons participated, of whom 44 provided reasonably complete diary and lung function records, and 34 provided useful heart rate records in both seasons. Collectively, the asthmatic volunteers reported spending at least 75% of their waking hours indoors and 10% in vehicles. Only 5%–7% of waking-hour activity was of "medium" intensity and only about 1% was "fast", in summer or in winter. The median ventilation rate estimated from heart rate records was 17 l/min, and the 99th-percentile estimated rate was 32 l/min. In summer, the subjects showed marked diurnal variation in lung function; the average forced expired volume in one second (FEV_1) was about 15% lower in the early morning than in the early afternoon. The average FEV_1 was significantly decreased when subjects took medication in response to chest symptoms, but FEV_1 values were not unusual at times when subjects took their regularly scheduled medication. Somewhat surprisingly, FEV_1 varied less in relation to temporal or clinical factors in winter than in summer.

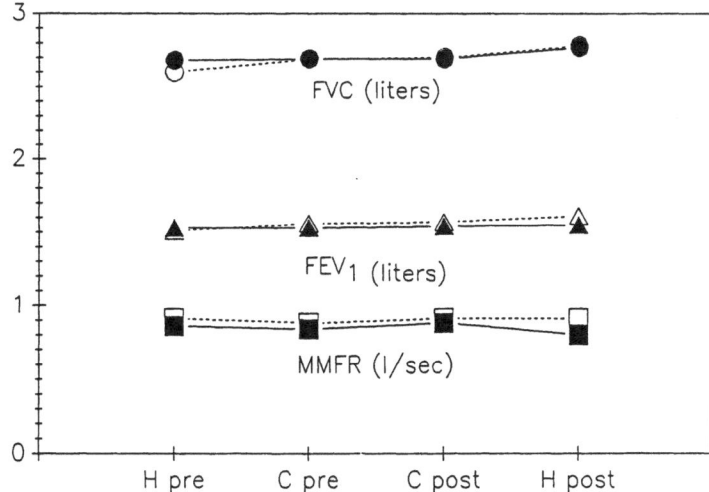

Fig. 1. Comparison of lung function test results between self-measurements at home (*H*) and technicians' measurements in chamber (*C*), pre- and postexposure. *FVC*, forced vital capacity; *FEV₁*, forced expired volume in one second; *MMFR*, maximal midexpiratory flow rate; *Open symbol*, clean air; *Solid symbol*, NO_2

Combining Field Self-Monitoring with Chamber Exposure Studies

More recently, we studied the effects of NO_2 in a panel of 26 volunteer Los Angeles area residents with chronic obstructive pulmonary disease (COPD), combining chamber exposures with field monitoring (Hackney et al. 1991b). The subjects monitored themselves for 2-week periods during autumn or winter (low-ozone, high-NO_2 season) using diaries, home spirometry systems, and Yanagisawa NO_2 badges to estimate personal exposure. In the middle of each week, every subject underwent a chamber exposure, once with clean air and once with 0.3 ppm NO_2. The exposures lasted 4 h and included four 7-min periods of exercise, in which the average ventilation rate was about 25 l/min.

Fig. 1 shows mean lung function results measured by the subjects at home in the morning before chamber exposures, by technicians in the laboratory just before and at the end of exposure, and by the subjects at home in the afternoon or evening after exposure. These results apply to the 23 subjects who had complete home spirometry data before and after exposures. As the figure indicates, there were no significant differences between home and chamber measurements or between clean air and NO_2 exposure studies.

Fig. 2 shows a fairly typical set of lung function test results for a complete 2-week period, obtained in a 52-year-old woman volunteer, 163 cm tall

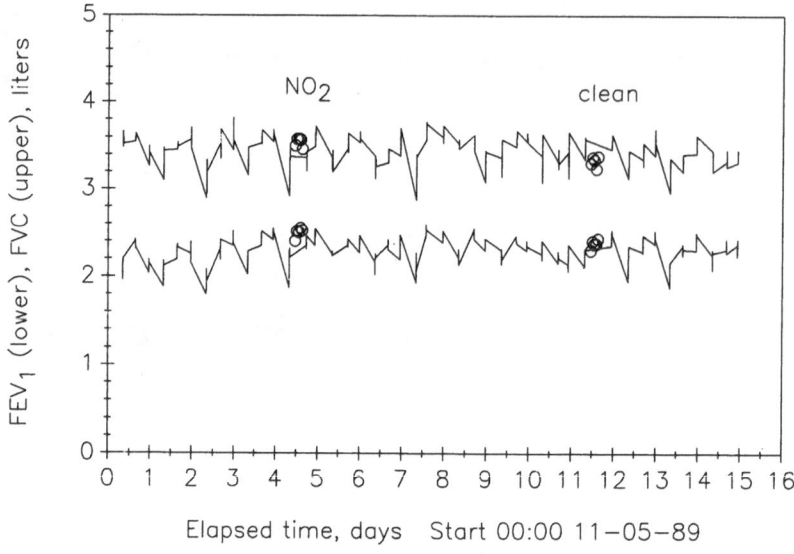

Fig. 2. Plot of all home (*line*) and chamber (*circles*) lung function measurements for a typical subject, see text for explanation

and weighing 57 kg, with normal forced vital capacity (FVC) and modestly reduced FEV_1. The solid lines represent home testing results: The vertical segments indicate the range of FVC or FEV_1 during a test session (usually involving 5 blows over approximately 5 min), and the diagonal segments indicate intervals between test sessions. The circles represent hourly measurements immediately before and during chamber exposures, each a mean of 3–5 blows. The home data show a diurnal pattern similar to asthmatics', with lowest function in the morning and no consistent change from day to day. The chamber data generally fall within the range of the home data.

Data from monitoring badges indicated that personal 24-h average NO_2 exposures were significantly correlated with 24-h average outdoor concentrations measured at the air monitoring stations nearest to the subjects' homes. Individual subjects' correlation coefficients relating their personal and monitoring-station NO_2 levels ranged from 0.12 to 0.90, averaging 0.68. Even though most subjects were smokers living in homes with gas stoves, only one – who worked in a machine shop – appeared to have experienced indoor personal exposures at concentrations substantially above outdoor ambient levels. Overall 2-week average estimated personal exposure concentrations ranged from 0.031 to 0.125 ppm and averaged 0.054 ppm. Corresponding overall average concentrations at nearby monitoring stations ranged from 0.045 to 0.089 ppm and averaged 0.066 ppm. No subject showed a significant negative correlation of daily average lung function measurements with NO_2 exposure level on the same day or with NO_2

exposure level on the previous day. For the majority of individuals, increasing NO_2 exposure was associated with better lung function, but the correlation was not statistically significant. Thus, both the chamber data and the field data from this study indicated that, in general, the subjects experienced no meaningful short-term effects on lung function from the NO_2 exposure. This negative result is consistent with our previous experience; however, others have reported slight lung function decrements in similar chamber exposures of volunteers with COPD (Morrow and Utell 1990).

Conclusions

All the new methodology discussed here promises significant advances in the capability to assess short-term effects of air pollution exposure. It also promises help in judging the public-health importance of findings from conventional chamber exposures and epidemiologic investigations. For example, suppose that conventional studies show statistically significant temporary lung dysfunction from exposure to a given pollutant. Regulatory officials must decide whether this effect is truly adverse to health (deserving high priority in prevention efforts) or is only a minor nuisance. Detailed field monitoring may contribute importantly to the decision, by documenting typical day-to-day lung function variability independent of pollution exposure. The larger the specific pollutant effect is in comparison with typical day-to-day variability, the more reason there is to consider it adverse to health.

Further progress is needed in this field, both in personal exposure monitoring and in health monitoring. Specific technological goals should include more compact, rugged, and inexpensive instruments for frequent self-testing of lung function and unobtrusive, inexpensive, personal exposure monitors for common pollutants which can document short-term peak exposures, i.e., can determine average concentrations over periods of 1 h or less. In addition, biostatisticians need to develop new procedures for testing exposure/health associations, applicable to data sets containing numerous closely-spaced longitudinal measurements of multiple atmospheric and biological variables in comparatively small experimental populations.

References

Folinsbee LJ, McDonnell WF, Horstman DH (1988) Pulmonary function and symptom responses after 6.6-hour exposure to 0.12 ppm ozone with moderate exercise. J Air Pollut Control Assoc 38:28–35

Hackney JD, Linn WS, Avol EL (1985) Assessing health effects of air pollution. Environ Sci Technol 18:115a–122A

Hackney JD, Linn WS, Johnson TR (1991a) Response to ozone in the population: individual and seasonal factors. 8th Health Effects Institute Annual Conference, Colorado Springs, 21–24 April 1991

Hackney JD, Linn WS, Avol EL, Shamoo DA, Anderson KR, Solomon JC, Little DE, Peng RC (1991b) Effects of nitrogen dioxide exposure on volunteers with chronic obstructive pulmonary disease (COPD): a combined field survey and exposure chamber study. Am Rev Respir Dis 143:A94

Koutrakis P, Wolfson JM, Lamborg CH, Brauer M, Spengler JD, Slater L (1990) Measurements of personal exposures to ozone, acid aerosols and gases, and fine particles. In: Total exposure assessment methodology: a new horizon. Air and Waste Management Association, Pittsburgh, pp 360–367

Linn WS, Shamoo DA, Trim SC, Solomon JC, Hackney JD (1990) New techniques to survey activity patterns and short-term respiratory health changes in populations exposed to ambient pollution. In: Total exposure assessment methodology: a new horizon. Air and Waste Management Association, Pittsburgh, pp 565–576

Morrow PE, Utell MJ (1990) Responses of susceptible subpopulations to nitrogen dioxide. Health Effects Institute, Cambridge (Health Effects Institute Research Report no. 23)

Raizenne ME, Spengler JD (1989) Dosimetric model of acute health effects of ozone and acid aerosols in children. In: Schneider T, Lee SD, Walters GJR, Grant LD (eds) Atmospheric ozone research and its policy implications. Elsevier, Amsterdam, pp 319–329

Shamoo DA, Linn WS, Trim SC, Peng RC, Little DE, Webb TL, Hackney JD (1991) Determination of activity patterns in asthmatics for air pollution risk assessment purposes. Am Rev Respir Dis 143:A272

Sheppard D, Saisho A, Nadel JA, Boushey HA (1981) Exercise increases sulfur dioxide-induced bronchoconstriction in asthmatics. Am Rev Respir Dis 123:486–491

Stram DO, Linn WS, Shamoo DA, Peng RC, Solomon JC, Little DE, Trim SC, Webb TL, Hackney JD (1991) Temporal patterns of respiratory status in a panel of asthmatic Los Angeles residents. Am Rev Respir Dis 143:A272

Yanagisawa Y, Nishimura H (1982) A badge-type personal sampler for measurements of personal exposure to NO_2 and NO in ambient air. Environ Int 8:235-242

Susceptible Populations: Lessons from Controlled Exposure Studies of Inhaled Pollutants

M.J. UTELL

Departments of Medicine and Environmental Medicine, Pulmonary and Critical Care Unit, Univ. of Rochester Medical Center, 601 Elmwood Avenue, Rochester, NY 14642-8692, USA

Introduction

With the persistent concerns about adverse effects of polluted air on the lungs, a new emphasis is pervasive; the focus has shifted from the avoidance of clinical disease among highly exposed individuals toward the protection of the general population from an unacceptable burden of disease at much lower exposures, and an attempt to ensure that even the most susceptible persons are not adversely affected (Samet and Utell 1991). These concerns extend equally to other environmental exposures and to diseases other than those affecting the lungs. This shift in emphasis from higher exposures producing clinical disease to lower levels projected to increase population risks has raised difficult questions and challenges for research on environmental lung disease. In assessing risks from exposure to low-level environmental pollutants, the need to more thoroughly identify and characterize susceptible populations has assumed increasing importance.

The framework for determining health risks from environmental agents arises from three approaches: toxicological studies, epidemiological research, and controlled exposures of human volunteers. In the controlled clinical study, the investigators create laboratory atmospheric conditions which are considered relevant to ambient pollutant atmospheres, and document any health-related effects resulting from breathing the atmospheres (Utell 1988). Advantage is taken of the highly controlled environment to identify responses to individual pollutants and characterize exposure-response relations as well as to examine interactions among pollutants per se or with other environmental variables such as exercise, humidity, or temperature. In selecting populations of volunteers for a clinical study, consideration is given to the population at greatest risk: individuals with acute and chronic respiratory disease, the elderly, children, or individuals with coronary artery disease. This approach, however, also has limitations: for practical and ethical reasons, studies must be limited to small groups presumably representative of larger populations, to short durations of exposure, and to pollutant

U. Mohr et al. (Eds.)
Advances in Controlled Clinical
Inhalation Studies
© Springer-Verlag Berlin Heidelberg 1993

concentrations that are expected to produce only mild and reversible responses. Even in populations with chronic respiratory illnesses, it is never the individuals with the most severe disease that comprise the study group. Although inflammation (injury) induced by pollutants is being evaluated by nasal and bronchoalveolar lavage in clinical studies of healthy volunteers (Frampton et al. 1989), for the susceptible populations endpoint assessment has been limited to pulmonary mechanics.

It should be recognized that concern for the most sensitive or susceptible groups within the population drives the setting of air quality standards. This paper briefly reviews current knowledge about susceptible populations derived from clinical studies and discusses strategies for future research. Two recent publications review these areas in detail (Utell and Frank 1989; Brain et al. 1988).

Susceptible Populations

There are large numbers of compounds in the ambient air that at some concentration are highly toxic. The likelihood of an adverse response to an inhaled pollutant depends on the degree of exposure to the pollutant and individual characteristics of the exposed person that determine susceptibility. The concept of susceptibility is highly relevant to public health protection and to the delivery of health care. Human response to environmental agents that affect the respiratory system depend upon many factors, which include genetic differences in the way in which agents are metabolized, differences in target sites in the lung and airways, and in the defense mechanisms of the respiratory system. Also important are preexisting diseases, airways reactivity, age, gender, pregnancy, and nutritional status (Last 1989). Exposure to other agents such as cigarette smoke or combinations of environmental agents may also influence susceptibility to certain air pollutants. Cigarette smokers may prove to be the largest susceptible subpopulation when the interactive role of cigarette smoking and air pollution is taken into account.

The term "susceptible" has been most often applied to groups who share one or more characteristics that place them at increased risk compared to people without those characteristics (Table 1). The United States Clean Air Act mandated that the national ambient air quality standards for the criteria pollutants were to be set low enough to protect the health of all susceptible groups within the population. However, the Act does not require that every member of the subpopulation be protected; that is, it does not require protection of the most susceptible individual. For example, those requiring life-support systems, namely, patients in intensive care units and newborn infants in nurseries, are presumably excluded. In relating susceptible groups to the Clean Air Act, it is relevant to inquire as to whether the group size is in the thousands, hundreds of thousands, or

Table 1. Populations considered susceptible to air pollution

Population	Potential mechanism	Consequences
Infants	Immature defense mechanisms of the lung	Increased risk for respiratory infection
Elderly	Impaired respiratory defenses; reduced functional reserve	Increased risk for infection; increased risk for clinically significant effects on function
Asthmatics	Increased airways responsiveness	Increased risk for exacerbation of respiratory symptoms
Persons with COPD	Reduced level of lung function	Increased risk for clinically significant effects on function
Persons with IHD	Impaired myocardial oxygenation	Increased risk for myocardial ischemia
Cigarette smokers	Impaired defense and clearance; lung injury	Increased damage through synergism

COPD, Chronic obstructive pulmonary disease; IHD, ischemic heart disease.

millions. However, in addition to the number of individuals involved is the question of whether a distinctive biological trait can be identified in the hyperresponsive subpopulation. Are we looking at two distinct populations, normal individuals and a "discrete" susceptible group? Or, alternatively, does the subpopulation simply represent the tail of a continuous distribution of responses for a larger population? Understanding the distribution of responses is essential in the risk assessment process.

Measuring Responses in Susceptible Populations

For some pollutants susceptible individuals are distinguished by certain medical characteristics. Airways responsiveness exemplifies a characteristic influencing responses to inhaled materials. Asthmatics have increased airway reactivity in response to histamine, methacholine, or cold air challenge; the distributions of airway reactivity in asthmatics and nonasthmatics are distinct and only slightly overlapping (Cockcroft et al. 1983). Airways responsiveness reflects both genetic and environmental factors. In clinical studies, asthmatics exhibit exaggerated responses to sulfur dioxide, acidic aerosols, and perhaps nitrogen dioxide whereas individuals with chronic obstructive lung disease (COPD) may have increased responsiveness to NO_2.

In the laboratory, the most striking effect of acute exposure to SO_2 at concentrations less than or equal to 1.0 ppm is the induction of bronchoconstriction in asthmatics after exposures lasting only 5 min (Sheppard et al. 1981). In contrast, inhalations of concentrations in excess of 5.0 ppm causes only small decrements in airway function in normal subjects. Similarly, clinical studies have identified exercising adolescent asthmatics (Koenig et al. 1988) and adult asthmatics (Morrow et al. in press) as susceptible to sulfuric acid aerosols at high ambient concentrations, levels which do not affect healthy volunteers. Although several controlled human studies have found asthmatics responsive to low levels of NO_2, the findings have not been consistent (Samet and Utell 1990). The conflicting results among these several studies are probably related to differences in subject selection and exposure protocols.

Effects of inhaled pollutants in COPD have not been extensively examined. To determine whether low-level NO_2 induces changes in pulmonary function, we investigated responses to inhalation of 0.3 ppm NO_2 for 4 h in 20 COPD subjects, all with a history of cigarette smoking, and with a mean age of 60 years and 20 elderly normals of comparable age (Morrow et al. 1992). Criteria for inclusion included dyspnea on exertion, obstructive airways disease ($FEV_1/FVC = 0.58 \pm 0.09$ (SD)), and a lack of response to inhaled bronchodilators. During intermittent light exercise, COPD subjects demonstrated progressive decrements in forced vital capacity (FVC) and FVC in 1s (FEV_1) compared to baseline with NO_2 but not with Air (Fig. 1). Subgroup analyses suggested that responsiveness to NO_2 decreased with severity of COPD. In the cohort of elderly normals, NO_2-induced reduction in FEV_1 was greater among smokers than non-smokers. A comparison of COPD and elderly normal subjects also revealed distinctions in NO_2-induced responsiveness; no changes in lung function were observed in the elderly normal group.

Low-level exposures to carbon monoxide have focused on subpopulations with ischemic heart disease and peripheral vascular disease. In patients with exertional angina, earlier onset of angina pectoris and ST segment depression have been consistently observed at carboxyhemoglobin (COHb) levels of 2%–4% by several investigative teams. In the largest of these studies, the Health Effects Institute multicenter CO study, 5% and 12% decreases in the time to onset of ST segment depression were observed at COHb levels of 2% and 4%, respectively (Allred et al. 1989). Significant decreases in time to onset of angina were also demonstrated at these respective COHb levels. The objective EKG endpoint and subjective endpoint of chest pain yielded consistent results and are compatible with the hypothesis that an elevated COHb level impairs the response of the myocardium to increased metabolic demands.

For other pollutants, such as ozone, the individual exhibiting exaggerated alterations in pulmonary function following exposure do not share any identifiable physiological or pathological characteristics, at least as can be ascertained with the methods presently available. An obvious need is to identify factors that may contribute to susceptibility to ozone. In the final sections of this paper, several recent approaches to identify markers linked with ozone sensitivity in animal and clinical studies are examined.

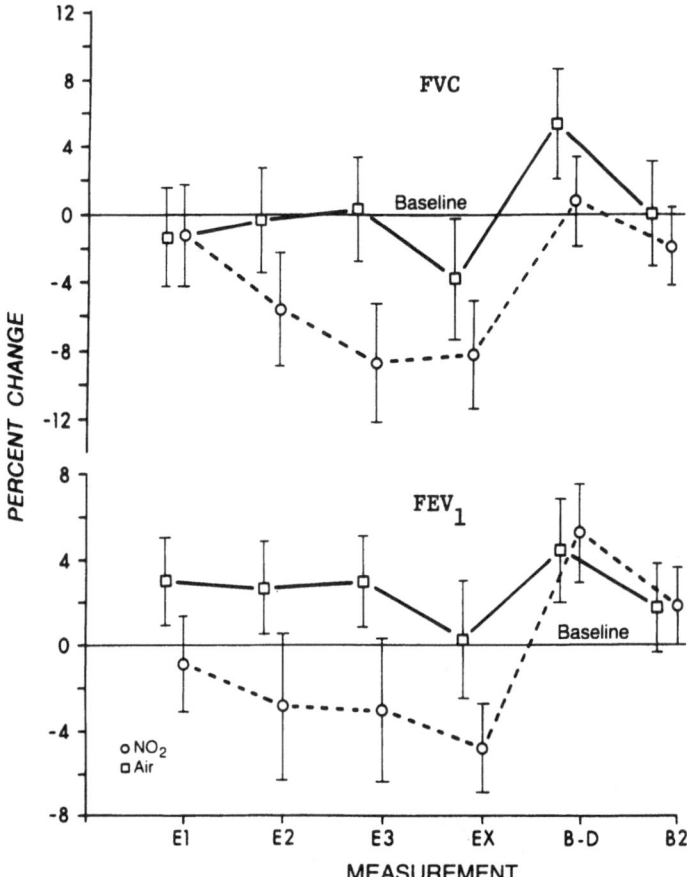

Fig. 1. Percentage change in FVC (*above*) and FEV_1 (*below*) between baseline measurements and measurements during NO_2 and air exposures for 20 subjects with COPD. *E1–E3*, exercise measurements; *EX*, final measurement at 4h; *B–D*, response to inhaled bronchodilator; *B2*, baseline 24-h after exposure. By crossover *t* test, the COPD group showed significant reductions ($p < 0.05$) in FVC at E3 and EX and in FEV_1 at EX, during NO_2 exposure but not in air. Data are mean ± SEM

Responsiveness to Ozone and Susceptible Populations

It is surprising that controlled clinical studies have yet to demonstrate that ozone dramatically affects lung function in asthmatic subjects, atopic non-asthmatic subjects, or individuals with COPD (Bromberg 1988). Several possible explanations exist. In contrast to studies with healthy volunteers, studies of asthmatic subjects have not been performed using many-hour exposures or repeated daily exposures. Furthermore, few studies with asthmatic subjects have incorporated multiple periods of exercise, an essential factor in provoking changes in airway function with low-level ozone exposure in healthy volunteers. Thus, the issue of ozone sensitivity will not be resolved until populations of normal and asthmatic subjects are compared using protocols of similar design.

However, several recent clinical studies provide some evidence that asthmatics may ultimately prove to be hyperresponsive to ozone. Aris and coworkers (1991) have observed a relationship between baseline airway hyperreactivity to methacholine and responsiveness to ozone, a finding of considerable interest but not in agreement with earlier studies. Their observations suggested that airway hyperresponsiveness may be a risk factor for ozone sensitivity even among healthy, asymptomatic athletes. Using an imaginative approach to study environmental interactions, Molfino et al. (1991) investigated whether inhalation of 0.12 ppm ozone for 1 h potentiates the airway allergic response in asthmatics with seasonal symptoms. Although ozone did not significantly alter baseline function, reactivity to inhaled allergen was significantly enhanced by prior ozone inhalation. Ozone has been shown to increase airway permeability using a variety of markers; it is conceivable that prior ozone exposure increased access of allergen to subepithelial mediator secreting cells.

The findings of Molfino et al. (1991) emphasize the potential for interactions between ozone and other relevant environmental pollutants. In our laboratory we are completing studies to determine whether prior exposure to low-level sulfuric acid sensitizes human airways to ozone (Frampton et al. 1992). Exposure-response relationships are examined using three levels of ozone ranging from below the current United States standard to 1.5 times the ambient air quality standard (0.08, 0.12, and 0.18 ppm ozone) with preexposure 24 h earlier to $100 \mu g/m^3$ H_2SO_4 or sodium chloride (NaCl) aerosol. The acidic aerosol and oxidant exposures are for 3 h; each subject is exposed to two of the three ozone concentrations using an incomplete block design. Since the study design includes exposure of 30 healthy and 30 asthmatic volunteers, the analyses will permit comparisons of responsiveness between the two groups as well as potentiation of the ozone response by prior particle exposure. The results should extend our understanding of ozone responses in asthmatics.

Finally, it is well recognized that clinical studies report a wide range of individual responses among subjects exposed to the same concentration of ozone (McDonnell et al. 1983). Despite the wide range of responses, individual responses are found to be highly reproducible, suggesting that there are determinants of susceptibility; to date, the nature of these determinants is unknown. One of the potentially most important effects of exposure to ozone is distal airway inflammation, a response which also shows considerable variability between subjects. Studies have been initiated to determine whether decrements in FEV_1 and lower airway inflammatory events are related. If these events are correlated, strong responders may represent a distinct susceptible subpopulation with identifiable characteristics rather than the "tail" of the population in a bell-shaped distribution.

Conclusions

Much attention has been given recently to identifying risk factors that predispose persons to the potentially harmful effects of pollutant gases and particles found in the environment. Human research has focused on identifying sensitivity, pollutant by pollutant; in this role, the clinical study has made significant contributions. To further determine the responsiveness of these sensitive groups, emphasis needs to be placed on more intensively mimicking natural exposures. Protocols to examine realistic mixtures, either in combination or sequence, and to study repeated exposures over multiple days are needed. Furthermore, efforts to relate the study polulation to the general population are warranted.

At the most fundamental levels of research, there is interest in determining the mechanisms for specific forms of sensitivity. The recent report by Kleeberger et al. (1990) of a genetic model for evaluating susceptibility to ozone-induced inflammation is exciting. The airways inflammatory response to ozone of inbred mice and their progeny was assessed. Known susceptible and resistant strains were crossed to produce F1 progeny, and then back-crossed with parent strains and litter mates to produce F2 progeny. Inflammatory indices of lavagable neutrophils and proteins were followed. The ratios of susceptible and resistant phenotypes in the segregating generations were consistent with a single-locus autosomal recessive inheritance. This unique model for investigating ozone susceptibility may have immediate extensions into the clinical arena. For example, a genetic contribution to the marked variability in ozone responsiveness could be addressed in family studies of twins and siblings. As with the mouse model, inheritable traits may be linked with responsiveness to ozone. Although it is unlikely that the relative contributions of heredity versus environment can be determined, the interaction of both factors would be established.

There is a growing awareness among the public, scientists, and regulators that individuals vary in their susceptibility and that the differences must be measured and translated into environmental and occupational policy. In addressing these needs, clinical studies will require special attention to experimental design for quantifying variations in susceptibility and improved statistical methods in data analyses. Ultimately, this will lead to more rational regulation and improved protection of the public.

Acknowledgements. Supported in part by grant no. RO1 ESO2679 from the National Institutes of Health, by grant no. RR0004 from the Division of Research Resources, by contract no. 88-8 from the Health Effects Institute, and by contract no. RP3009-1 from the Electric Power Research Institute.

References

Allred EN, Bleecker ER, Chaitman BR, Dahms TE, Gottlieb SO, Hackney JD, Pagano M, Selvester RH, Walden SM, Warren J (1989) Short-term effects of carbon monoxide exposure on the exercise performance of subjects with coronary artery disease. N Eng J Med 321:1426–1432

Aris R, Christian C, Sheppard D, Balmes JR (1991) The effects of sequential exposure to acidic fog and ozone on pulmonary function in exercising subjects. Am Rev Respir Dis 143:85–91

Brain JD, Beck BD, Warren AJ, Shaikh R (eds) (1989) Variations in susceptibility to inhaled pollutants – identification, mechanism, and policy implications. The Johns Hopkins Press, Baltimore

Bromberg PA (1988) Asthma and automotive emissions. In: Watson AY, Bates RR, Kennedy D (eds) Air pollution, the automobile, and public health. National Academy Press, Washington, DC, pp 465–498

Cockcroft DW, Berscheid BA, Murdock KY (1983) Unimodal distribution of bronchial responsiveness to inhaled histamine in a random human population. Chest 83:751–754

Frampton MW, Finkelstein JN, Roberts NJ Jr, Smeglin AM, Morrow PE, Utell MJ (1989) Effects of nitrogen dioxide exposure on bronchoalveolar lavage proteins in humans. Am J Respir Cell Mol Biol 1:499–505

Frampton MW, Morrow PE, Cox C, Levy PC, Speers DM, Gibb FR, Condemi JJ, Utell MJ (1992) Does pre-exposure to acidic aerosols alter airway responses to ozone in humans? Am Rev Respir Dis 145:A428

Kleeberger SR, Bassett DJP, Jakab GJ, Levitt RC (1990) A genetic model for evaluation of susceptibility to ozone-induced inflammation. Am J Physiol 258:L313–L320

Koenig JQ, Covert DS, Pierson WE (1989) Effects of inhalation of acidic compounds on pulmonary function in allergic adolescent subjects. Environ Health Perspect 79:173–178

Last JA (1989) Nutritional status and oxidants. In: Utell MJ, Frank R (eds) Susceptibility to inhaled pollutants. ASTM STP 1024, American Society for Testing and Materials, Philadelphia, pp 162–173

McDonnell WF, Horstman DH, Hazucha MH, Seal E, Haak ED, Abdul-Salaam S, House DE (1983) Pulmonary effects of ozone exposure during exercise: dose-response characteristics. J Appl Physiol: Respir Environ Exercise Physiol 54:1345–1352

Molfino NA, Wright SC, Katz I, Tarlo S, Silverman F, McClean PA, Szalai JP, Raizenne M, Slutsky AS, Zamel N (1991) Effect of low concentration of ozone on inhaled allergen responses in asthmatic subjects. Lancet 338:199–203

Morrow PE, Utell MJ, Bauer MA, Smeglin AM, Frampton MW, Cox C, Speers DM, Gibb FR (1992) Pulmonary performance of elderly normals and subjects with chronic obstructive pulmonary disease exposed to 0.3 ppm nitrogen dioxide. Am Rev Respir Dis 145:291–300

Morrow PE, Utell MJ, Bauer MA, Speers DM, Gibb FR (1993) Effects of near ambient levels of sulfuric acid aerosol on lung function in exercising subjects with asthma and COPD. Ann Occup Hyg (in press)

Samet JM, Utell MJ (1991) The environment and the lung. JAMA 266:670–675

Samet JM, Utell MJ (1990) The risk of nitrogen dioxide: what have we learned from epidemiological and clinical studies? Toxicol Industrial Health 6:247–262

Sheppard D, Saisho A, Nadel JA, Boushey HA (1981) Exercise increases sulfur dioxide-induced bronchoconstriction. Am Rev Respir Dis 123:486–491

Utell MJ (1988) Human clinical exposure studies: body box or Pandora's box. In: Mohr U (ed) Inhalation toxicology: the design and interpretation of inhalation studies and their use in risk assessment. Springer, Berlin Heidelberg New York, pp 273–286

Utell MJ, Frank R (eds) (1989) Susceptibility to inhaled pollutants. ASTM STP 1024, American Society for Testing and Materials, Philadelphia

Inhalation of Pollutants and Pollutant Mixtures in Subjects with Bronchial Hyperresponsiveness

H. Magnussen and R. Jörres

Krankenhaus Großhansdorf, Zentrum für Pneumologie und Thoraxchirurgie, Wöhrendamm 80, W-2070 Großhansdorf, FRG

Airway Hyperresponsiveness

Subjects with asthma are supposed to represent the segment of our population which is most sensitive to the potential harmful effects of air pollution. One of the characteristic features of asthma is airway hyperresponsiveness, which is phenomenologically defined as an abnormally high responsiveness to unspecific test stimuli like histamine and methacholine. The underlying cellular and biochemical processes are currently under intensive investigation (e.g., Djukanovic et al. 1990). In accordance with that, in recent times the experimental investigation of the effects of air pollutants on human subjects has utilized the analysis of cellular processes in the airways, especially by performing bronchoalveolar lavage.

Air Pollutants

Sulfur Dioxide

The airway response to low concentrations of SO_2 has been studied by numerous authors in healthy subjects and in patients with bronchial asthma. It is known that in healthy subjects inhalation of SO_2 in concentrations up to 3 ppm during acute exposure and during tidal breathing does not cause airway obstruction (Sheppard et al. 1980). In patients with asthma, short-term inhalation of 0.5 ppm SO_2 or less may elicit bronchoconstriction only at increased ventilation rates (Sheppard et al. 1981). Due to the high absorption of SO_2, the rate of ventilation and the route of inhalation are essential in determining the bronchoconstrictive effect (Bethel et al. 1983). Tolerance to repeated exposures of SO_2 has been observed (Sheppard et al. 1983) but no change of airway responsiveness to methacholine after inhaling SO_2 (Hazucha et al. 1984). The degree of intrinsic bronchial responsiveness to SO_2 does not correlate to the airway responsiveness to histamine (Magnussen

U. Mohr et al. (Eds.)
Advances in Controlled Clinical
Inhalation Studies
© Springer-Verlag Berlin Heidelberg 1993

et al. 1990) or methacholine (Horstman et al. 1986). Evaluation of the bronchoalveolar lavage fluid after exposure to SO_2 of normal subjects revealed induction of an inflammatory response, with an increase in the numbers of lymphocytes and mast cells (Sandström et al. 1989).

Nitrogen Dioxide

Several investigations have demonstrated that short-term exposure to low concentrations of NO_2 (0.1–0.5 ppm) may enhance airway responsiveness to histamine (Bylin et al. 1988), methacholine or carbachol (Orehek et al. 1976; Kleinman et al. 1983; Ahmed et al. 1982; Mohsenin 1987), exercise, and hyperventilation of cold air (Bauer et al. 1986) in asthmatic subjects. These findings could not, however, be confirmed by others (Hazucha et al. 1983; Jörres and Magnussen 1991). The type of cellular and biochemical effects of NO_2 on the lung has been investigated mainly in normal subjects. At concentrations of 4 ppm significant increases in the numbers of lymphocytes and mast cells were found in the bronchoalveolar lavage fluid up to 24 h after exposure (Sandström et al. 1990). A decrease in the activity of α_1-protease inhibitor has been found at concentrations of 3–4 ppm NO_2 (Mohsenin and Gee 1987) but not at lower concentrations up to 1.5 ppm (Johnson et al. 1990). However, the level of the antiprotease α_2-macroglobulin in the bronchoalveolar lavage fluid was changed after exposure to 0.6 ppm NO_2 (Frampton et al. 1989).

Ozone

In the past decade a large amount of data has been published about the effects of O_3 on pulmonary function. The general outcome is that exposure produces significant airway obstruction and increases in bronchial responsiveness in O_3-sensitive subjects. In healthy, nonhyperresponsive subjects, inhalation of O_3 may induce bronchial hyperresponsiveness (Golden et al. 1978; Seltzer et al. 1986). During prolonged exposure and moderate to heavy exercise, even concentrations as low as 0.08 ppm O_3 produced significant airway obstruction and significant increases of nonspecific airway responsiveness (Horstman et al. 1990). During shorter exposures, the threshold concentration in healthy human subjects lies between 0.2 and 0.4 ppm O_3 (Dimeo et al. 1981). Adaption to repeated inhalation of O_3 has been described, which was shortest for the most sensitive subjects (Horvath et al. 1981). This adaptation, however, may be of little importance in a public health sense, since it is commonly lost within a 7-day interval (Linn et al. 1982).

Despite the large intersubject variability which can be derived from all the published data, the individual airway response to O_3 is well reproducible

(McDonnell et al. 1985). Thus, the observed variability seems to be based on differences in the individual intrinsic responsiveness to O_3. Sensitivity to O_3 seems not to require airway hyperresponsiveness as one of its prerequisites. Nevertheless, even in normal subjects, those with higher unspecific airway responsiveness are more likely to be adversely affected by inhaling O_3 than those with lower responsiveness. Kreit et al. (1989) found that patients with asthma showed greater airway obstruction than normal subjects after inhaling 0.4 ppm O_3. Also, in the subjects investigated by Aris et al. (1991), a correspondence between the sensitivity to O_3 and the airway responsiveness to methacholine was found. The response to O_3 depends on ventilation, exposure duration, and concentration, with concentration being more influential than ventilation (Hazucha 1987) and duration (Horstman et al. 1990).

The functional impairment after breathing O_3 is attributed to a restriction of inspired volume, possibly due to a reflex inhibition of a maximal inspiratory effort (Horstman et al. 1990). The increase of bronchial responsiveness is coupled to an influx of inflammatory cells, e.g., polymorphonuclear leukocytes, changes of the levels of some cyclooxygenase metabolites of arachidonic acid, and an increase of soluble factors capable of producing damage in the lower airways. These variables have been determined from the bronchoalveolar lavage fluid (Seltzer et al. 1986; Koren et al. 1989). Few experimental data exist on the possible effect of O_3 on the allergic state of the human airways. Bascom et al. (1990) performed nasal challenges with antigen after exposure to 0.5 ppm O_3 and found no alteration of the acute response to antigen. Despite some evidence that the integrity of the cellular immune system may be altered by O_3 (e.g., T lymphocytes), no adverse effect of the inhalation of O_3 on the immune response to an experimentally induced rhinovirus infection could be found (Henderson et al. 1988).

Aerosols

Most investigations have shown that short-term exposure to sulfuric acid or sulfate aerosols did not cause airway obstruction in normal subjects at concentrations up to 1 mg/m^3 (Sackner et al. 1978). Adverse effects in asthmatic subjects could be demonstrated at concentrations of 0.1 mg/m^3 (Koenig et al. 1983) or higher (Utell et al. 1983b), whereas others did not find significant effects (Avol et al. 1990). Inhalation of sulfuric acid aerosols at a concentration of 0.45 mg/m^3 may produce latent development of airway hyperreactivity to carbachol in normal subjects (Utell et al. 1983a). In patients with asthma, the specific reactivity to inhalation of sulfuric acid correlates well with the subjects unspecific airway reactivity to carbachol (Utell et al. 1983b). The effect of acid aerosols may be mediated not only by their pH value but also by their titratable acidity and the specific chemical composition (Fine et al. 1987). Short-term exposure to nitrate aerosols at a concentration of $7 \, mg/m^3$ has been found not to alter significantly pulmonary function in normal and mildly asthmatic subjects (Utell et al. 1979). However, during acute respiratory disease, previously healthy subjects may exhibit airway obstruction after inhalation of nitrates at these concentrations (Utell et al. 1980).

Mixtures of Pollutants

Nitrogen Dioxide and Sulfur Dioxide

Very few studies have addressed the issue of interactions between NO_2 and the response to SO_2 in asthmatic subjects. It has been shown that inhalation of 0.25 ppm NO_2 for 30 min increases the responsiveness to subsequent hyperventilation of 0.75 ppm SO_2 in nonsmoking (Jörres and Magnussen 1990) but not in smoking subjects. When producing dose-response curves with increasing concentrations of SO_2 after breathing 0.3 ppm NO_2 for 30 min, no NO_2-induced shift was noted (Rubinstein et al. 1990). Breathing 0.3 ppm SO_2 and 0.5 ppm NO_2 simultaneously for 2 h during intermittent exercise did not exert significant effects on lung function parameters (Linn et al. 1980). There may be a small effect of NO_2 on the response to SO_2; however, this effect is probably not specific to SO_2 but due to enhancement of the hyperventilation response. This hypothesis would be in accordance with the results of Bauer et al. (1986).

Sulfur Dioxide and Aerosols

In order to mimic the simultaneous occurrence of SO_2 in the community air together with hygroscopic aerosols, Koenig and coworkers (1981) tested asthmatic adolescents by exposing them to 1 ppm SO_2 plus $1 \, mg/m^3$ sodium chloride aerosol. Significant airway obstruction was measured. However, this effect was not compared with inhalation of SO_2 alone. When investigating nonasthmatic subjects (Koenig et al. 1982), no difference in the response between exposure to SO_2 alone and SO_2 plus sodium chloride aerosol was found. After repeatedly inhaling aerosols of either saline, ammonium sulfate, or sulfuric acid, patients with bronchial asthma did not show significant changes of their bronchial response to subsequent inhalation of SO_2 (Jörres et al. 1990).

Ozone and Nitrogen Dioxide or Nitric Acid Fog

Only data on healthy subjects are available. During exercise, the presence of 0.6 ppm NO_2 did not evoke additive effects beyond those induced by

0.3 ppm O_3 (Adams et al. 1987). The effect of combining both pollutants at low concentrations (0.15 ppm) on lung function, if present, may be very weak (Kagawa 1983). Possibly, there is also a weak interaction between inhalation of peroxyacetyl nitrate (PAN) and O_3 with respect to its effect on pulmonary function (Drechsler-Parks et al. 1984). Pre-exposure to fog containing nitric acid did not potentiate, rather possibly attenuated, the airway response to O_3 during exercise (Aris et al. 1991).

Ozone and Sulfur Dioxide or Sulfate Aerosols

Most studies done in healthy subjects do not indicate the presence of a significant O_3-SO_2 interaction. In presence of O_3, the response to SO_2 has even found to be slightly decreased (Folinsbee et al. 1985). Pre-exposure to 0.3 ppm O_3 did not cause airway reaction to subsequent inhalation of 0.1 mg/m^3 sulfuric acid aerosol (Kulle et al. 1982). On the other hand, combined exposure to 0.37 ppm O_3, 0.37 ppm SO_2, and 0.1 mg/m^3 sulfuric acid aerosol has been reported to induce significant reductions in pulmonary function (Kleinman et al. 1981). Few data are available in patients with asthma. Recently, Koenig and coworkers (1990) demonstrated that asthmatic subjects developed a significant reaction to 0.1 ppm SO_2 during exercise after inhaling 0.12 ppm O_3. The same concentration of SO_2 did not cause airway obstruction without prior breathing of O_3 in these patients. Thus, these data support the hypothesis of a sensitizing effect of O_3 on the response to SO_2 in patients with asthma. This effect, however, may be only a manifestation of the general increase of unspecific airway responsiveness induced by inhaling O_3.

Acknowledgement. Financial support for this research was provided by the Bundesministerium für Forschung und Technologie, FRG.

References

Adams WC, Brookes KA, Schelegle ES (1987) Effects of NO_2 alone and in combination with O_3 on young men and women. J Appl Physiol 62:1698-1704
Ahmed T, Marchette B, Danta I et al. (1982) Effect of 0.1 ppm NO_2 on bronchial reactivity in normals and subjects with bronchial asthma (abstract). Am Rev Respir Dis 125 [Suppl 2]:152
Aris R, Christian D, Sheppard D, Balmes JR (1991) The effects of sequential exposure to acidic fog and ozone on pulmonary function in exercising subjects. Am Rev Respir Dis 143:85-91
Avol EL, Linn WS, Shamoo DA et al. (1990) Respiratory responses of young asthmatic volunteers in controlled exposures to sulfuric acid aerosol. Am Rev Respir Dis 142:343-348
Bascom R, Naclerio RM, Fitzgerald TK, Kagey-Sobotka A, Proud D (1990) Effect of ozone inhalation on the response to nasal challenge with antigen of allergic subjects. Am Rev Respir Dis 142:594-601

Bauer MA, Utell MJ, Morrow PE, Speers DM, Gibb FR (1986) Inhalation of 0.30 ppm nitrogen dioxide potentiates exercise-induced bronchospasm in asthmatics. Am Rev Respir Dis 134:1203–1208

Bethel RA, Erle DJ, Epstein J et al. (1983) Effect of exercise rate and route of inhalation on sulfur-dioxide-induced bronchoconstriction in asthmatic subjects. Am Rev Respir Dis 128:592–596

Bylin G, Hedenstierna G, Lindvall T, Sundin B (1988) Ambient nitrogen dioxide concentrations increase bronchial responsiveness in subjects with mild asthma. Eur Respir J 1:606–612

Dimeo MJ, Glenn MG, Holtzman MJ et al. (1981) Threshold concentration of ozone causing an increase in bronchial reactivity in humans and adaptation with repeated exposures. Am Rev Respir Dis 124:245–248

Djukanovic R, Roche WR, Wilson JW et al. (1990) Mucosal inflammation in asthma: state of the art. Am Rev Respir Dis 142:434–457

Drechsler-Parks DM, Bedi JF, Horvath SM (1984) Interaction of peroxyacetyl nitrate and ozone on pulmonary functions. Am Rev Respir Dis 130:1033–1037

Fine JM, Gordon T, Thompson JE, Sheppard D (1987) The role of titratable acidity in acid aerosol-induced bronchoconstriction. Am Rev Respir Dis 135:826–830

Folinsbee LJ, Bedi JF, Horvath SM (1985) Pulmonary response to threshold levels of sulfur dioxide (1.0 ppm) and ozone (0.3 ppm). J Appl Physiol 58:1783–1787

Frampton MW, Finkelstein JN, Roberts NJ Jr, Morrow PE, Utell MJ (1989) Effects of nitrogen dioxide exposure on bronchoalveolar lavage proteins in humans. Am J Respir Cell Mol Biol 1:499–505

Golden JA, Nadel JA, Boushey HA (1978) Bronchial hyperirritability in healthy subjects after exposure to ozone. Am Rev Respir Dis 118:287–294

Hazucha MJ (1987) Relationship between ozone exposure and pulmonary function changes. J Appl Physiol 62:1671–1680

Hazucha MJ, Ginsberg JF, McDonnell WF et al. (1983) Effects of 0.1 ppm nitrogen dioxide on airways of normal and asthmatic subjects. J Appl Physiol 54:730–739

Hazucha MJ, Kehrl HR, Roger LJ, Horstman DH (1984) Airway responsiveness to methacholine of asthmatics exposed to 0.25, 0.5 and 1.0 ppm SO$_2$. Am Rev Respir Dis 129 [Suppl 2]:A145 (abstr)

Henderson FW, Dubovi EJ, Harder S, Elston S Jr, Graham D (1988) Experimental rhinovirus infection in human volunteers exposed to ozone. Am Rev Respir Dis 137:11248–1128

Horstman DH, Roger LJ, Kehrl H, Hazucha M (1986) Airway sensitivity of asthmatics to sulfur dioxide. Toxicol Environ Health 2:289–298

Horstman DH, Folinsbee LJ, Ives PJ, Abdul-Salaam S, McDonnell WF (1990) Ozone concentration and pulmonary response relationships for 6.6-hour exposures with five hours of moderate exercise to 0.08, 0.10, and 0.12 ppm. Am Rev Respir Dis 142:1158–1163

Horvath SM, Gliner JA, Folinsbee LJ (1981) Adaptation to ozone: duration of effect. Am Rev Respir Dis 123:496–499

Johnson DA, Frampton MW, Winters RS, Morrow PE, Utell MJ (1990) Inhalation of nitrogen dioxide fails to reduce the activity of human lung alpha-1-proteinase inhibitor. Am Rev Respir Dis 142:758-762

Jörres R, Magnussen H (1990) Airways response of asthmatics after a 30 min exposure, at resting ventilation, to 0.25 ppm NO$_2$ or 0.5 ppm SO$_2$. Eur Respir J 3:132–137

Jörres R, Magnussen H (1991) Effect of 0.25 ppm nitrogen dioxide on the airway response to methacholine in asymptomatic asthmatic patients. Lung 169: 77–85

Jörres R, Boerger S, Templin K, Magnussen H (1990) Effect of short-term inhalation of sulphate aerosols on lung function and response to SO$_2$ in patients with asthma. Eur Respir J 3 [Suppl 10]:172s (abstr)

Kagawa J (1983) Respiratory effects of two-hour exposure with intermittent exercise to ozone, sulfur dioxide and nitrogen dioxide alone and in combination in normal subjects. Am Ind Hyg Assoc J 44:14–20

Kleinman MT, Bailey RM, Chang YTC et al. (1981) Exposures of human volunteers to a controlled atmospheric mixture of ozone, sulfur dioxide and sulfuric acid. Am Ind Hyg Assoc J 42:61–69

Kleinman MT, Baily RM, Linn WS et al. (1983) Effect of 0.2 ppm nitrogen dioxide on pulmonary function and response to bronchoprovocation in asthmatics. J Toxicol Environ Health 12:815–826

Koenig JQ, Pierson WE, Horike M, Frank R (1981) Effects of SO_2 plus NaCl aerosol combined with moderate exercise on pulmonary function in asthmatic adolescents. Environ Res 25:340–348

Koenig JQ, Pierson WE, Horike M, Frank R (1982) Bronchoconstrictor responses to sulfur dioxide or sulfur dioxide plus sodium chloride droplets in allergic, nonasthmatic adolescents. J Allergy Clin Immunol 69:339–344

Koenig JQ, Pierson WE, Horike M (1983) The effects of inhaled sulfuric acid on pulmonary function in adolescent asthmatics. Am Rev Respir Dis 128:221–225

Koenig JQ, Covert DS, Hanley QS, Van Belle G, Pierson WE (1990) Prior exposure to ozone potentiates subsequent response to sulfur dioxide in adolescent asthmatic subjects. Am Rev Respir Dis 141:377–380

Koren HS, Devlin RB, Graham DE et al. (1989) Ozone-induced inflammation in the lower airways of human subjects. Am Rev Respir Dis 139:407–415

Kreit JW, Gross KB, Moore TB et al. (1989) Ozone-induced changes in pulmonary function and bronchial responsiveness in asthmatics. J Appl Physiol 66:217–222

Kulle TJ, Kerr HD, Farrell BP, Sauder LR, Bermel MS (1982) Pulmonary function and bronchial reactivity in human subjects with exposure to ozone and respirable sulfuric acid aerosol. Am Rev Respir Dis 126:996–1000

Linn WS, Jones MP, Bailey RM et al. (1980) Respiratory effects of mixed nitrogen dioxide and sulfur dioxide in human volunteers under simulated ambient exposure conditions. Environ Health 22:431–438

Linn WS, Medway DA, Anzar UT et al. (1982) Persistence of adaptation to ozone in volunteers exposed repeatedly for six weeks. Am Rev Respir Dis 125:491–495

Magnussen H, Jörres R, Wagner HM, von Nieding G (1990) Relationship between the airway response to inhaled sulfur dioxide, isocapnic hyperventilation, and histamine in asthmatic subjects. Int Arch Occup Environ Health 62:485–491

McDonnell III WF, Horstman DH, Abdul-Salaam S, House DE (1985) Reproducibility of individual responses to ozone exposure. Am Rev Respir Dis 131:36–40

Mohsenin V (1987) Airway responses to nitrogen dioxide in asthmatic subjects. J Toxicol Environ Health 22:371–380

Mohsenin V, Gee JBL (1987) Acute effect of nitrogen dioxide exposure on the functional activity of alpha-1-protease inhibitor in bronchoalveolar lavage fluid of normal subjects. Am Rev Respir Dis 136:646–650

Orehek J, Massari JP, Gayrard P, Grimaud C, Charpin J (1976) Effect of short-term, low-level nitrogen dioxide exposure on bronchial sensitivity of asthmatic patients. J Clin Invest 57:301–307

Rubinstein I, Bigby BG, Reiss TF, Boushey HA Jr (1990) Short-term exposure to 0.3 ppm nitrogen dioxide does not potentiate airway responsiveness to sulfur dioxide in asthmatic subjects. Am Rev Respir Dis 141:381–385

Sackner MA, Ford D, Fernandez R et al. (1978) Effects of sulfuric acid aerosols on cardiopulmonary function of dogs, sheep, and humans. Am Rev Respir Dis 118:497–510

Sandström T, Stjernberg N, Andersson MC, Kolmodin-Hedman B, Lindström K, Rosenhall L (1989) Cell response in bronchoalveolar lavage fluid after sulfur dioxide exposure. Scand J Work Environ Health 15:142–146

Sandström T, Andersson MC, Kolmodin-Hedman B, Stjernberg N, Ångström T (1990) Bronchoalveolar mastocytosis and lymphocytosis after nitrogen dioxide exposure in man: a time-kinetic study. Eur Respir J 3:138–143

Seltzer J, Bigby BG, Stulbarg M et al. (1986) O_3-induced change in bronchial reactivity to methacholine and airway inflammation in humans. J Appl Physiol 60:1321–1326

Sheppard D, Wong WS, Uehara CF, Nadel JA, Boushey HA (1980) Lower threshold and greater bronchomotor responsiveness of asthmatic subjects to sulfur dioxide. Am Rev Respir Dis 122:873–878

Sheppard D, Saisho A, Nadel JA, Boushey HA (1981) Exercise increases sulfur dioxide-induced bronchoconstriction in asthmatic subjects. Am Rev Respir Dis 123:486–491

Sheppard D, Epstein J, Bethel RA, Nadel JA, Boushey HA (1983) Tolerance to sulfur dioxide-induced bronchoconstriction in subjects with asthma. Environ Res 30:412–419

Utell MJ, Swinburne AJ, Hyde RW et al. (1979) Airway reactivity to nitrates in normal and mild asthmatic subjects. J Appl Physiol 46:189–196

Utell MJ, Aquilina AT, Hall WJ et al. (1980) Development of airway reactivity to nitrates in subjects with influenza. Am Rev Respir Dis 121:233–241

Utell MJ, Morrow PE, Hyde RW (1983a) Latent development of airway hyperreactivity in human subjects after sulfuric acid aerosol exposure. J Aerosol Sci 14:202–205

Utell MJ, Morrow PE, Speers DM, Darling J, Hyde RW (1983b) Airway responsiveness to sulfate and sulfuric acid aerosols in asthmatics. Am Rev Respir Dis 128:444–450

Section 5. New Methodologies

Controlled Clinical Inhalation Studies with Environmental Air Pollutants at Concentrations Commonly Found in the Ambient Air

T.O.F. Wagner, W.H.T. Schürmann, and H. Fabel

Medizinische Hochschule Hannover, Abteilung Pneumologie, Konstanty-Gutschow-Straße 8, W-3000 Hannover 61, FRG

Introduction

People are becoming increasingly aware of environmental health hazards. Air pollutants have long been at the center of interest for both the public and the scientific community. Scientific interest has concentrated mainly on acute effects of high concentrations of pollutants. This has led to relatively strict governmental regulations and, for example, maximum allowable workplace concentrations, on the one hand, and decreasing mean and peak concentrations of some of the classical pollutants such as sulfur dioxide and nitrogen dioxide, on the other (von Boehmer and Fabel 1987). This must not lead to neglect of the specific problems arising from chronic exposure to the same pollutants or the health hazard of low concentrations for groups of patients at high risk. As long as we and our volunteers or patients do not live in an ideal ("synthetic" = well-defined) atmosphere, all studies must consider the fact that only rough approximations of effects can be obtained and must be seen against the background of the atmosphere and the ambient pollutant load at the facility where the studies are performed. Nevertheless, our knowledge of the health effects of pollutants at concentrations commonly found in the ambient air is insufficient, and particularly the effects of such pollutants on the respiratory or other body functions of patients with lung or other diseases must be studied. This is true not only from the aspect of prophylaxis and prevention of disease caused by chronic exposure to pollutants but also to help in early detection of symptoms indicative of deterioration of lung or other functions due to pollutants and to provide patients with the information of the specific risks that air pollutants carry for their body.

For example, patients with chronic obstructive lung disease or with bronchial asthma seem likely to have an increased risk of suffering from pollutants, even at concentrations commonly found in the air which would not obviously cause symptoms in man without prior damage to the lung. It is

U. Mohr et al. (Eds.)
Advances in Controlled Clinical
Inhalation Studies
© Springer-Verlag Berlin Heidelberg 1993

not necessarily true that the effects observed at high concentrations over short periods of time can be extrapolated to low concentrations over long periods of time. We therefore consider controlled clinical inhalation studies with environmental air pollutants at concentrations commonly found in the ambient air to be not only important but also indispensible, and we describe clinical, ethical, and methodological considerations for obtaining the most information from such exposures.

Clinical Aspects

There are many clinical problems in which environmental influences are thought to be of major importance. During the summer months high ozone concentrations have been shown to increase bronchial reactivity and to induce increased manifestation of asthma attacks. For most of the health problems usually observed or supposed in the context of air pollutants, convincing evidence for a causal relation is lacking. Early studies made use mainly of lung function tests which are so insensitive, that high concentrations of pollutants had to be used to see any effects at all. Chronic exposure to such high concentrations is not feasable. Only with the introduction of much more sensitive research tools has it become possible to detect pollutant effects even at very low concentrations, i.e., at concentrations commonly found in the ambient air. These investigative tools (e.g., fiberoptic bronchoscopy with bronchoalveolar lavage) are of course much more invasive, which means that the clinical relevance of such research must be proven before ethical consideration of such studies is positive. We therefore provide some examples of meaningful research in clinical inhalation with reasonable chances for significant contributions to our hitherto insufficient knowledge.

Effects of SO_2 and Acid Fog on Pulmonary Function

Asthmatic reactions triggered by inhalation of cold air and fog are well-known phenomena that have great impact on the well-being of asthmatics during the winter. Based on current understanding of the pathomechanisms of cold-induced asthma, it can be hypothesized that air pollution increases this effect (Hahn et al. 1984). Increased concentrations of O_3 and H_2SO_4 are rarely seen in Europe during winter, but the coincidence of low outside temperature and increased SO_2 concentrations is a common feature. Studies on the combined effect of cold air and SO_2 uniformly show an increase in the SO_2-induced asthmatic reaction by cold air as well as by exercise (Bethel et al. 1984). The kinetics of this combined effect – different levels of relatve humidity and the transition from a typical warm indoor atmosphere to a cold, SO_2-containing outdoor situation have not been studied so far.

Cold and fog are typical features of the German climate. During their formation, fog droplets incorporate gaseous and particulate components from ambient air. This may generate considerable amounts of sulfuric and nitric acid, occasionally lowering the pH value of fog water to below 2 (Hoffmann et al. 1986). Epidemiologic studies suggest a positive correlation between asthmatic complaints and increased H_2SO_4 concentrations in the ambient air (Speizer 1989). Only one controlled clinical trial on the effects of acid fog on lung function has been carried out so far (Mackney 1989). Neither in normal subjects nor in asthmatics was a significant change detected in pulmonary function tests. The fog used in this study represents one of many possible types of acid fog. The impact of droplet size, aging of the fog atmosphere, ion species, and acidity must be clarified in further investigations.

Effects of Acid Aerosols on Nonspecific Cellular Defense Mechanisms of the Lung

Clinical experience indicates a strong influence of both climate and airborne pollutants on the prevalence of repiratory infections (Scherrer 1985). Epidemiologic studies suggest a connection between increased concentrations of NO_2, O_3, SO_2, and total particle count and an increased prevalence or worsened course of respiratory diseases (Bates and Sizto 1987a). Such studies also provide evidence for a positive correlation between respiratory infections and SO_2 or O_3 concentrations (Dodge et al. 1985). Recent studies seem to indicate a negative impact of acid aerosols on pulmonary infections (Bates and Sizto 1987b). So far virtually no investigations have been made on the effects of acid aerosols on the elements of the specific or nonspecific cellular defense mechanisms, especially macrophage, granulocyte and lymphocyte, or natural killer cell functions.

Effects of Airborne Pollutants on Pulmonary Surfactant

Pulmonary surfactant is exposed to respirable airborne pollutants. Lining the alveolar surface, it is hit directly by inhaled materials. Similarly, the surfactant film between sol and gel phases of the bronchial mucus is separated from inhaled materials only by a thin overlying mucus layer. Type II alveolar cells are synthesizing and reabsorbing surfactant components: they are constituents of the alveolar wall and thus are also directly exposed to pollutants. Pulmonary surfactant is involved in multiple basic aspects of lung physiology, such as lung compliance, bronchial and alveolar clearance mechanisms, and various defense mechanisms. A number of studies has shown enhancement of macrophage migration, phagocytosis, and intracellular killing by pulmonary surfactant material (Baughman et al. 1987). A recent preliminary study by Oosting and coworkers indicated that apoprotein SP-A mediated enhancement of intracellular killing by alveolar macrophages may be reduced by ozone exposure in vivo and in vitro (Oosting et al. 1989). Thus it seems worthwhile to study in detail the effects of air pollutants at concentrations commonly found in the air on surfactant itself and on the surfactant interaction with the cellular defense mechanisms.

Ethical Considerations

Clinical inhalation studies raise an ethical problem. Human subjects must be submitted to studies that do not immediately address therapeutic or diagnostic problems on an individual basis. The subjects do not necessarily benefit individually from the studies. Therefore, one must consider the ethical legitimacy of such studies. Agreement is necessary to be able to explain the studies conclusively to the subjects, the public, and the scientific community (Deutsch 1979). In the first place, advantages and dangers must be balanced against one another with regard to the individual and the community. Since patients are taking part in the studies, their specific risk must be thoroughly evaluated. Weighing the advantages and dangers does not make sense unless the scientific importance of a given study objective has been proven (Beecher 1966). Therefore, ways must be found to make this importance understandable even to a nonscientist. Once these basic demands are fulfilled, the modalities of the studies (voluntariness, explanation, consent, carefulness, etc.) must be defined and steps taken to make these modalities definitive constituents of the design of each single study (Schimikowski 1980). Each study must of course be submitted to the local ethics committee to verify that these criteria are fulfilled.

Advantages and Dangers

The studies contribute to a better understanding of respiratory diseases and of the pathogenic effects of air pollutants, thus leading to substantial progress for both medical science and practive. The subject taking part in the study may not necessarily benefit from this progess, although on a more general basis the increase in medical knowledge may help him at some time to be able to protect himself from possible harm. An immediate advantage for participating subjects may result from the thorough medical and especially pulmonary examination preceding each such study. Patients and subjects may learn more about their reserve in capacity (controlled exercise with thorough observation of changes in lung functions) than they would in usual medical examinations. With pollutant concentrations in the exposure atmosphere that do not exceed levels commonly found in the ambient air, the danger linked to the exposure itself can be defined for participating subjects and patients. Under controlled study conditions usually one but sometimes two air pollutants are applied at the same time. Therefore the risk of a negative reaction is rather low compared to outdoor conditions.

High technical standards must be implemented to guarantee safety for the subjects at all times during the studies. Regardless of the objective danger of the study design, it must be ensured that all subjects are able to analyze for themselves at all times the risk which they are running, and that they definitively agree with the procedures.

Possible danger may arise from the methods used for detecting pollutant effects. There are no known risks in carrying out lung function tests when simple hygiene measures are taken (one-way mouthpieces, bacterial filters, etc.). Physical exercise during exposure, as part of many studies, must be effectd only below individual work load limits that have been fixed during preexamination under medical supervision. Risks during exposure are negligible because subjects or patients presenting with clearly pathologic or borderline findings at preexamination can be excluded from the study. Such considerations must be made for all specific and nonspecific tests performed during such a study, and with increasing invasiveness of such measures the possible risks must be weighed against the possible dangers. If patients instead of normal volunteers are studied, these risks may be very substantial, and evaluation must take into account the very specific situation of each single patient.

Scientific Relevance

There is no doubt that better understanding is needed of the role of air pollutants in the pathogenesis of pulmonary disease. To confirm the usefulness of the planned studies alongside the need for such studies, the probability must exist that the tests will achieve a desired result and yield the information needed. In other words, the studies must be of scientific relevance and offer a real gain in knowledge as a basis for improving diagnosis or therapy. This scientific importance must be checked at several levels. The group of scientists carrying out the studies make an initial check into this question and do not continue unless they are convinced that scientific relevance is present. Then the project should be presented to a team of experts (as in the grant application process) who look particularly into the queston of scientific importance. In addition, the ethics committee, before which each such project must be presented, also considers the scientific significance.

Precise Definitions of the Modalities

Even when the benefit clearly outweighs the risk in a scientific study, and there is no doubt as to its scientific relevance, the study itself can only go ahead if certain further conditions are met. One of these conditions is an absolute voluntariness. Since in the selection of suitable subjects or patients a voluntary basis must not be automatically restricted, an independent third-party should operate between the scientific group and the test subjects or patients. This means, for instance, that the supervising physician and the head of a series of experiments should not be the same person. In extreme cases, the voluntary basis may be restricted by considering students from the Medical School as test subjects. This aspect loses significance when it is guaranteed that nonparticipation can in no way lead to disadvantages. Explanation of the dangers involved is a particularly important task for the head of the experiment group to ensure that the decision made by both subjects and patients is completely voluntary. All tests and modalities of the study must be described in detail. Should certain information carry with it the risk of influencing the result, a policy of "nondeception" must be observed. In other words, if may be allowed not to specify to a subject whether he will be exposed to a pollutant on day 1 or day 2 if he is aware that on one of those two days exposure to a certain pollutant will be carried out. After receiving relevant and adequate information, a subject or patient must at any time be able to decide to withdraw from the tests, without giving his reasons and without prejudice or disadvantage. Consent to the tests must be given in writing with notice of the subject's right of withdrawal. Thus the conditions laid down in the Helsinki Agreement as well as further stipulations set out under local law must be fulfilled.

Methodological Considerations

Over the past 20 years interactions between environmental factors and human health have gained increasing public attention. For a long time, epidemiologic and clinical studies have indicated that increased concentrations of NO_2, O_3, SO_2, and particles correlate positively with an increased prevalence or aggravation of respiratory diseases. For most inhaled materials sizeable test populations must be investigated because in individual cases the question hardly can be answered of whether or not environmental factors are inducing respiratory ailments.

Looking through the literature on clinical inhalation studies, it is evident that the majority of studies deals with normal subjects, using pulmonary function testing as the only parameter for measuring biological effects of the inhaled material. Most of these studies have been performed with high concentrations of air pollutants. Only a small number of studies have examined patients with respiratory or cardiovascular diseases. Furthermore, data are scarce on the effects of combinations of pollutants or on the impact of cold and wet weather and climate, which is typically found, for example, in central Europe, on such effects.

Deposition, retention, and resorption of airborne pollutants take place in different areas of the respiratory tract depending on the physicochemical properties of the pollutants. Therefore, the parameters measuring the biological effects of pollutants must be adequate. The ideal test would combine high specificity and sensitivity for lesions at the site in the respiratory tract typically affected by a given pollutant with the least possible invasiveness.

Since the bronchial tree is the probable site of action of a given pollutant, quite a few noninvasive and invasive parameters may be used as indicators of pollutant-induced lesions. These include:

Bronchial compartment
Reactivity	(local, general)
Size	(lung function measurements)
Inflammation	(markers/cells or cell function/mediators)
Mucus secretion	(quantitative/qualitative physicochemical measurements)
Clearance	(direct/indirect measurements)
Perfusion	(invasive/noninvaslve methods)
Permeability	

Alveolar compartment
Diffusion capacity	(CO, O_2, multiple inert gas method)
Surfactant	(production, synthesis, storage and reuptake, physiochemical, biochemical composition, interaction with immunocompetent cells)
Defense mechanisms	(macrophages, lymphocytes, granulocytes)
Biochemical properties	(enzymes, metabolic capacity)

Interstitial compartment
Elasticity	(lung function measurement, compliance)
Cellular infiltration	(bronchoalveolar lavage cells/spill-over, transbronchial biopsy (?))
Proliferation	(bronchoalveolar lavage cells, proliferation markers, computed tomography, high-resolution computed tomography, positron emission tomography)

Vascular compartment
Perfusion	(perfusion/ventilation scan)
Resistance	(right ventricle catheterization)

The availability of the noninvasive lung function tests has led to a preferential investigation of these effects, although a substantial amount of negative data might hint at insufficient sensitivity. Lesions in the alveolar region may be indicated by alterations in the diffusion capacity, although the huge physiologic reserve allows only major changes to be detected in this way and probably causes false-negative results. Biochemical parameters may be much more sensitive to toxic influences. Alterations in the interstitial and vascular compartments are detected only if invasive techniqes are employed (the transbronchial biopsy with the risk of pneumothorax or critical bleeding seems prohibited) unless very severe changes in compliance or pulmonary hypertension occur, which again must not be in human studies.

These few hints at possible markers of pollutant effects indicate that the available noninvasive techniques are most probably not sensitive enough to show effects of environmental air pollutants at concentrations commonly found in the ambient air on lung function in normal subjects. The sensitivity of these tests can of course be increased when patients with respiratory diseases or normal volunteers under exercise conditions (increased ventilation, i.e., increased exposure to air pollutants) are studied. With the invasive technique of the fiberoptic bronchoscopy combined with bronchoalveolar lavage and study of the retrieved material and cells, as well as bronchial epithelial biopsies, lesions in the bronchi or in the equilibrium of the system may be found even in the absence of clinical symptoms and complaints.

It must be considered, however, that the invasiveness of bronchoscopy and bronchoalveolar lavage (combined with local anesthesia) does not allow the retrieval cells or material of a "normal" and undisturbed state. Nevertheless, against the background of this artifact, changes caused by airborne pollutants can be found.

Summary

Diseases of the respiratory tract and the lungs present an eminent challenge to both medical research and health politics. Effects of environmental pollutants on induction and course of respiratory diseases are still poorly understood. Even with major air pollutants such as ozone, nitrogen dioxide, and sulfur dioxide at concentrations commonly found in the ambient air, insufficient data are available as to the chronic health effects. For studies in this field chronic exposure of volunteers and patients with diseases of the lung must be performed under strict experimental conditions. Ethical aspects must be thoroughly discussed to ensure scientific relevance and positive risk-benefit ratio. With increasingly invasive pulmonary research more sensitive techniques have become available so that in combination with exercise tests during exposure even minor effects of air pollutants may be distinguishable. In patients with pulmonary disease controlled clinical inhalation studies with environmental air pollutant concentrations commonly found in the ambient air may provide further information as to special risk of such patients under certain outdoor or indoor conditions.

References

Bates DV, Sizto R (1987a) Air pollution and hospital admissions in southern Ontario: the acid summer haze effect. Environ Res 43:317–331

Bates DV, Sizto R (1987b) The Ontario air pollution study: identification of the causative agent. Environ Health Perspect 79:69–72

Baughman RP, Mangels DJ, Strohofer S, Corser BC (1987) Enhancement of macrophage and monocyte cytotoxicity by the surface active material of lung lining fluid. J Lab Clin Med 109:692–697

Beecher HK (1966) Ethics and clinical research. N Engl J Med 274:1354

Bethel RA, Sheppard D, Epstein J, Tam E, Nadel JA, Boushey HA (1984) Interaction of sulfur dioxide and dry cold air in causing bronchoconstriction in asthmatic subjects. J Appl Physiol 57:419–423

Deutsch, E (1979) Das Recht der klinischen Forschung am Menschen. Lang Frankfurt

Dodge R, Solomon P, Moyers J, Hayes C (1985) A longitudinal study of children exposed to sulfur oxides. Am J Epidemiol 121:720–736

Hackney JD (1989) Acid fog: effects on respiratory function and symptoms in healthy and asthmatic volunteers. Environ Health Perspect 79:159–162

Hahn A, Anderson SD, Morton AR, Black JL, Fitch KD (1984) A reinterpretation of the effect of temperature and water content of the inspired air in exercise-induced asthma. Am Rev Respir Dis 130:575–579

Hoffmann MR, Waldman JM, Munger JW, Jacob DJ (1986) The chemistry and physics of acid fogs, clouds and haze aerosols. In: Lee SD, Schneider T, Grant LD, Verkerk PJ (eds) Aerosols. Lewis, Chelsea

Oosting RS, van Greevenbroek MMJ, van Bree L (1989) Inhibition of surfactant protein – A activity by ozone and hydrogenperoxide. Floating congress on the River Rhine, 11–77 Nov, 1989

Scherrer M (1985) Luftbelastung und Atem- und Kreislauferkrankungen. Schweiz Med Wochenschr 115:1042–1048

Schimikowski P (1980) Experiment am Menschen. Enke, Stuttgart

Speizer FE (1989) Studies of acid aerosols in six cities and in a new multi-city investigation: design issues. Environ Health Perspect 79:61–67

von Boehmer H, Fabel H (1987) Zur akuten Wirkung von Luftschadstoffen auf Lunge und Atemwege von Risikopatienten. Prax Klin Pneumol 41:108–117

Time- and Dose-Dependent Cellular and Biochemical Changes in Response to Ozone Exposure*

H.S. KOREN[1], S. BECKER[2], P.A. BROMBERG[3], and R.B. DEVLIN[1]

[1] Health Effects Research Laboratory (MD-58), US Environmental Protection Agency, Research Triangle Park, NC 27711, USA
[2] TRC Environmental Corporation, 6320 Quadrangle Drive, Chapel Hill, NC 27514, USA
[3] University of North Carolina, Center for Environmental Medicine and Lung Biology, Medical Research Building C, Chapel Hill, NC 27599–7310, USA

Introduction

Inflammation may play a key role in the development of lung disease (Hunninghake et al. 1981a; Wright et al. 1984; Cooper et al. 1986) and the severity of lung injury and may be directly related to the amount of subsequent chronic inflammation and fibrosis (Shen et al. 1988). The primary feature of the acute inflammatory response is an influx of neutrophils (PMN). An increase in PMN in the lower lung has been implicated in the development of emphysema (Janoff et al. 1977), idiopathic pulmonary fibrosis (Hunninghake et al. 1980), airway hyperactivity (Holtzman et al. 1983), and increased mucous secretion after irritant exposure (Harkema et al. 1988). Many air pollutants including ozone (O_3) have already been shown to induce a lung inflammatory response in multiple animal species (Hunninghake et al. 1981b; Luciano 1982; Castleman et al. 1980), but the effect in humans has been less well studied due to the difficulty of obtaining adequate samples for analysis.

Our understanding of the effects of inhaled pollutants on human health has improved in recent years, due in part to the ability to study bronchoalveolar lavage (BAL) and nasal lavage (NAL) fluids and cellular content. These studies allow us an insight into the inflammatory response of the lower and upper respiratory tracts, respectively.

---

* The research described in this article has been reviewed by the Health Effects Research Laboratory, United States Environmental Protection Agency, and approved for publication. Approval does not signify that the contents necessarily reflect the views and policies of the Agency nor does mention of trade names or commercial products constitute endorsement or recommendation for use.

U. Mohr et al. (Eds.)
Advances in Controlled Clinical
Inhalation Studies
© Springer-Verlag Berlin Heidelberg 1993

Seltzer and associates (1986) have shown increases (compared to air-exposed subjects) in the concentrations of PMN and of some arachidonic acid metabolites in BAL fluids obtained from human subjects approximately 3h after termination of a 2h exposure to 0.4 or 0.6ppm O_3. Seltzer and associates were also able to demonstrate an increase in airway responsiveness to methacholine challenge in the O_3-exposed subjects. We have shown that human exposure to 0.4ppm of O_3 for 2h induced an inflammatory response in the lung as determined by numerous cellular and biochemical changes detected in BAL 18h after O_3 exposure (Koren et al. 1989).

The nose is the primary portal of entry for inspired air in host humans and is generally the first region of the respiratory tract in contact with airborne pollutants, inert particles, and microbes. The number of PMN has been shown to increase by a factor of 10–100 during an upper respiratory tract viral infection (Henderson et al. 1988). A significant increase in the number of NAL PMN has also been shown to occur in response to acute exposure to ozone at 0.5ppm O_3 (Graham et al. 1988).

The NAL procedure allows measurements of the effect of a pollutant on a mucosal surface. The NAL is simple to perform, noninvasive, and atraumatic, allowing collection of multiple sequential samples from the same person. For these reasons and because no special equipment is required, the nasal lavage is an attractive and inexpensive approach for epidemiologic and occupational studies. Furthermore, the possibility exists that the NAL can be useful in determining which air pollutants are capable of inducing an inflammatory response in the human respiratory tract.

In addition to the in vivo exposures conducted in environmentally controlled exposure chambers, in vitro exposure studies performed with isolated cells can be useful in understanding mechanisms of cellular responses and in extrapolation issues between species.

The purpose of this paper is to review recent in vivo and in vitro studies with emphasis on the application of various assay techniques and potentially useful markers in inhalation exposure research.

Experimental Approach

This section briefly describes the methods used in the various studies.

Subject Population and Experimental Design

Healthy, nonsmoking male volunteers 18–35 years of age served as subjects. The screening procedure for the subjects was previously described in detail (Koren et al. 1989). The protocol and consent form were approved by the University of North Carolina School of Medicine Committee on the Protection of the Rights of Human Subjects.

Two experimental designs were used in the studies reviewed below. In one case, each subject was exposed on two occasions, once to filtered air and once to 0.4 ppm O_3, with at least 4 weeks between exposures. The exposure and training protocols were identical to those previously described (Koren et al. 1989). Briefly, exposures were of 2-h duration and consisted of alternating 15-min periods of rest and heavy treadmill exercise that was performed at a level to produce a minute ventilation (V_e) of approximately $35\, l\, min^{-1}\, m^{-2}$ body surface area. Lung function and symptoms were assessed before and 5 min after exposure. Subjects underwent BAL 1 h or 18 h following the 2-h exposure to O_3.

In the second study each of ten subjects was exposed on three separate occasions: once to filtered air, once to 0.08 ppm ozone, and once to 0.10 ppm ozone. Exposures were randomized and double blind, with at least 5 weeks between exposures. An additional ten subjects were exposed on two separate occasions: once to filtered air and once to 0.08 ppm ozone, with at least 5 weeks between exposures. The subjects exercised on either a treadmill or cycle ergometer set to produce a V_e of about 40 l/min per square meter. Exposure consisted of six sessions lasting a total of 6.5 h. Each exercise session lasted 50 min and was followed by a 10-min rest and lung function measurement period.

BAL and NAL Procedures

Bronchoscopies and BAL were performed as previously described in detail (Koren et al. 1989). The same procedures were used in all BAL studies (1 h and 18 h after exposure). The bronchoscope was wedged into a subsegmental bronchus of the lingula and right middle lobes. Each lobe was lavaged with 6 × 50 ml aliquots of sterile saline. Samples were put on ice immediately after aspiration and centrifuged at $300\, g$ for 10 min at 4°C. Supernatants from the first two aliquots of each lobe were pooled for analysis of BAL fluid components. Cell viability exceeded 85% as ascertained by trypan blue exclusion. Cell differentials were performed on cytocentrifuged slides stained with a modified Wright's stain (Leukostat Solution; Fisher Scientific).

The NAL procedure as used in our laboratory (Graham et al. 1988) was adapted from Powell et al. (1977). Ten milliliters of sterile phosphate-buffered saline without Ca^{2+} and Mg^{2+} (Gibco) warmed to 37°C was instilled, 5 ml in each nasal cavity, using a needleless syringe. By palatal pressure the saline was held in the nasopharyngeal region 10 s and then forcibly expelled into a sterile plastic specimen cup. The samples were centrifuged and the supernatant frozen at −70°C for later analyses. Cells were counted and calculated for the number of total cells per lavage, as well as the number of cells/ml of recovered fluid. The average amount of fluid recovered was 7.0 ± 0.2 ml. Cytocentrifuge-prepared slides were stained with Wright's stain for cell differentials.

In Vivo Exposure Chamber

Exposures and measurements were conducted in a $4 \times 6 \times 3.2$ m stainless steel Rochester-style chamber maintained at 22°C and 40% relative humidity. A detailed description of the chamber, ozone generating, delivery, monitoring, and control system has been previously published (Strong 1978; Glover et al. 1981).

In Vitro Exposure Chamber

The tissue culture dishes or plates were placed in a rocking platform exposure system (Bellco, Vineland, NJ) with controlled temperature and humidity (>95%) as previously described in detail (Becker et al. 1991). The plexiglass tissue culture box was equipped with 0.25-in. tube fittings for entry and removal of humidified 5% CO_2, air, and O_3. O_3 concentration in the culture box was monitored with a Dasibi 1003 AH O_3 analyzer connected to the lowest port and the concentration adjusted with a shield over the UV lamp. An identical box receiving only filtered air (control exposure) was placed in a separate but identical incubator.

Assays

The specific procedures used in the various studies have been published in detail elsewhere (Koren et al. 1989; Devlin et al. 1990). Tables 1 and 2 summarize the major endpoints (markers) used in the various studies based on materials obtained by BAL and NAL, respectively.

Results and Discussion

Effect of Duration between Exposure and BAL on the Levels of Biological Responses

While pulmonary function decrements can occur almost immediately after the start of an exposure to O_3 (0.4 ppm), it is not known how quickly the cellular and biochemical changes indicative of inflammation occur in humans. Changes in PMN and prostaglandin E_2 (PGE_2) have been observed in humans as early as 2–3 h (Seltzer et al. 1986) and as late as 18 h after exposure (Koren et al. 1989). The purpose of this study was to determine whether inflammatory changes occur relatively rapidly (within approximately

Table 1. Biomarkers of interest in BAL studies

Marker	Major activity/indication
Neutrophils	Inflammation; tissue damage
Prostaglandin E_2	Inflammation; immune system suppression
Interleukin 6	Inflammation; acute-phase response
Protein, albumin	Permeability increase
Leukotriene B_4	Neutrophil chemotaxis
Fibronectin	Fibroblast, epithelial cell chemotaxis; fibrosis
Lactate dehydrogenase	Tissue damage
Tissue factor	Fibrin deposition
Plasminogen activator	Fibrinolysis

Table 2. Biomarkers of interest in NAL studies

Marker	Indication
Neutrophils	Inflammatory response
Protein, albumin	Permeability
Eosinophils, mast cells	Allergic response
Histamine, tryptase, TAME esterase, serotonin, kinins, prostaglandin D_2	Mast cell degranulation/allergic response
Immunoglobulin E	Allergic response
Eicosanoids, C5a, C3a, antioxidants, kallikrein, kinins, substance P, cytokines	Inflammatory/allergic responses

1 h) following exposure to O_3, or whether the cascade of events which are initiated by O_3 and lead to inflammation take some time to develop. We exposed ten healthy volunteers twice: once to filtered air and once to 0.4 ppm ozone. Each exposure lasted for 2 h at an exercise level of 60 l/min, and BAL was performed 1 h following exposure. The data from this study were compared to those from a previous study in which ten subjects were exposed to O_3 under identical conditions except that BAL was performed 18 h following exposure.

The results of our study suggest that (a) several inflammatory indicators are elevated after exposure, and (b) they achieve their maximal levels in the lung at different times (Table 3). Several markers (PMN; interleukin 6, IL-6; PGE_2) were demonstrably higher at 1 h following exposure to O_3 than at 18 h. These markers seem to be associated with an acute and early stage of inflammatory response and may thus result from a direct effect of O_3 on pulmonary cells. Seltzer et al. (1986) also detected an increase in PMN and PGE_2 3 h following a 4-h exposure. Schelegle et al. (1991), however, did not

Table 3. Time-dependent changes in the level of inflammatory markers following exposure to ozone

Marker in BAL	Time of BAL post exposure	
	1 h	18 h
Protein	+	+
Tissue factor	+	+
Neutrophils	++	+
Interleukin 6	++	+
Prostaglandin E_2	++	+
Fibronectin	+	++
Plasminogen activator	+	++

Subjects were exposed to 0.4 ppm O_3 for 2 h with exercise. BAL was performed 1 h or 18 h after exposure.

observe an increase in PMN 1 h after exposure, which may be related to the fact that the exposure duration in their study was only 1 h. Since in our study pulmonary function tests such as that for forced expiratory volume in 1 s are depressed at this early time point (1 h after exposure), it is tempting to speculate that some or all of these markers may also be related to O_3-induced alteration in pulmonary function.

Indeed, a second group of markers, fibronectin and urokinase-plasminogen activator (u-PA), were detected at higher levels at the later time point (18 h). Only a slight increase in u-PA was detected after 1 h of exposure. Fibronectin and u-PA are known to be involved in the fibrotic and fibrinolytic processes, respectively (Rennard et al. 1981; Cooper et al. 1986; Chapman et al. 1984). Their higher levels at the later time point (18 h) support a role in less acute changes in the lung which could eventually lead to fibrosis. Protein and tissue factor (TF), although both were elevated after ozone exposure, did not show significantly different levels at early versus late time points. Total protein in BAL fluid is a nonspecific indicator of increased permeability of lung epithelia. The data obtained in animals where BAL fluid was sampled at different time points suggested that the level of protein was concentration-dependent, and that both in guinea pigs (Hu et al. 1982) and in other rodent species (Hatch et al. 1986) an increase in protein level was not observed shortly after exposure but rather 10–15 h later. TF is involved in reactions leading to fibrin formation (Coleman 1976; Nemerson and Bach 1982). It is unlikely that the increase in TF was due to increased permebility since TF is an integral component of cellular membranes (Nemerson and Bach 1982).

Further studies may elucidate the time course, duration, and mechanism of this process as well as determine whether causal relationship exists between the biochemical and cellular changes and the changes in lung function and airway reactivity.

Correlation between BAL and NAL in Response to Ozone Exposure

In a previous study, we determined that the NAL procedure could be used to detect an acute inflammatory reaction in the nasal passages of humans, as measured by an influx of PMN (Graham et al. 1988). Since humans are predominantly nose breathers, the cells lining the nasal passages are generally the first to come in contact with an air pollutant (Niinimaa et al. 1980). The relationship of the human cellular response in the nasal passages to events in the lower lung is not known.

To study the relationship between the responses in the upper and lower respiratory tracts, we investigated the correlation of the cellular changes detected in the NAL with those detected in the BAL from the same individual (Graham and Koren 1990). Subjects were exposed, while moderately exercising, to filtered air or 0.4 ppm ozone for 2 h (as described above). BAL was performed 18 h after exposure; NAL was performed prior to, immediately after, and 18 h after exposure. The PMN counts as well as the concentration of biochemical markers associated with acute inflammation were measured and compared.

An influx of PMN occurred in both the upper and lower airways in response to O_3. The PMN were increased in the NAL immediately after the ozone exposure and continued to increase at 18 h after exposure. At 18 h after the ozone exposure, the mean PMN counts for both the NAL and BAL were increased sixfold. This supports a strong qualitative correlation between the O_3-induced inflammatory responses of the nasopharyngeal region and of the lower lung. Although the PMN significantly increased in both the NAL and BAL from the same individual, the NAL PMN could not predict the total number of BAL PMN.

This lack of quantitative correlation within an individual following the O_3 exposure may be related to (a) a difference in the intensity of an inflammatory response in the upper airways versus the lung periphery, (b) the variability in nasopharyngeal clearance of this pollutant by different individuals, or (c) a difference in sampling of the PMN. The latter possibility is supported by the recent findings of Gerrity and colleagues (1981) showing that the nasopharyngeal clearance of O_3 ranged from 20% to 80% in different individuals. This would affect the actual dose of O_3 being delivered to each of the respiratory regions. Another factor affecting the distribution of O_3 may have been the degree to which individuals switched from nasal to oral breathing during the exercise periods.

This study demonstrates that PMN counts in the NAL can be a useful, inexpensive means of studying acute inflammatory effects of O_3 and monitoring those effects in the lower lung.

176   H.S. Koren et al.

Effect of Dose on Biological Responses to Ozone

The present air quality guidelines and the National Ambient Air Quality Standards (NAAQS) for ozone specify that the maximal hourly average ozone concentration may not exceed 0.12 ppm more than once a year. The design of these studies, upon which the NAAQS guidelines were set, was influenced by the typical ozone pattern occurring in the Los Angeles area beginning in the 1950s and 1960s, in which brief (1- to 3-h) peaks of high ozone concentrations were reached in the late morning or early afternoon (Rombout et al. 1986). However, recent monitoring data reveal that other areas of the United States (parts of the East Coast, suburbs of large cities, and even rural areas downwind from large cities) experience ozone levels that, while not as high as those found in southern California, remain elevated for several hours at a time (US EPA 1985). Therefore, a significant population, including sensitive subgroups, may be exposed to low ozone levels for several hours each day, even though the current hourly ozone standard may not be exceeded.

Our objective in the following study was to determine whether these cellular and biochemical changes also occur in humans exposed to very low levels of ozone for several hours as opposed to the previous studies which were carried out at higher concentrations of ozone (Seltzer et al. 1986; Koren et al. 1989). In addition to allowing an assessment of significant cellular and biochemical changes occurring in the lung at levels approximating the current as well as the proposed standard, exposing humans to these near-ambient levels of ozone may also allow us to determine whether there is a threshold level of ozone below which no changes can be measured with the assays described in this report.

Nonsmoking men were randomly exposed to filtered air and either 0.10 or 0.08 ppm ozone for 6.6 h with moderate exercise (40 l/min per BSA). BAL was performed 18 h after each exposure, and cells and fluid were analyzed. As shown in Table 4, the BAL fluid of volunteers exposed to 0.10 ppm ozone had significant increases in PMN, protein, PGE$_2$, fibronectin, IL-6, and lactate dehydrogenase (LDH) compared with BAL fluid from the same volunteers exposed to filtered air. In addition, there was a decrease in the ability of alveolar macrophages (AM) to phagocytize yeast via the complement receptor. Exposure to 0.08 ppm ozone resulted in significant increases in PMN, PGE$_2$, IL-6, alpha-1-antitrypsin, and decreased phagocytosis via the complement receptor. However, BAL fluid protein and fibronectin were no longer significantly elevated.

In general, exposure to 0.08 ppm ozone resulted in smaller increases in inflammatory mediators than did exposure to 0.10 ppm ozone. Taken together, these results indicate a clear difference in response after exposure to the two concentrations of ozone.

The finding that IL-6 levels are increased in subjects exposed to ozone has not been reported previously. This cytokine is of potential importance

Table 4. Comparative effects of different levels of ozone exposure on markers in human BAL

Marker in BAL	Exposure dose (PPM)	
	0.1 (6.7 h)	0.08 (6.7 h)
Neutrophils	+ +	+
Prostaglandin E_2	+ +	+
Lactate dehydrogenase	+	+
Interleukin 6	+ +	+
Protein	+	−
Fibronectin	+	−
Phagocytosis (C-mediated)	+	+

Subjects were exposed to 0.1 or 0.08 ppm for 6.7 h; BAL was performed 18 h after exposure.

because of its involvement in the body's acute-phase response to inflammation (Gauldie et al. 1987; Helfgott et al. 1989). Injury to a local site such as the lung caused by trauma, inflammation, or infection can lead to a systemic response resulting in leukocytosis, fever, increased vascular permeability, and the production of several acute-phase plasma proteins by the liver (Koz 1985).

The magnitude of these differences in response compared with the relatively small differences in total exposure suggest that either ozone concentration, V_e, or both are more important determinants of response than is duration of exposure. However, future studies measuring effects at several ozone concentrations and altering both the duration of exposure and ventilatory rate will be necessary to confirm these findings.

In Vitro Exposure Studies

In parallel with the in vivo exposures to O_3, a decrease in immune mechanisms involving T, B, and natural killer cells have been measured in vitro (Becker et al. 1989, 1991; Harder et al. 1990). Recently, we have investigated the effects of in vitro exposure to O_3 on several AM functions which are important in host defense. The functions studies were selected to gain an understanding of O_3 effects on human AM-mediated antimicrobial activity under nontoxic conditions as well as to enable a comparison of results with human cells to those obtained from animal experiments (Table 5).

Exposure of AM to O_3 resulted in the release of increased amounts of arachidonic acid and an increased production of PGE_2. These results are in agreement with previous work with rat and rabbit AM which were induced to release PGE_2 by exposure to O_3 both in vivo and in vitro (Driscoll and

Table 5. Ozone-induced immunomodulation (in vitro)

Alveolar macrophages function	Effect
Fc receptor phagocytosis (EA)	↓
Complement receptor phagocytosis (EAC)	NC
Inhibition of fungal growth (*Cryptoccus neoformans*)	NC
FcR1, FcR2, FcR3 expression	NC
CR1, CR3, CR4 expression	NC
PGE_2 release	↑
Superoxide production	↓
Monokine production:	
lipopolysaccharide-induced tumor necrosis factor-α, IL-1β, IL-6	↓
spontaneous IL-6, colony-stimulating factor-1	NC

Alveolar macrophages obtained by BAL from normal subjects were exposed to 1.0 ppm O_3 for 2 h in vitro and then assayed for different functions. NC, no change.

Schlesinger 1987; Madden et al. 1991) as well as with studies with O_3-exposed humans who showed increase in PGE_2 in their lavage fluids (Seltzer et al. 1986; Koren et al. 1989).

Phagocytosis of sheep erythrocytes coated with antibody (EA) was inhibited by O_3. This process is mediated mainly by FcR1 on the AM cell surface, with minor involvement of FcR2 (Unkeless 1989). However, the expression of these receptors was not affected by O_3, suggesting that the affinity or signal transduction by the receptors was inpaired.

Phagocytosis of opsonized *Cryptococcus neoformans* was not affected by O_3 (CR3-mediated), nor was there a change in the number of membrane complement receptors which are required for phagocytosis of the yeast. In addition, neither intra- nor extracellular growth inhibition of the yeast was inhibited by exposure of AM to O_3.

Freshly isolated AM are relatively poor producers of oxygen radicals (Fels et al. 1987). We found that if the cells were adhered to tissue culture dishes, they "spontaneously" released O_2^- and did not respond to stimulation with PMA by additional O_2^- release. Upon short-term (2 h) culture of the cells the "spontaneous" O_2^- production subsided, and the cells became responsive to stimulation with phorbol myristate acetate (PMA). Maximum responsiveness to PMA appeared only after overnight culture (16–18 h). Therefore, we exposed AM to O_3 immediately after isolation and after 2 and 18 h of culture. O_3 only downregulated O_2^- production in the cells cultured for 2 h which were in transition form a PMA-unresponsive to a PMA-responsive state.

The production of reactive oxygen intermediates by in vitro and in vivo O_3-exposed rodent macrophages has previously been shown to be significantly reduced (Goldstein et al. 1970; Amoruso et al. 1981; Ryer-Power et al. 1988).

Upon stimulation by microorganisms, injury, or interaction with toxic particles macrophages release a number of inflammatory mediators whcih interact in recruitment and activation of other inflammatory cells. IL-1, tumor necrosis factor, and IL-6 are polypeptide mediators with pleiotropic effects on a wide variety of host defense processes which ensue upon infection or injury (Le and Vilcek 1987, 1989). Low to undetectable levels of these cytokines were found in both O_3-exposed and control AM supernatants. However, O_3-exposed AM produced decreased levels of cytokines in response to a strong activating signal such as endotoxin. The release of colony-stimulating factor-1, which is constitutively produced by AMs and not induced by lipopolysaccharide, was not affected by O_3.

Although O_3 may attack and cause alterations in the cell membrane (Mudd and Freeman 1977; Menzel 1984), it appears that in vitro O_3 exposure of AM causes very few changes in AM proteins. This can be seen by two-dimensional gel analysis, in which we found that the rate of synthesis of only 11 proteins was altered by the exposure in vitro. These results contrast with those obtained with AM removed from humans exposed to 0.4 ppm O_3 in vivo. In these studies the rate of synthesis of 123 different proteins was altered (Devlin et al. 1990). Therefore, it seems likely that most of the protein changes seen after an in vivo O_3 exposure are secondary effects on the AM resulting from airway injury and inflammation rather than a direct effect of O_3 on the AM.

It is not known how the in vitro O_3 concentrations in the exposure chamber and the delivered dose to the cells relate to the dose delivered to the AM in in vivo exposure studies (Koren et al. 1989; Devlin et al. 1990). However, this dosimetry issue is currently being investigated in our laboratory in both in vivo and in vitro exposures using the non-radiolabeled $^{18}O_3$ isotope.

Summary and Conclusions

Human studies with inhaled pollutants are of utmost importance for assessing the effects of the various toxic gases and particles on the respiratory tract. These data are important from regulatory and mechanistic points of view. Studies of mechanisms provide us with a better understanding of how pollutants exert their effects. The studies in this paper summarize data obtained from controlled human exposures to O_3 and from in vitro exposure of human AM.

A key question that was addressed in this paper is whether one can detect indicators of an inflammatory response as early as 1 h after a 2-h exposure to 0.4 ppm ozone. The results of this study were compared to those of an earlier study which was conducted under the same conditions but in which the subjects underwent BAL 18 h after exposure. The study has demonstrated that indicators of inflammation can already be detected 1 h after exposure. PMN, PGE_2, and IL-6 were higher after 1 h than after 18 h. In contrast, fibronectin and u-PA were higher at the latter time point. Two other markers of inflammation, protein and TF, were the same at both time points. One can speculate as to why these differences were observed relative to the inflammatory response and lung tissue damage resulting form the exposure to ozone. Of practical importance, however, is the fact that different markers have a different time course, which may be very important in determining when to perform the BAL. This decision may depend on the type of question addressed in a particular study.

The studies described in this paper also demonstrate that low exposures to ozone (0.1 and 0.08 ppm) for an extended period of time are sufficient to induce an inflammatory response in human lung. The importance of this finding is twofold. First, it supports the argument that an extended ozone standard based on a less than 1 h exposure time (as opposed to a 1 h standard) may be reasonable. Second, the comparative data obtained at the two different concentrations of O_3 suggest that at the lower concentration of ozone (0.08 ppm) one approaches a dose that has relatively mild inflammatory effects following an acute exposure to the pollutant.

It has long been speculated that the nose may be a "window" to the lower airways. Experiments described in this paper attempting to correlate the data obtained form BAL and NAL, performed on the same volunteers that were exposed to 0.4 ppm ozone from 2 h, suggest that there exists a correlation between the change detected in the nose and that in the bronchoalveolar region of the respiratory tract. Even though one cannot directly extrapolate from the nose to the lower airways, one can obtain a qualitative estimate as far as the number of PMN is concerned. A quantitative correlation can, however, be obtained when comparing the number of PMN in the noses and lungs of normal air-exposed subjects. It is tempting to speculate that the subjects with higher PMN counts following exposure to air may be the ones who respond more vigorously to irritation by pollutants than those that have very low numbers of these cells. This hypothesis will have to be studied more extensively before this knowledge can be applied in a meaningful way.

The ability to expose primary cells to a particular pollutant in vitro and then extrapolate to the in vivo effects of that pollutant is very important especially when one needs to study pollutants to which humans cannot be ethically or safely exposed. Since O_3 toxicology can be studied with both in vivo and in vitro exposure, we have used this gas to establish an in vitro exposure model. Exposing human AM to ozone in vitro resulted in various changes, some of which resembled those obtained in BAL from ozone-exposed subjects. Most notably, the phagocytic activity and superoxide release of these cells were depressed following both in vivo and in vitro exposures. Interestingly, however, two-dimensional gel analysis performed on in vitro exposed AM indicated only very minor changes in the protein synthesis of these cells when compared to in vivo exposed AM, where about 10% of the total proteins were modulated. These data are intriguing and suggest that some of the observed changes in cells obtained from in vivo exposed subjects may be a result of secondary changes related to the inflammatory response. Experiments testing this hypothesis are currently under investigation in our laboratory.

It can be concluded that for a thorough understanding of the health effects of a particular pollutant on the respiratory tract one needs to take a comprehensive approach that includes both in vivo and in vitro exposures, using a broad spectrum of cellular and biochemical endpoints relevant to the questions addressed. Ideally, these studies also need to be carried out in animals to enable species-to-species extrapolation. Establishing optimal animal and in vitro models is essential to achieve improved risk assessment and to study mechanisms of toxicity in human studies.

Acknowledgements. The authors thank Drs. Terry Noah and Michael Madden for their review of the manuscript. We would also like to thank Vickie Worrell and Grace Coats for their skilled assistance in the preparation of the manuscript.

References

Amuroso MA, Witz G, Goldstein BD (1981) Decreased superoxide anion radical production by rat alveolar macrophages following inhalation of ozone or nitrogen dioxide. Life Sci 28:2215–2221

Becker S, Jordan RL, Orlando GS, Koren HS (1989) In vitro ozone exposure inhibits mitogen-induced lymphocyte proliferatin and IL-2 production. J Toxicol Environ Health 26:469–483

Becker S, Quay J, Koren HS (1991) Decrease in IgG production induced by ozone in vitro. Toxicol Environ Health 34:353–366

Castleman WL, Dungworth DL, Schwartz LW, Tyler WS (1980) Acute respiratory bronchiolitis: an ultrastructural and autoradiographic study of epithelial cell injury and renewal in rhesus monkeys exposed to ozone. Am J Pathol 98:811–840

Chapman HA Jr, Stone OL, Vavrin Z (1984) Degradation of fibrin and elastin by intact human alveolar macrophages in vitro. Characterization of a plasminogen activator and its role in matrix degradation. J Clin Invest 73:806–815

Coleman RW (1976) Factor VI. In: Spect TH (ed) Progress in hemostatis and thrombosis. Grune and Stratton, New York, pp 109–143

Cooper JA, Buck MG, Gee JB (1986) Vegetable dust and airway disease: inflammatory mechanisms. Environ Health Perspect 66:7–15

Devlin RB, McDonnell WF, Mann R, Becker S, House DE, Schreinemachers D, Koren HS (1990) Exposure of humans to ambient levels of ozone for 6.6 hours causes cellular and biochemical changes in the lung. Am J Respir Cell Mol Biol 4:72–81

Driscoll KE, Schlesinger RB (1987) Exposure to ambient air pollutant ozone stimulates arachidonic acid metabolism by rabbit alveolar macrophages. J Toxicol Environ Health 21:27–43

Fels AOS, Nathan CF, Cohn ZA (1987) Hydrogen peroxide release by alveolar macrophages from sarcoid patients and by alveolar macrophages from normals after exposure to recombinant interferon alpha, beta, and gamma, and 1,25-dihydroxyvitamin D3. J Clin Invest 80:381–387

Gauldie J, Richards C, Harnish D, Lansdorp P, Baumann H (1987) Interferon β_2/B-cell stimulatory factor type 2 shares identity with monocyte-derived hepatocyte-stimulating factor and regulates the major acute phase protein response in liver cells. Proc Natl Acad Sci USA 84:7251–7255

Gerrity TR, Weaver RA, Berntsen JH, O'Neil JJ (1981) Nasopharyngeal and lung removal of ozone during tidal breathing in man. Physiologist 29:173

Glover DE, Hernsten JH, Crider WL, Strong AA (1981) Design and performance of a system to control concentrations of common gaseous air pollutants within environmental laboratories used for human exposure studies. J Environ Sci Health 16:501–522

Goldstein E, Tyler WS, Hoeprich PD, Eagle C (1970) Adverse influence of ozone on pulmonary bacterial activity of murine lung. Nature 229:202–203

Graham DE, Henderson FW, House D (1988) Neutrophil influx measured in nasal lavages of humans exposed to ozone. Arch Environ Health 43:228–233

Graham ED, Koren HS (1990) Biomarkers of inflammation in ozone-exposed humans. Comparison of the nasal and bronchoalveolar lavage. Am Rev Respir Dis 142:152–156

Harder SD, Harris TD, House D, Koren HS (1990) Inhibition of human natural killer cell activity following in vitro exposure to ozone. Inhal Toxicol 2:161–173

Harkema JR, Hotchkiss JA, Harmsen AG, Henderson RF (1888) In vivo effects of transient neutrophil influx on nasal respiratory epithelial mucosubstances. Am J Pathol 130:605–615

Hatch GE, Slade R, Stead AG, Graham JA (1986) Species comparison of acute inhalation toxicity of ozone and phosgene. J Toxicol Environ Health 19:43–53

Helfgott DC, Tatter BS, Santhanam U et al. (1989) Multiple forms of IFN-β_2/IL-6 in serum and body fluids during acute bacterial infection. J Immunol 142:948–953

Henderson FW, Dubovi EJ, Harder S, Seal E, Graham DE (1988) Experimental rhinovirus infection in human volunteers exposed to ozone. Am Rev Respir Dis 137:1124

Holtzman MJ, Fabbri LM, O'Bryne PM et al. (1983) Importance of airway inflammation of hyperresponsiveness induced by ozone. Am Rev Respir Dis 127:686–690

Hu PC, Miller FJ, Daniels MJ et al. (1982) Protein accumulation in lung lavage fluid following ozone exposure. Environ Res 29:377–88

Hunninghake GW, Gadek J, Crystal R (1980) Smoke attracts polymorphonuclear leukocytes to lung. Chest 77:273

Hunninghake GW, Gadek JE, Lawley TJ (1981a) Mechanisms of neutrophil accumulation in the lungs of patients with idiopathic pulmonary fibrosis. J Clin Invest 68:259–269

Hunninghake GW, Kawanami O, Ferrans FJ, Young RC, Roberts WC, Crystal RG (1981b) Characterization of the inflammatory and immune effector cells in the lung parenchyma of patients with interstitial lung disease. Am Rev Respir Dis 123:407–412

Janoff A, Sloan B, Weinbaum G (1977) Experimental emphysema induced with purified human neutrophil elastase. Am Rev Respir Dis 115:461–478

Koren HS, Devlin RB, Graham DE, Mann R, McGee MP, Horstman DH, Kozumbo WJ, Becker S, House DE, McDonnell WF, Bromberg PA (1989) Ozone-induced inflammation in the lower airways of human subjects. Am Rev Respir Dis 139:407–415

Koj A (1985) The acute phase response to injury and infection. In: Gordon AH, Kolj A (eds) The roles of interleukin I and other mediators. Elsevier, Amsterdam, pp 139–144

Le J, Vilcek J (1987) Tumor necrosis factor and interleukin 1: cytokines with multiple overlapping biological activities. Lab Invest 56:234–248

Le J, Vilcek J (1989) Interleukin 6: a multifunctional cytokine regulating immune reaction and the acute phase protein response. Lab Invest 62:588–602

Luciano EM (1982) Acute experimental silicosis. Am J Pathol 109:27–36

Madden MC, Eling TE, Dailey LA, Friedman M (1991) The effect of ozone exposure on rat alveolar macrophage arachidonic acid metabolism. Exp Lung Res 17:47–63

Menzel DB (1984) Ozone: an overview of its toxicity in man and animals. J Toxicol Environ Health 13:183–204

Mudd JB, Freeman BA (1977) Reaction of ozone with biological membranes. In: Lee SD (ed) Biochemical effects of environmental pollutants. Arbor, New York, pp 97–127

Nemerson Y, Bach R (1982) Tissue factor revisited. Prog Hemost Thromb: 6:237–261

Niinimaa V, Cole P, Mintz S, Shephard RJ (1980) The switching point from nasal to oronasal breathing. Respir Physiol 42:61–71

Powell KR, Shorr R, Cherry JD, Hendley JD (1977) Improved method for collection of nasal mucus. J Infect Dis 136:1

Rennard SI, Hunninghake GW, Bitterman PB, Crystal RB (1981) Production of fibronectin by human alveolar macrophages: mechanisms for the recruitment of fibroblasts to sites of tissue injury in interstitial lung diseases. Proc Natl Acad Sci USA 78:7147–7151

Rombout P, Lioy PJ, Goldstein BD (1986) Rationale for an eight hour ozone standard. JAPCA 36:913–917

Ryer-Powder JE, Amoruso MA, Czerniecki B, Witz G, Golstein BD (1988) Inhalation of ozone produces a decrease in superoxide anion radical production in mouse alveolar macrophages. Am Rev Respir Dis 138:1128–1123

Schelegle ES, Siefkin AD, McDonald RJ (1991) Time course of ozone-induced neutrophilia in normal humans. Am Rev Respir Dis 143:1353–1358

Seltzer J, Bigby BG, Stulborg M et al. (1986) O_3 induced change in bronchial reactivity in methacholine and airway inflammation in humans. J Appl Physiol 60:1321–1326

Shen AS, Haslett C, Feldstein DC, Henson PM, Cherniack RM (1988) The intensity of chronic lung inflammation and fibrosis after bleomycin is directly related to the severity of acute injury. Am Rev Respir Dis 137:564–571

Strong AA (1978) Description of the CLEANS human exposure system. EPA-600/1-78-064. US Environmental Protection Agency, Research Triangle Park

Unkeless JC (1989) Function and heterogeneity of human Fc receptors for immunoglobulin G. J Clin Invest 83:355–361

US Environmental Protection Agency (1985) Air quality criteria for ozone and other photochemical oxidants, vol II. EPA 600-8-84-0206. US Environmental Protection Agency, Research Triangle Park

Wright JL, Lawson LM, Pare PD, Kennedy S, Wiggs B, Hogg JC (1984) The detection of small airways disease. Am Rev Respir Dis 129:989–994

Regeneration, Differentiation, and Neoplastic Transformation of Type II Alveolar Epithelial Cells

K.-U. Thiedemann[1], I. Paulini[2], N. Lüthe[1], A. Kreft[3], U. Abel[4], U. Heinrich[1], U. Glaser[5], and U. Mohr[2]

[1] Fraunhofer-Institut für Toxikologie und Aerosolforschung, Nikolai-Fuchs-Straße 1, W-3000 Hannover 61, FRG
[2] Medizinische Hochschule Hannover, Inst. für Experimentelle Pathologie, Konstanty-Gutschow-Straße 8, W-3000 Hannover 61, FRG
[3] Zentrum Pathologie und Rechtsmedizin, Pathologisches Institut, Konstanty-Gutschow-Str. 8, W-3000 Hannover 61, FRG
[4] Krankenhaus Stade Abt. HNO, Bremervörder Str. 111, W-2160 Stade
[5] Kali Chemie AG, Hans Böckler-Allee 20, W-3000 Hannover 1

Introduction

In humans, the majority of lung tumors are of bronchiogenic origin, while peripheral, bronchiolo-alveolar tumors occur with a considerably lower frequency (about 5%; Greenberg 1987). As implied by the term, "bronchiogenic" these tumors are thought to originate from cells of the bronchial epithelium per se, although it is still controversial whether this applies to all neoplasms of this category. Studies of the histogenesis of lung tumors in man have until now focused on the development of neoplastic formations from the bronchial epithelium (e.g., McDowell et al. 1978; Barrett et al. 1978; Becci et al. 1978, Nasiell et al. 1987), while peripheral lung tumors have received less attention. The results of ultrastructural examinations of peripheral lung tumors in humans suggest that bronchiolo-alveolar cell carcinomas may arise from: (a) bronchiolar Clara cells; (b) type II alveolar epithelial cells, and (c) metaplastic bronchiolar mucous cells (for review, see Greenberg 1987). However, relatively few efforts have been directed toward the systematic ultrastructural investigation of the mechanisms leading to the development of peripheral lung tumors in man. In domestic animals and the commonly used laboratory animals, neoplasms of peripheral origin represent the largest group of spontaneous as well as induced pulmonary tumors. Experimental evidence in animals suggests both Clara cells and alveolar type II epithelial cells to be the cells of origin of bronchiolo-alveolar adenomas and adenocarcinomas (for review, see Schüller 1987).

In an inhalation carcinogenicity study with various cadmium compounds we studied the epithelial damage, regeneration, and differentiation after

U. Mohr et al. (Eds.)
Advances in Controlled Clinical
Inhalation Studies
© Springer-Verlag Berlin Heidelberg 1993

short-term and chronic exposure in rats and Syrian golden hamsters. From our observations we concluded that hyperplastic type II alveolar epithelial cells under certain conditions and in certain species give rise to a population of poorly differentiated epithelial cells from which peripheral lung tumors can originate.

Materials and Methods

Short-Term Inhalation Study

Rats (Han: WIST) and Syrian golden hamsters (Han:AURA), three animals per group, were exposed to aerosolized (mass median aerodynamic diameter $<0.5 \mu m$) CdO dust, $CdCl_2$, or CdS at a concentration of $270 \mu g \, Cd/m^3$ for 18 h/day, 5 days/week for 3 days, 10 days (8 days Cd), 4 weeks (22 days Cd), and 4 weeks (22 days Cd) plus 20 weeks clean air (recovery group) in whole-body horizontal flow inhalation chambers.

Chronic Inhalation Study

Small numbers of rats (Bor:W) and Syrian golden hamsters [Hoe:SYHK (SPF Ars)] were derived from the experimental groups of the long-term study (Heinrich et al. 1986; Oldiges et al. 1989). Hamsters were exposed to CdO $(10 \mu g \, Cd/m^3)$, $CdCl_2$ $(30 \mu g \, Cd/m^3)$, $CdSO_4$ $(30 \mu g \, Cd/m^3)$, or CdS $(90 \mu g \, Cd/m^3)$ 19 h/day, 5 day/week, for 15 months or to CdO $(90 \mu g \, Cd/ m^3, 270 \mu g \, Cd/m^3)$ or CdS $(270 \mu g \, Cd/m^3)$ 8 h/day, 5 days/week, for 6–15 months. After termination of the exposure, animals were kept in clean air and sacrificed at 20–30 months of age. Rats were exposed to CdO $(10 \mu g \, Cd/m^3, 30 \mu g \, Cd/m^3, 90 \mu g \, Cd/m^3)$ or $CdCl_2$ $(30 \mu g \, Cd/m^3)$ for 22 h/day, 5 days/week, for 18 months or to CdO $(90 \mu g \, Cd/m^3)$ or CdS $(270 \mu g \, Cd/m^3)$ for 8 h/day, 5 days/week for 6 months. After termination of the exposure, animals were kept in clean air and sacrificed at 21–30 months of age.

Immediately after sacrifice, the lungs of the animals were fixed by intratracheal instillation of a modified Karnovsky fixative (0.53% paraformaldehyde, 0.66% glutaraldehyde in $0.08 M$ sodium cacodylate buffer, pH 7.4) at a pressure of 20 cm H_2O and simultaneous immersion in the same fixative solution. Tissue samples were dissected from the right middle lobe of the lung, routinely postfixed with 1% OsO_4 in sodium cacodylate buffer, and embedded in Epon according to a routine procedure. Appropriate areas for ultrastructural evaluation were selected by light microscopy from semithin sections (1 μm) of the embedded tissue samples. The ultrathin sections were stained with uranyl acetate and lead citrate and were examined in a Zeiss EM 10C or a Philips EM 420 electron microscope.

Results

In general, the nonneoplastic tissue reaction caused by the exposure to cadmium was qualitatively similar after inhalation of all compounds used. Quantitatively, however, differences were observed with regard to the Cd compound administered, length of exposure or total dose of cadmium, and sex of the animals (Aufderheide et al. 1990). Additionally, marked differences were observed concerning the carcinogenic effect of cadmium in different species: while all compounds caused a significant increase in the incidence of tumors in rats, no tumors were observed in hamsters (Heinrich et al. 1989; Glaser et al. 1990).

The present communication is limited to the results obtained from rats and hamsters exposed to CdO. The effects of other Cd compounds will be described in another publication (I. Paulini et al., in preparation).

Observations in the Rat

Short-Term Inhalation Studies

In rats exposed to CdO dust for 3 days, a focal thickening of interalveolar septae was visible in the centroacinar region by light microscopy. This thickening was due partly to the emergence of a large number of pale-staining, rounded cells with large, light-staining nuclei exhibiting a slim margin of heterochromatin. In addition, a mild inflammatory interstitial infiltration was observed.

By transmission electron microscopy (TEM), the surface of the light cells was rounded and bulged into the alveolar lumen. Their cytoplasm was electron lucent and relatively undifferentiated with numerous polyribosomes, short strands of rough endoplasmic reticulum (r-ER), few mitochondria of variable size and shape, a very small Golgi apparatus, and occasionally small electron-dense inclusions that resembled condensed lamellar bodies (Fig. 1). The surface of these cells was smooth or exhibited few short microvilli. Because of their juvenile, relatively undifferentiated morphologic appearance these cells are referred to as "undifferentiated cells" here.

With increasing distance from the bronchiolo-alveolar border, undifferentiated cells occurred less frequently and were located in the neighborhood of injured or necrotic type I alveolar epithelial cells. The injured cells exhibited a swollen, electron-lucent cytoplasm and commonly showed signs of vacuolar degeneration. Necrotic cells had a wavy course and were partly detached from the basal lamina or were overlapping neighboring cells (Fig. 2). Detachment of necrotic cells was always accompanied by the presence of undifferentiated cells so that in no instance were denuded stretches of basal lamina observed. Therefore, undifferentiated cells were considered to represent juvenile cells that arose from the regeneration process.

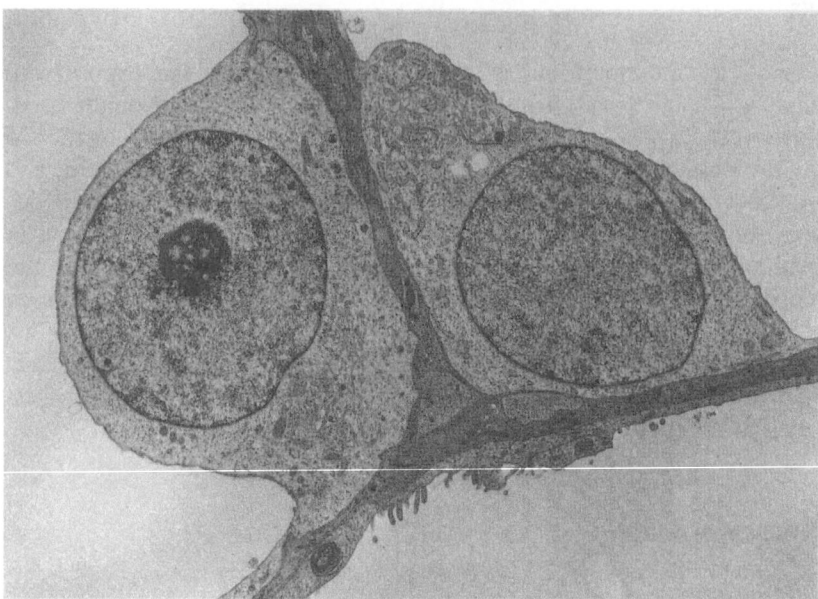

Fig. 1. TEM micrograph showing two light cells in the epithelium of two neighboring alveoli of a rat exposed to CdO for 3 days. The cells bulge distinctly into the alveolar lumen. The cytoplasm is relatively undifferentiated. The luminal surface is smooth. An elongated cell in the epithelial lining of an adjacent alveolus contains a lamellar body and bears numerous microvilli. This cell presumably represents a juvenile cell differentiating into a type I alveolar epithelial cell

Besides injured or necrotic type I pneumocytes and undifferentiated cells a broad spectrum of cells that, as judged by their ultrastructural characteristics, were in different stages of differentiation, were present in the altered centroacinar regions. These cells varied in their shape, the electron density of their cytoplasm, and their content in cellular organelles. Lighter cells that contained few organelles tended to have a rounded surface with few short microvilli while more electron-dense cells appeared flattened, exhibited more and longer microvilli, and contained more numerous organelles such as lysosomes or lamellar bodies.

After 10 days of exposure, the intensity of the tissue reaction was increased but was still confined to the centroacinar region. The differentiation of the regenerating cells had progressed so that a distinct type II cell hyperplasia had replaced the type I pneumocytes in the central areas. More distally in the alveolar duct, flat cells bearing microvilli and small knoblike surface protrusions were observed. By TEM these cells were seen to have long flat cytolasmic processes, an electron-lucent cytoplasm containing few organelles and only occasionally contained lamellar bodies. By their ultra-

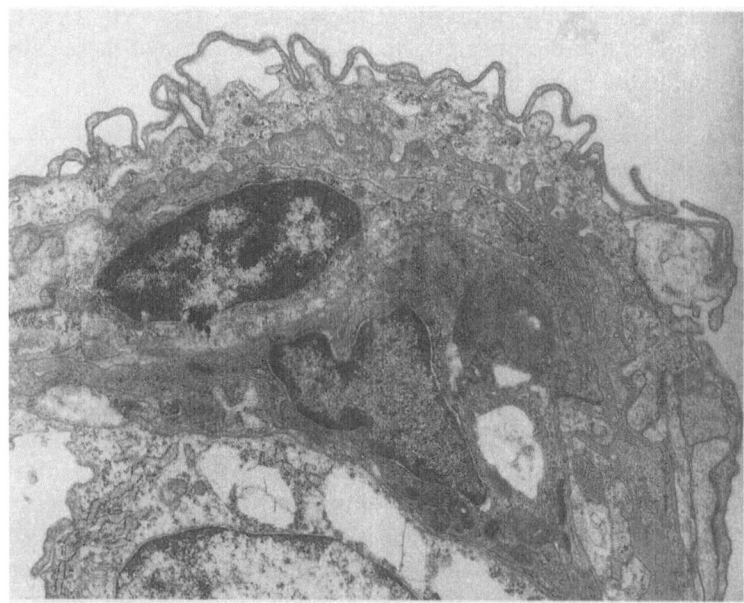

Fig. 2. TEM micrograph showing a detaching injured type I alveolar epithelial cell in a rat exposed to CdO for 3 days. A relatively thick, elongated epithelial cell underlies the detaching cell, presumably representing a juvenile cell differentiating into a type I cell. *Right*, cytoplasmic processes of a swollen epithelial cell are visible. In the neighboring alveolus (*lower border*) a vacuolated epithelial cell is present

structural appearance, these cells were considered to represent juvenile cells in an intermediate stage of differentiation into type I pneumocytes.

After 30 days of exposure the tissue reaction had progressed further and involved larger portions of the acini. The epithelial alterations and the massive interstitial inflammatory reaction, however, were more or less confined to the centroacinar region. In the central portion of the altered tissue area a massive type II cell hyperplasia consisting of relatively electron dense cuboidal cells was present. Many of these cells were elongated and contained only few lamellar bodies while their surface was covered by a dense coat of microvilli. The bronchiolo-alveolar border was shifted distally, so that alveoli of the proximal alveolar duct were lined by bronchiolar epithelium. Furthermore, groups of bronchiolar epithelial cells that lacked continuity with the epithelium of terminal bronchioli were present in alveoli and on epithelial ridges of alveolar duct bifurcations in the centroacinar region.

After 30 days of exposure and 20 weeks of recovery the extent of the epithelial alterations had decreased slightly while the interstitial inflammatory infiltration persisted or was even increased. In the centroacinar region the alveolar bronchiolization persisted, and the bronchiolo-alveolar border was shifted distally into the alveolar duct. The extensive type II cell hyperplasia had disappeared; however, the number of these cells present in the epithelial lining was still somewhat increased.

Chronic Inhalation Study

In rats chronically exposed to CdO, a marked alveolar bronchiolization was observed. The hyperplastic epithelium consisted of bronchiolar epithelial cells (ciliated cells, Clara cells) in the centroacinar region. In the periphery of hyperplastic areas, the epithelial lining of former alveoli commonly consisted of a mixed population of bronchiolar epithelial cells and cuboidal or elongated, dark-staining cells, which by TEM exhibited structural features of mature type II pneumocytes. Commonly, alveoli entirely lined by hyperplastic type II cells were observed. In such locations the alveolar lumen often contained large amounts of surfactant and macrophages laden with surfactant and lipid, and cellular detritus.

In some animals cells that morphologically resembled type II pneumocytes but lacked the characteristic lamellar bodies were present in the hyperplastic epithelium (Fig. 3). These cells had about the same size as hyperplastic type II cells (Fig. 4) but tended to be more elongated. Their surface was commonly lined by a dense coat of microvilli. The electron-dense cytoplasm of these cells contained strands of r-ER, a relatively large and often lobulated nucleus, a prominent Golgi apparatus, and in some instances bundles of cytoplasmic filaments. Occasionally a few dark granules were present. When compared to hyperplastic type II pneumocytes, these cells were connected to neighboring cells by a slightly increased number of desmosomes.

The nature of this latter cell population, which is morphologically different from any specific type of pulmonary epithelium, is not clear. We speculate, however, that these cells may be derived from hyperplastic type II pneumocytes and may represent transitional stages in the development of metaplastic or neoplastic lesions. This assumption is supported by immunohistochemical observations by T. Nolte et al. (in preparation) and Thiedemann et al. (1991). In a different experimental setup, these authors observed morphologically similar cells to express cytokeratins. Thus the cells observed represent transitional forms in the development of squamous metaplasias.

Observations in the Hamster

Short-Term Inhalation Studies

After 3 days of exposure to CdO, the tissue reaction observed in hamsters was qualitatively similar to that seen in the rat. Quantitatively, however, it was much less intense and was restricted to small epithelial areas in the

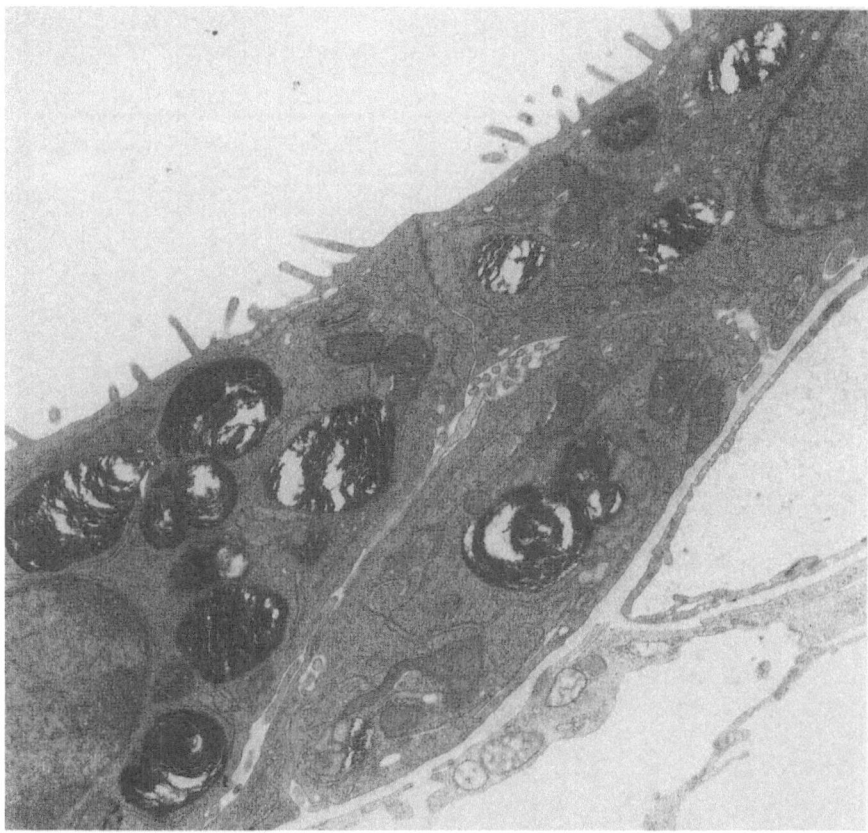

Fig. 3. TEM micrograph of hyperplastic type II alveolar epithelial cells filled with lamellar bodies in the alveolar epithelium of a rat chronically exposed to CdO

centroacinar region and to the epithelium of the first bifurcation of alveolar ducts. In these locations small foci consisting of pale-staining cells and mature hyperplastic type II pneumocytes were observed. By TEM the light cells exhibited ultrastructural features similar to those of the undifferentiated cells observed in the rat.

Therefore, these cells were considered to represent juvenile cells that were the result of cellular proliferation occurring as a result of epithelial damage and regeneration. Occasionally, solitary ciliated cells bearing small numbers of cilia of variable length were observed in these foci.

On epithelial ridges of bifurcations of the proximal part of alveolar ducts, groups of cells that by SEM exhibited structural features of Clara cells were occasionally present. These cells bore a central apical surface protrusion while short, knoblike microvilli were present in the cellular periphery.

After 10 days of exposure, the changes had increased only slightly. In addition to a slightly increased number of mature hyperplastic type II

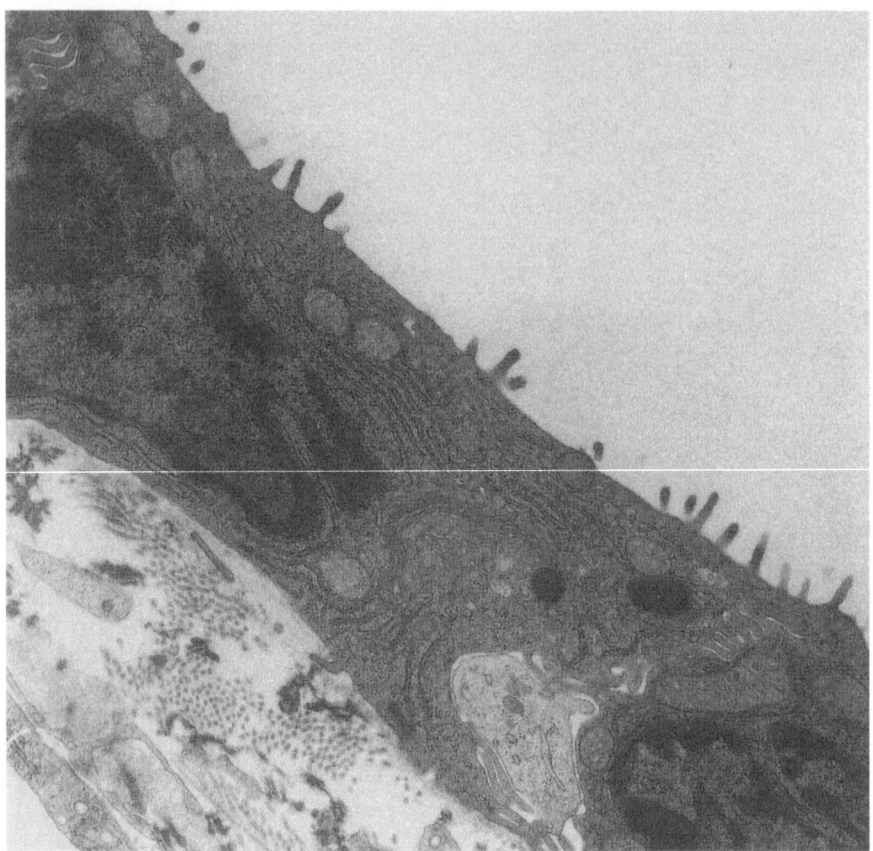

Fig. 4. TEM micrograph of a poorly differentiated cell presumably derived from hyperplastic type II alveolar epithelial cells in the epithelial lining of a bronchiolized alveolar region in a rat chronically exposed to CdO. These cells may represent transitional stages in the development of metaplastic or neoplastic lesions

pneumocytes, very few undifferentiated cells, occasionally bearing knoblike surface protrusions, were observed. Mature type II cells often contained numerous large and very dense lamellar bodies. A very mild inflammatory infiltration of the interstitium was found in the centroacinar region.

After 30 days of exposure to CdO a mild but distinct type II cell hyperplasia containing solitary or small groups of undifferentiated cells was present in the centroacinar region. In addition, a distinct alveolar bronchiolization was observed. Groups of Clara cells and brush cells (type III pneumocytes), sometimes mixed with undifferentiated cells, were often seen distal to the bronchiolo-alveolar border.

After 30 days of exposure and 20 weeks of recovery the extent of alveolar bronchiolization had increased while virtually no inflammatory infiltrate was present in the interstitium of the centroacinar region.

Chronic Inhalation Study

After chronic exposure to CdO a marked alveolar bronchiolization was present in the centroacinar region of all hamsters. The extent of the bronchiolization varied with the exposure concentration and duration (i.e., with the total Cd dose; Aufderheide et al. 1990).

The epithelial lining of the bronchiolized areas was composed of ciliated cells and Clara cells in proportions that are normally present in terminal bronchioli (Fig. 5). Clara cells in the hyperplastic areas frequently contained lamellar bodies, organelles normally characteristic of type II alveolar epithelial cells. In the border zone between bronchiolized areas and alveolar epithelium, cells exhibiting structural features of both type II pneumocytes and Clara cells were occasionally observed. In hamsters of the clean air control group such cells were observed very rarely and were always confined to the bronchiolo-alveolar border. In the epithelial lining of terminal bronchioli of exposed or unexposed hamsters, Clara cells containing lamellar bodies or cells that exhibited structural features of type II pneumocytes and Clara cells were never found.

Discussion

Our observations show that short-term exposure to Cd compounds causes an acute injury and necrotization of type I alveolar epithelial cells in the centroacinar region of the lung. For unknown reasons, the toxicity of cadmium compounds seems to be more pronounced in rats than in hamsters. The epithelial damage gives rise to a surge of epithelial proliferation and regeneration. From earlier studies it is known that alveolar type II pneumocytes represent the proliferative cell pool of the alveolar region, while type I alveolar epithelial cells are postmitotic and thus are incapable of proliferating (Evans et al. 1973; Adamson and Bowden 1974; for review, see Plopper and Dungworth 1987). Juvenile and proliferating type II pneumocytes can easily be recognized by their pale-staining cytoplasm in the light microscope. By TEM they exhibit ultrastructural features that are characteristic of undifferentiated cells as well as remnants of lamellar bodies typical for the mature cell type. These observations lead us to the assumption that the pale-staining cells are juvenile cells derived from type II pneumocytes.

The regenerative proliferation of type II pneumocytes initially leads to formation of a centroacinar hyperplasia of juvenile type II cells. However, these cells soon differentiate into type I alveolar epithelial cells (epithelial regeneration) or mature type II cells. This process starts very early after the onset of cellular proliferation. After only 3 days of exposure to Cd compounds cells were found to be in various stages of this differentiation process.

194   K.-U. Thiedemann et al.

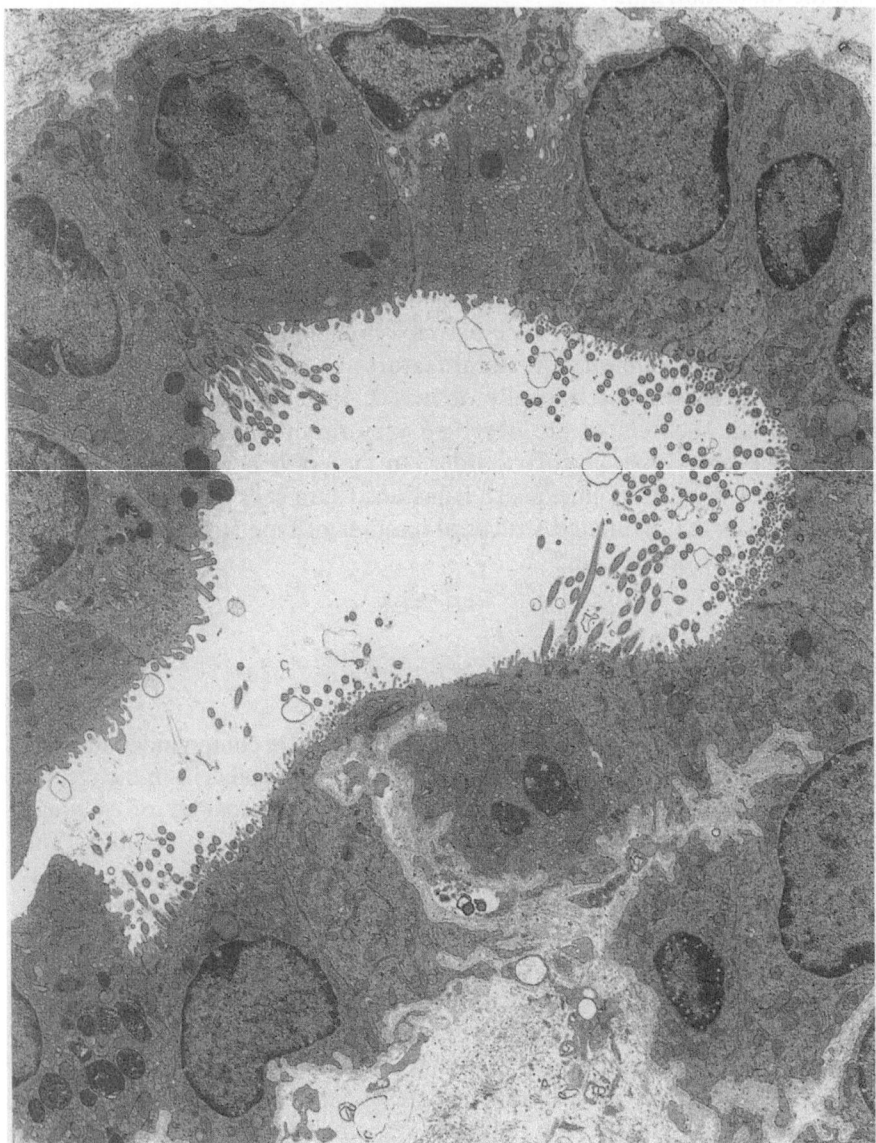

Fig. 5. TEM micrograph of a bronchiolized alveolar region in a hamster chronically exposed to CdO. The epithelial lining consists of Clara cells, ciliated cells, and occasional brush cells. Some of the cells with Clara cell morphology contain lamellar bodies

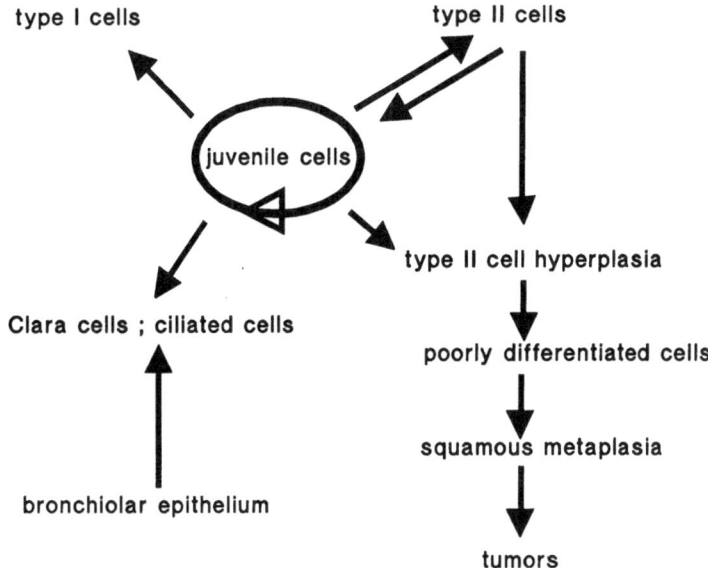

Fig. 6. Schematic representation of the differentiational pathways juvenile type II cells may pursue during epithelial regeneration

However, differentiation into type I alveolar epithelium and type II pneumocytes is not the only differentiational pathway that juvenile type II cells can persue. Our observations suggest that this cell pool may also give rise to bronchiolar epithelial cells (Fig. 6). This process evokes the occurrence of a distinct alveolar bronchiolization in the centroacinar region that, in early stages of the experiment, was lined by hyperplastic juvenile type II epithelial cells.

Alveolar bronchiolization is generally believed to be the result of a peripheral extension of bronchiolar epithelial cells (Nettesheim and Szakal 1972; for review, see Plopper and Dungworth 1987). Although we cannot exclude that proliferation of bronchiolar epithelial cells occurred during our experiment, we suggest that the time course of the alterations in the centroacinar region as well as the occurrence of Clara cells containing lamellar bodies and cells that exhibit morphologic features intermediate between type II cells and Clara cells in the epithelium of bronchiolized areas in hamsters are indications for a transdifferentiation of juvenile type II pneumocytes into bronchiolar epithelial cells.

The bronchiolar epithelium in the hamster seems to represent a stable cell type that is no longer susceptible to the carcinogenic action of Cd compounds, although Clara cells are known to represent the proliferative cell pool of the bronchioli. This is suggested by the lack of an increase in the tumor incidence in this species.

In the chronic experiment with hamsters, the transdifferentiation of type II pneumocytes into bronchiolar epithelial cells led to a complete disappearance of type II cell hyperplasias in the centroacinar region. In contrast, this pathway of cellular differentiation, although occurring initially, seemed to be impeded in the chronic experiment in rats. This is suggested by the occurrence of large numbers of hyperplastic type II cells in the bronchiolized areas in this species. The reason for this species difference is completely unknown at present. However, an altered composition of the interstitial matrix and differences in the cell/matrix interaction must be considered as a possible mechanism.

As persisting hyperplastic type II cells represent a proliferative cell pool, these cells may be subject to the action of mutagenic or carcinogenic substances. In rats we observed a population of morphologically poorly differentiated cells in areas of persisting type II cell hyperplasia. Although these cells do not show morphologic criteria of any specific population of lung epithelial cells, they reminded of hyperplastic type II cells by their size, shape, surface structure, and cytoplasmic organization. Therefore, we assume that these cells may be derived from type II pneumocytes by an as yet unknown mechanism. We speculate that these cells undergo or may already have undergone transformation and thus potentially may give rise to the formation of metaplasias or neoplasias. The occurrence of these poorly differentiated cells in the rat lung after chronic inhalation of Cd compounds may thus explain the species difference observed in the incidence of lung tumors.

As mentioned earlier, only few ultrastructural studies have described morphologic alterations of the human lung under pathologic conditions. Thus, little is known about the histogenesis of preneoplastic and neoplastic alterations of the peripheral lung. From the study of human lung tumors it was concluded that at least some of these neoplasms may arise from type II cells. This, however, must be regarded as mere speculation, as these investigations only described the tumors to consist of cells exhibiting the morphologic features of type II pneumocytes and did not study the differentitation pathways of possible tumor precursor cells. Furthermore, a study by Kawanami et al. (1982) presented evidence that proliferation of type II alveolar epithelial cells occurs in the majority of patients with fibrotic lung disorders where these cells were restricted to focal areas with less severe fibrosis. We therefore speculate that mechanisms of cellular damage, proliferation, differentiation, and transformation similar to those observed in our experimental animals may also take place in the human lung under pathologic conditions. There is no doubt that further careful studies are necessary and need to be initiated to increase the insight into the pathogenetic mechanisms of tumor development in humans.

Acknowledgements. The authors gratefully acknowledge the expert technical assistance of R. Griebel, A. von Malotki, and F. Müller. Supported by BMFT/DFVLR-HdA Nr. 01 KD 1838.

References

Adamson IYR, Bowden DH (1974) The type II cell as progenitor of alveolar epithelial regeneration. A cytodynamic study in mice after exposure to oxygen. Lab Invest 30:35–42

Aufderheide M, Mohr U, Thiedemann K-U, Heinrich U (1990) Quantitation of hyperplastic areas in hamster lungs after chronic inhalation of different cadmium compounds. Toxicol Environ Chem 27:173–180

Becci PJ, McDowell EM, Trump BF (1978) The respiratory epithelium:IV. Histogenesis of epidermoid metaplasia and carcinoma in situ in the hamster. J Natl Cancer Inst 61:577–586

Evans MJ, Cabral LJ, Stephens RJ, Freeman G (1973) Renewal of alveolar epithelium in the rat following exposure to NO_2. Am J Pathol 70:175–178

Glaser U, Hochrainer D, Otto FJ, Oldiges H (1990) Carcinogenicity and toxicity of four cadmium compounds inhaled by rats. Toxicol Environ Chem 27:153–162

Greenberg SD (1987) Carcinomas of the peripheral airways. In:McDowell EM (ed) Lung carcinomas. Churchill Livingstone, Edinburgh, pp 286–309

Heinrich U, Pott F, Dasenbrock C, König H, Peters L, Takenaka S (1986) Carcinogenicity studies in rats, hamsters, and mice using various cadmium compounds. In:Israel G (ed) Aerosols, formation and reactivity:Proceedings Second International Aerosol Conference, 22–26 September 1986, Berlin, Pergamon Press, Oxford, pp 290–294

Heinrich U, Peters L, Ernst H, Rittinghausen S, Dasenbrock C, Koenig H (1989) Investigation on the carcinogenic effects of various cadmium compounds after inhalation exposure in hamsters and mice. Exp Pathol 37:253–258

Kawanami O, Ferrans VJ, Crystal RG (1982) Structure of alveolar epithelial cells in patients with fibrotic lung disorders. Lab Invest 46:39–53

McDowell EM, Becci PJ, Barrett LA, Trump BF (1978) Morphogenesis and classification of lung cancer. In: Harris CC (ed) Pathogenesis and therapy of lung cancer. Dekker, New York, p 445

Nasiell M, Auer G, Kato H (1987) Cytological studies in man and animals on development of bronchogenic carcinoma. In: McDowell EM (ed) Lung carcinomas. Churchill Livingstone, Edinburgh, pp 207–242

Nettesheim P, Szakal AK (1972) Morphogenesis of alveolar bronchiolization. Lab Invest 26:210–219

Oldiges H, Hochrainer D, Glaser U (1989) Long-term inhalation study with Wistar rats and four cadmium compounds. Toxicol Environ Chem 19:217–222

Plopper CG, Dungworth DL (1987) Structure, function, cell injury and cell renewal of bronchiolar and alveolar epithelium. In: McDowell EM (ed) Lung carcinomas. Churchill Livingstone, Edinburgh, pp 94–128

Schüller HM (1987) Experimental carcinogenesis in the peripheral lung. In: McDowell EM (ed) Lung carcinomas. Churchill Livingstone, Edinburgh, pp 243–254

Thiedemann K-U, Nolte T, Rittinghausen S, Ernst H (1991) Immunohistochemistry and morphology of particle-induced pulmonary lesions. In: Graumann W, Drukker J (eds) Histo- and cytochemistry as a tool in environmental toxicology. Fischer, Stuttgart, pp 200–212 (Progress in histo- and cytochemistry, vol 23)

Trump BF, McDowell EM, Glavin F et al. (1978) The respiratory epithelium: III. Histogenesis of epidermoid metaplasia and carcinoma in situ in the human. J Natl Cancer Inst 61:563–575

Infectivity Models in Clinical Inhalation Studies

M.W. FRAMPTON

Assistant Professor of Medicine, University of Rochester Med. Center, Department of Medicine, Pulmonary and Critical Care Unit, 601 Elmwood Avenue, Box 692, Rochester, NY 14642-8692, USA

Introduction

The respiratory tract, because of its role in gas exchange, has a very large surface area in continuous contact with the atmosphere. Both atmospheric pollutants and infectious microorganisms gain access to the respiratory membrane, and it is reasonable to expect that inhaled toxic substances may interfere with the ability of the airways to defend against inhaled micro-organisms. In fact, evidence exists from both epidemiologic observations and animal exposure studies supporting this hypothesis. However, questions remain about which pollutants and what levels of exposure are important, who is most susceptible, what kinds of infections are involved, and the mechanisms by which susceptibility is altered. This paper will examine the role of clinical inhalation studies in providing answers to these and other questions.

Importance of Respiratory Infections

Despite the use of antibiotics, antisepsis, and vaccination, infectious diseases remain a major cause of morbidity and mortality, with respiratory infections leading the list. It was estimated in 1985 that respiratory tract infections were responsible for 1 250 000 hospital admissions at a direct cost of more than 4 billion dollars in the USA alone (Dixon 1985). Costs of treating the more than 78 million respiratory infections seen in the ambulatory setting exceeded 10 billion dollars. This does not include the cost in productivity of days lost to illness. Although most respiratory infections are of viral etiology and self-limited, viral infections increase the susceptibility to subsequent bacterial infections through changes in mucosal adherence and humoral and cell-mediated immunity (Welliver and Ogra 1988). Thus, increases in the incidence of viral infections related to pollutant exposure could lead to increases in fatal pneumonia and other long-term complications of infection such as bronchiectasis and airways hyperreactivity. Given the large number

U. Mohr et al. (Eds.)
Advances in Controlled Clinical
Inhalation Studies
© Springer-Verlag Berlin Heidelberg 1993

of people exposed to both atmospheric pollution and respiratory viruses, even brief impairment of a single component of respiratory host defense by exposure to a pollutant could have major public health implications. For these reasons, the development of sensitive methods to detect even minor pollutant effects on host defense is of paramount importance.

Nature of the Evidence

The evidence supporting a relationship between exposure to atmospheric pollutants and respiratory infection comes from two sources: epidemiologic studies and animal exposure studies. Pennington (1988) has reviewed this evidence for pollutants related to automotive emissions. Consideration of these data forms the basis on which hypotheses are generated, and the design of human clinical studies is directed at testing those hypotheses.

One example of the need for human studies to address hypotheses derived from the previous database is exposure to nitrogen dioxide (NO_2). Studies of children residing in homes near a munitions plant in Chattanooga described a relationship between atmospheric NO_2 levels and the incidence of respiratory illness (Shy et al. 1970; Pearlman et al. 1971). Subsequent studies suggested a link between childhood respiratory infection and use of gas stoves for cooking (Speizer et al. 1980; Melia et al. 1977). These studies have been criticized (Pennington 1988; Samet et al. 1987), and other studies have failed to confirm a relationship between indoor NO_2 levels and respiratory infection (Melia et al. 1982; Florey et al. 1979; Keller et al. 1979). However, the data have provided an impetus for the development of animal models to study the impact of NO_2 exposure on host defense.

The relationship between NO_2 exposure and increased susceptibility to infection has been most clearly established using the mouse model (reviewed in Frampton and Roberts 1989). NO_2 exposure increases the mortality of mice challenged with bacterial aerosols, and the mechanisms include decreased killing of organisms within the lung parenchyma, presumably by alveolar macrophages (AM). However, the ability to extrapolate from these animal infectivity models to human exposure has been limited by a number of problems. These include (1) use of exposure levels well above that commonly found in human exposure, (2) use of microorganisms that are not common pathogens in humans, (3) the questionable relevance of mortality as an endpoint, and (4) differences between murine and human mechanisms of host defense. Improving the design of animal studies including the use of relevant exposure levels and challenge with common pathogenic organisms will help to overcome these limitations. However, human clinical studies are needed to determine whether findings from animal studies have relevance to human respiratory defense. Pennington (1988) has recently recommended that such studies receive a high research priority.

Experimental Approaches Using Clinical Studies

Studies examining the effects of pollutants on host defense in humans can be categorized according to experimental design as follows: (1) effects of in vivo pollutant exposure on individual mechanisms of host defense, (2) effects of in vivo pollutant exposure on responses to infectious challenge in vivo, and (3) effects of in vivo pollutant exposure on infectious challenge in vitro. Each of these approaches will be discussed in turn, using examples from reported studies.

Effects of In Vivo Pollutant Exposure on Individual Mechanisms of Host Defense

In this approach, humans are exposed to the pollutant, and the effects on one or more specific elements of host defense are then assessed, such as airway clearance mechanisms, local inflammatory responses, or various measures of immunologic competence. This approach avoids the risk, discomforts, and technical difficulties of exposing volunteers to infectious agents. The primary disadvantages of this approach are two. First, pollutant exposure may alter mechanisms of host defense that are unknown, poorly understood, or untestable. Measuring the measurable may not provide an accurate assessment of effects on host defense. Second, observations of effects on isolated mechanisms of defense neglect the integrated functioning of the organism in response to the infectious challenge. Alterations in one or more measured responses do not necessarily prove the existence of a deficit in host defense for the whole organism. These limitations underscore the importance of using data from animal models to target specific defense mechanisms for study.

An example in which human clinical studies have been used to explore the effects on a specific mechanism of host defense is that of exposure to acid aerosols on mucociliary clearance. Mechanical clearance of inhaled microorganisms that deposit on the respiratory mucous layer is an important element of respiratory host defense (Green et al. 1977). Ciliary movement propels particles and organisms to the oropharynx where they are swallowed or expectorated. Mucociliary clearance can be assessed in humans using timed clearance of radiolabelled particles; careful control of tracer particle size determines the relative deposition in various regions of the respiratory tract and thus the region of the lung in which clearance is being measured. Schlesinger (1990) has reviewed techniques for the measurement of respiratory clearance.

Leikauf et al. (1981) and Spektor et al. (1989) demonstrated a reduction in the clearance rate of radiolabelled aerosols following 1- and 2-h exposure to H_2SO_4 aerosols at a level of $100 \, \mu g/m^3$. These data confirmed observations in animals (Schlesinger 1989). It is logical to assume that decreases in clearance rates could increase susceptibility to infection by prolonging the opportunity for contact between inhaled infectious agents and respiratory epithelial cells. However, increased susceptibility to infections in response to exposure levels that alter mucociliary clearance has not been established in animals or humans, leaving unclear the implications of these observations for human health.

Effects of In Vivo Pollutant Exposure on Responses to Infectious Challenge In Vivo

In designing experiments to study pollutant effects on infectivity, the most direct approach combines pollutant exposure with infectious challenge in vivo. This model has been explored extensively in animals, most notably for NO_2 exposure using the mouse model as discussed previously. For human studies, the challenging infectious organism should have the potential to infect regions of the respiratory tract most susceptible to the effects of the pollutant under study and yet must be sufficiently benign so that resulting infections are self-limited and without potential for serious complications. In addition, accurate methods for assessing the presence of infection, quantitating the shedding of infectious organisms, and assessing specific immune responses should be available. An example is the study of infections caused by *Mycoplasma*. They are common causes of respiratory infections in humans, and animal data exist suggesting that exposure to NO_2 is associated with an increase in susceptibility to infection with *M. pulmonis* (Parker et al. 1989). However, the difficulties involved in culturing these organisms from secretions derived from infected subjects, as well as the risk for developing pneumonia, limit the possibility of investigating their role in the human setting.

Table 1 lists the three studies that have used in vivo infectious challenge in humans to assess the effects of pollutant exposure. Two of these studies examined effects of pollutant exposure (SO_2 and ozone) on experimental rhinovirus infection; a third studied effects of NO_2 exposure on infection with a reassortant, cold-adapted influenza virus. None of these studies demonstrated unequivocal impairment in host defense against the challenge agent. Exposure to SO_2 was associated with a decrease in symptoms and virus shedding in infected individuals. It is important to consider that the viruses used in these studies, including the cold-adapted influenza virus, were incapable of infecting the lower respiratory tract. Thus, possible alterations in defense mechanisms at the alveolar level, which has particular relevance for NO_2 exposure, were not tested. The use of wild-type influenza virus to induce experimental infection in humans has already been tried in studies evaluating the efficacy of vaccines (Clements et al. 1984), and the use of such viruses in studies of NO_2 exposure, similar to those of Goings et al. (1989), should be considered.

Table 1. Human clinical studies utilizing infectious challenge in vivo

Reference	Pollutant	Agent	Endpoints	Findings
Andersen et al. 1977	SO_2 5 ppm, 4 h × 2	Rhinovirus	• Symptoms • Virus shedding • Nasal clearance • Systemic antibody	• Decreased symptoms • Decreased virus shedding
Henderson et al. 1988	O_3 0.3 ppm, 6 h × 5	Rhinovirus	• Virus shedding • Nasal inflammation • Nasal interferon • Lymphocyte proliferation • Nasal and systemic antibodies	• No effect
Goings et al. 1989	NO_2 1–3 ppm, 2 h × 3	Cold-adapted influenzavirus	• Symptoms • Virus shedding • Nasal and systemic antibodies	• No definite effect

A corollary to in vivo infectious challenge as described above is the study of individuals with naturally acquired infections. Subjects with uncomplicated viral infections represent an important opportunity to study pollutant effects on host defense. Utell et al. (1980) observed that volunteers with uncomplicated influenza A infection exposed to nitrate aerosols demonstrated decreases in specific airway conductance. This occurred at a level of nitrate exposure that did not cause airway constriction in normal or asymptomatic asthmatic subjects. Similar studies utilizing oxidant exposure and focussing on mechanisms of host defense may prove enlightening.

Effects of In Vivo Pollutant Exposure on Responses to Infectious Challenge In Vitro

This approach requires the sampling of tissue or cells from subjects following exposure, with assessment in vitro of effects on those tissues or cells caused by infectious agents. This model has become useful because the growth in our understanding of immunological responses to infectious challenge permits the study of specific cellular effects. It avoids the difficulties associated with infecting volunteers directly. This approach is similar to the first one described above in that only the role of the cells or tissues being challenged is evaluated, and the potential cellular and tissue interactions that comprise the response to infectious challenge in vivo are not evaluated.

The development of bronchoalveolar lavage (BAL) to sample distal airway cells from humans has provided an opportunity to obtain immunocompetent cells from the lungs of subjects exposed to environmental pollutants. This technique has been used to characterize the inflammatory response to ozone exposure (Seltzer et al. 1986; Koren et al. 1989; Graham and Koren 1990). The predominant cell recovered by BAL is the AM, believed to have a central role in phagocytosis and the killing of organisms that reach the alveoli, as an accessory cell in the cellular immune response, and in the release of chemotactic and activating cytokines for inflammatory cells (Sibille and Reynolds 1990). It is likely that AM play an important role in the defense against viral infections, since one of the histological features of viral pneumonia is accumulation of macrophages in the alveoli (Jakab et al. 1983). Frampton et al. (1989) used BAL to obtain AM from subjects exposed to NO_2 and then challenged the AM with infectious influenza virus in vitro. The rate of decline in the quantity of infectious virus over a 5-day period was measured, after exposure to both air and 0.6 ppm NO_2. In addition, interleukin-1 (IL-1) activity released by AM was quantitated at baseline and after challenge with influenza virus. Exposure to NO_2 was associated with a reduced inactivation of influenza virus when compared with air exposure (1.96 vs 1.25 $\log_{10}$ plaque-forming units on day 2 of incubation, $P < 0.07$). Four of nine subjects accounted for the observed difference, and cells from these four subjects demonstrated an increase in IL-1 production after NO_2 vs air, whereas the five remaining subjects exhibited decreased IL-1 production after NO_2. These findings suggested the possibility that differences exist between individuals in the effect of NO_2 exposure on AM-virus interactions. Whether such differences correspond to differences in host defense has yet to be established, but studies such as these may have a role in identifying subgroups of individuals for further study.

Future Directions

The design of human clinical studies should address three areas of particular importance. First, there is a need for deliberate coordination between animal and human studies of pollutant effects on host defense. Studies specifically designed to compare effects in animals and in humans following similar exposures and using similar response measures will help to overcome the difficulties in extrapolating from animal studies to human exposures. Such studies, using brief exposures, will help to identify the most appropriate animal models for the study of a given issue. These animal models can then be utilized to study the effects of prolonged exposures to provide clues about chronic health effects.

Second, human clinical studies should be directed toward the identification of individuals most susceptible to effects of pollutants on host defense. Populations likely to have altered host defenses should be targeted for study, including patients with chronic obstructive pulmonary disease, chronic bronchitis, and normal elderly subjects. Individuals with naturally acquired viral infections such as rhinovirus, influenza virus, and respiratory syncytial virus should be studied to determined if pollutant exposure potentiates the virus-mediated immune suppression or alters the inflammatory response to the infection. These studies should include assessment of effects on clearance mechanisms, local and systemic antibody responses, and cell-mediated immunity. One goal of such studies should be to identify markers of susceptibility that can be used to target groups of individuals for subsequent study.

Third, human clinical studies need to be coordinated with in vitro exposure of cells and tissues. Findings from clinical studies should be used to guide the design of in vitro exposure systems that best reflect the changes seen in vivo. Such systems could then be used in working out mechanisms of pollutant effect.

Clinical studies of exposure to atmospheric pollutants have traditionally been descriptive in nature, with effects on pulmonary function being the primary response indicator. With regard to effects on host defense, we are ready to move beyond the descriptive phase and utilize clinical exposure studies to answer some specific questions about pollutant effects on human respiratory defense. Accomplishing this will require careful integration of data from human studies with that from animal, epidemiologic, and in vitro exposure studies.

Acknowledgements. This work was supported by: National Institutes of Health grant RO1 ESO2679; Division of Research Resources grant RR00044; and Health Effects Institute contract no. 91-2.

References

Andersen I, Jenson PL, Reed SE, Craig JW, Proctor DF, Adams GK (1977) Induced rhinovirus infection under controlled exposure to sulfur dioxide. Arch Environ Health 32:120-126

Clements ML, Betts RF, Murphy BR (1984) Advantage of live attenuated cold-adapted influenza A virus over inactivated vaccine for A/Washington/80 (H3N2) wild-type virus infection. Lancet i:705-708

Dixon RE (1985) Economic costs of respiratory tract infections in the United States. Am J Med 78 [Suppl 6B]:45-51

Florey CduV, Melia RJW, Chinn S et al. (1979) The relation between respiratory illness in primary school children and the use of gas for cooking. III. Nitrogen dioxide, respiratory illness and lung infection. Int J Epidemiol 8:347-353

Frampton MW, Roberts NJ Jr (1989) Respiratory infection and oxidants. In: Utell MJ, Frank R (eds) Susceptibility to inhaled pollutants. American Society for Testing and Materials, Philadelphia, pp 182-191

Frampton MW, Smeglin AM, Roberts NJ Jr, Finkelstein JN, Morrow PE, Utell MJ (1989) Nitrogen dioxide exposure in vivo and human alveolar macrophage inactivation of influenza virus in vitro. Environ Res 48:179-192

Goings SAJ, Kulle TJ, Bascom R et al. (1989) Effect of nitrogen dioxide exposure on susceptibility to influenza A virus infection in healthy adults. Am Rev Respir Dis 139:1075-1081

Graham DE, Koren HS (1990) Biomarkers of inflammation in ozone-exposed humans. Comparison of the nasal and bronchoalveolar lavage. Am Rev Respir Dis 142:152-156

Green GM, Jakab GJ, Low RB, Davis GS (1977) Defense mechanisms of the respiratory membrane. Am Rev Respir Dis 115:479-514

Henderson FW, DuBovi EJ, Harder S, Seal E Jr, Graham D (1988) Experimental rhinovirus infection in human volunteers exposed to ozone. Am Rev Respir Dis 137:1124-1128

Jakab GJ, Astry CL, Warr GA (1983) Alveolitis induced by influenza virus. Am Rev Respir Dis 128:730-739

Keller MD, Lanese RR, Mitchell RI, Cote RW (1979) Respiratory illness in households using gas and electricity for cooking. I. Survey of incidence. Environ Res 19:495-503

Koren HS, Devlin RB, Graham DE et al. (1989) Ozone-induced inflammation in the lower airways of human subjects. Am Rev Respir Dis 139:407-415

Leikauf G, Yeates DB, Wales KA, Spektor D, Albert RE, Lippmann M (1981) Effects of sulfuric acid aerosol on respiratory mechanics and mucociliary particle clearance in healthy nonsmoking adults. Am Ind Hyg Assoc J 42:273-282

Melia RJW, Florey CduV, Altman DG, Swan AV (1977) Association between gas cooking and respiratory disease in children. Br Med J 2:149-152

Melia RJW, Florey CduV, Morris RW et al. (1982) Childhood respiratory illness and the home environment. II. Association between respiratory illness and nitrogen dioxide, temperature and relative humidity. Int J Epidemiol 11:164-169

Parker RF, Davis JK, Cassell GH et al. (1989) Short-term exposure to nitrogen dioxide enhances susceptibility to murine respiratory mycoplasmosis and decreases intrapulmonary killing of *Mycoplasma pulmonis*. Am Rev Respir Dis 140:502–512

Pearlman ME, Finklea JF, Creason JP, Shy CM, Young MM, Horton RJM (1971) Nitrogen dioxide and lower respiratory illness. Pediatrics 47:391–398

Pennington JE (1988) Effects of automotive emissions on susceptibility to respiratory infections. In: Watson AY, Bates RR, Kennedy D (eds) Air pollution, the automobile, and public health. Health Effects Institute, National Academy Press, Washington, DC, pp 499–518

Samet JM, Marbury MC, Spengler JD (1987) Health effects and sources of indoor air pollution. Part I. Am Rev Respir Dis 136:1486–1508

Schlesinger RB (1989) Factors affecting the response of lung clearance systems to acid aerosols: role of exposure concentration, exposure time and relative acidity. Environ Health Perspect 79:121–126

Schlesinger RB (1990) The interaction of inhaled toxicants with respiratory tract clearance mechanisms. CRC Crit Rev Toxicol 20:257–286

Seltzer J, Bigby BG, Stulbarg M et al. (1986) O_3-induced change in bronchial reactivity to methacholine and airway inflammation in humans. J Appl Physiol 60:1321–1326

Shy CM, Creason JP, Pearlman ME, McClain KE, Benson FB (1970) The Chattanooga schoolchildren study: effects of community exposure to nitrogen dioxide. II. Incidence of acute respiratory illness. J Air Pollut Control Assoc 20:582–588

Sibille Y, Reynolds HY (1990) Macrophages and polymorphonuclear neutrophils in lung defense and injury. Am Rev Respir Dis 141:471–501

Speizer FE, Ferris B Jr, Bishop YMM, spengler J (1980) Respiratory disease rates and pulmonary function in children associated with NO_2 exposure. Am Rev Respir Dis 121:3–10

Spektor DM, Yen BM, Lippmann M (1989) Effect of concentration and cumulative exposure of inhaled sulfuric acid on tracheobronchial particle clearance in healthy humans. Environ Health Perspect 79:167–172

Utell MJ, Aquilina AT, Hall WJ et al. (1980) Development of airway reactivity to nitrates in subjects with influenza. Am Rev Respir Dis 121:233–241

Welliver RC, Ogra PL (1988) Immunology of respiratory viral infections. Annu Rev Med 39:147–162

Does the Pulmonary Surfactant System Yield Meaningful Parameters in Inhalation Toxicity Studies? A Review

R. Klingebiel and U. Heinrich

Fraunhofer-Institut für Toxikologie und Aerosolforschung, Nikolai-Fuchs-Straße 1, W-3000 Hannover 61, FRG

Introduction

The existence of a surface active agent (surfactant) in the lung was first postulated by von Neergard in 1929. He himself did not seem to recognize the importance of his discovery, and it was up to other investigators (Clements and Chambers 1957; Pattle 1955) to supply experimental evidence for such a substance, almost 30 years later. Soon afterwards (Avery and Mead 1959) the pathophysiological importance of an immature surfactant system for the respiratory distress syndrome of the newborn (IRDS) was described. The therapeutic implication of this was successfully assessed by Fujiwara et al. (1980), who demonstrated that endotracheal replacement therapy with surfactant reduced the severity and mortality of IRDS. A historical review on the advances of surfactant research was published by Tierney in 1989.

In the meantime numerous investigations have confirmed that the effects of pulmonary surfactant comprise not only modification of alveolar surface tension but also modulation of the alveolar immune response (Baugham and Strohofer 1989; Catanzaro et al. 1988), participation in alveolar and bronchial clearance mechanisms (Morgenroth 1986), and impact on deposition and clearance of inhaled material even in the upper airways (Gehr et al. 1990a,b; Schürch et al. 1990). Furthermore, pulmonary surfactant is a characteristic metabolic product of the type II pneumocyte and should yield some information about its morphologic and functional integrity.

Thus the pulmonary surfactant system is of interest in pulmonary toxicology because of its effects on respiratory mechanics and nonspecific defense mechanisms and because it is closely associated with the type II pneumocyte.

U. Mohr et al. (Eds).
Advances in Controlled Clinical
Inhalation Studies
© Springer-Verlag Berlin Heidelberg 1993

Composition and Metabolism

Some important aspects of surfactant biochemistry are mentioned below. For more detailed information the reader is referred to the comprehensive reviews on the topic by other authors (Harwood 1987; Rooney 1985, 1987; Van Golde 1985; Van Golde et al. 1988; J.R. Wright 1990).

The pulmonary surfactant system is constituted predominantly by phospholipids (about 90%) and glycoproteins, the so-called apoproteins. Also present are small amounts of cholesterol, neutral lipids, and carbohydrates.

Pulmonary surfactant is synthesized characteristically in the endoplasmatic reticulum of type II pneumocytes, from where it is transported via the Golgi field to the lamellar bodies. The lamellar body secretes its content via exocytosis into the alveolar space, where it is reconstructed to the surfactant monolayer, passing through an intermediate form called tubular myelin. Recently Hills (1990) questioned what he called the "conventional" theory regarding the mechanisms of actions of surfactant and suggested a different model, featuring a discontinuous alveolar fluid layer with the surfactant being absorbed directly to the epithelial surface.

The phospholipid constituents of surfactant are subdivided into phosphatidylcholine (PC; 60%–70%) and phosphatidylglycerol (PG; 7%–10%) as well as phosphatidylinositol (PI), phosphatidylserine (PS), phosphatidylethanolamine (PE), and sphingomyelin (SPH), these amounting each to about 3%–5% of surfactant by weight. Phospholipids are suited for covering interfaces because of their amphiphilic character. They have a polar, hydrophilic head with the phosphatidic aminoacid residue and lipophilic fatty acid tails directed toward the alveolar space. Phospholipids are part of cell membranes and can also be found in serum. Nevertheless, the high percentage of phosphatidylglycerol seems to be specific for surfactant. PC consists mainly of disaturated dipalmitoylphosphatidylcholine (DPPC), which is responsible for lowering surface tension at end-expiration. This composition of pulmonary surfactant is not restricted to man but seems to be about the same in all adult mammalians investigated up to now (Harwood 1987; Harwood et al. 1975).

Associated with the surfactant phospholipids is a group of glycoproteins called SP-A (28–36 kDa, reduced), SP-B (8–9 kDa, reduced), and SP-C (4–5 kDa, reduced). More recently Persson et al. described a further glycoprotein to be synthesized by the type II pneumocyte which they called SP-D (43 kDa, reduced) (Persson et al. 1989, 1990). In 1991 Singh et al. released a report about a hydrophilic, 7.5-kDa surfactant-associated protein, indicating that our knowledge concerning the constituents of the pulmonary surfactant system is still somewhat incomplete. SP-B and especially SP-C are hydrophobic proteins, being isolated in the chloroform phase with the phospholipids during lipid extraction. Lately the current understanding of surfactant protein functions has been reviewed by Possmayer (1990).

Obviously SP-A is not a necessary constituent for surfactant replacement therapy, but new experimental evidence suggests that it may support the biophysical activities of SP-B and SP-C (Cockshutt et al. 1990). SP-A plays a role in surfactant turnover as it suppresses secretion from the type II cells and enhances surfactant uptake. It also protects the intraalveolar surfactant from inhibition by transudated plasma proteins such as fibrinogen degradation products as may occur during the course of the adult respiratory distress syndrome (ARDS) (Cockshutt et al. 1990; O'Brodovich et al. 1990; Venkitaraman et al. 1990). Furthermore, SP-A seems to interact with alveolar macrophages, stimulating oxygen radical generation and phagocytosis of viruses and bacteria (Tenner et al. 1989; Van Iwaarden et al. 1990, 1991). SP-B is important for refinement of the surfactant monolayer during expiration in terms of increasing the concentration of the disaturated PC (Possmayer 1990). This is thought to be necessary for the end-expiratory surface tension reduction to values near 0 mN/m as known from the intact alveolus. SP-C enhances the adsorption of phospholipids to the alveolar air/water interface (Possmayer 1990). SP-B and SP-C also seem to play a role in the regulation of intraalveolar surfactant recycling (Rice et al. 1989).

Phospholipids and apoproteins are synthesized in the type II pneumocyte microsomes, stored in lamellar bodies and secreted together into the alveolar space. As some enzymes involved in PG biosynthesis are associated with mitochondria, PG formation may not be restricted to the endoplasmatic reticulum (Van Golde et al. 1988). New experimental evidence suggests that compared to the microsomes the intracellular storage granule, the lamellar body, is highly enriched with the most surface-active surfactant components, i.e., DPPC and the hydrophobic apoproteins (Longmuir and Haynes 1991; Oosterlaken-Dijksterhuis et al. 1991).

Surfactant synthesis and secretion are subject to stimulation by a number of hormones and mediators (adrenergic stimuli, thyroxine, estrogen, adenosine, etc.) as well as by simple mechanical extension of the alveolus during deep inspiration (Hildebran et al. 1981; Nicholas et al. 1982). The alveolar turnover time varies among phospholipids from 4 h (PG) to 8 h (PC). Studies performed with labeled substrates indicate a reutilization of intraalveolar surfactant by the type II pneumocyte of up to 90% (Van Golde et al. 1988). Other factors contributing to the alveolar surfactant clearance are uptake by other alveolar and airway epithelial cells, intra-alveolar degradation, phagocytosis by macrophages and loss into the bronchi and further upwards via the ciliary escalator (Wright 1990).

Functional Aspects

Surfactant and Respiratory Mechanics

Surfactant may reduce end-expiratory surface tension in the alveolus to values near 0 mN/m as determined in vitro by the Wilhelmy balance

(Clements and Chambers 1957; Goerke 1974). This prevents alveolar collapse, as would occur if surface tension values of water (72 mN/m) existed in the alveolus. On the other hand, surfactant increases surface tension in the expanded state thus supporting expiration and protecting the tissue from excessive expansion (Van Golde et al. 1988). Alveolar surface tension and the retractive forces of the lung tissue are the two constituents determining pulmonary compliance or distensibility (Mathe et al. 1974). Liu et al. (1991) concluded from studies with glass capillaries creating pressure and flow characteristics similar to those in the respiratory bronchiole that surfactant also secures airflow in the airways adjoining to the alveolus.

Predominantly the disaturated fraction of PC is responsible for the surface activity, due to the rigidity of its fatty acid chains supported by the hydrophobic apoproteins in terms of spreading and formation of the monolayer (Possmayer 1990; Van Golde et al. 1988). By reducing the surface tension the transudation pressure from the vascular system into the alveolar space is decreased, which may be of special interest in disease processes leading to alveolar edema (Van Golde et al. 1988). A further function of surfactant covering the watery hypothase is minimizing the pulmonary water evaporation, which in the nondiseased state may amount to almost 20% of the physiological daily water loss. It can be speculated whether this represents even the principal surfactant function in species not showing alveolar structures, such as snakes.

Surfactant and the Nonspecific Local Infection Defense

As a continuous layer on the alveolar air-water interface, surfactant inhibits adhesion and tissue penetration of foreign bodies in the lung periphery. It may coat the intruder and subsequently facilitate the recognition and phagocytosis by macrophages. It is thought to protect the ciliary system from sticking induced by the mucus (Morgenroth and Newhouse 1988), and in vitro investigations suggest a promotion of ciliary beat frequency by surfactant (Kakuta et al. 1991). Recently it was demonstrated that surfactant is also important for the displacement of inhaled particles from the airway surface to the aqueous subphase and further down to the epithelium in the upper airways (Gehr et al. 1990a,b; Schürch et al. 1990). There the particles would be cleared slowly by phagocytosis rather than by the quickly operating mucociliary escalator.

Accumulating evidence suggests that surfactant exerts immunomodulatory effects in the alveolar space. Phospholipids by themselves seem to act antimicrobially toward pneumococci (Coonrod 1987). Proliferation (Ansfield and Benson 1980; Ansfield et al. 1979; Catanzaro et al. 1988; Rich 1990; Wilsher et al. 1988a,b,c) and cytotoxicity (Coonrod 1987) of lymphocytes as well as the natural killer cell activity against tumor cells

(Baugham and Strohofer 1989) were shown to be reduced by the pulmonary surfactant system. Suppression of lymphocyte proliferation has been attributed to PC and PG whereas PE seemed to exert inductive effects on this cell type. In contrast, surfactant may enhance the local infection defense by stimulating alveolar macrophage functions. Migration, phagocytosis, and intracellular killing of bacteria (O'Neill et al. 1984a) as well as the tumor cytotoxicity (Baugham et al. 1987) of alveolar macrophages were enhanced by surfactant.

Among the first investigators in this area of research, La Force et al. showed in 1973 that staphylococci were killed intracellularly by alveolar macrophages of rats only after coincubation with alveolar lining fluid. Similar findings were reported by Juers et al. (1976) and Webb and Jeska (1986). Jonsson et al. (1986) did not obtain comparable results in their experiments with human alveolar macrophages and *Staphylococcus aureus* and *Haemophilus influenzae*. In 1987 Baugham et al. presented evidence that PC, SPH, and PG may increase cytotoxicity of macrophages and monocytes whereas PI proved to have the opposite effect.

The major apoprotein, SP-A, seems to participate in the immuno-modulatory effects of the pulmonary surfactant system as well (Schlepper-Schäfer et al. 1989; Tenner et al. 1989; Van Iwaarden et al. 1990, 1991). In 1989 Wright and Tenner reported that phagocytosis of antibody-labeled sheep erythrocytes was enhanced by SP-A, and van Iwaarden et al. (1990, 1991) observed increased oxygen radical production and enhanced phago-cytosis of bacteria and viruses by rat alveolar macrophages subsequent to coincubation with SP-A. In contrast, Weber et al. (1990) found a decrease in the superoxide anion production of canine alveolar macrophages coincubated with canine SP-A and subsequently stimulated with phorbol-12-myristate-13-acetate. By a still unknown cause canine SP-A seems to act differently in terms of macrophage activation compared to rat and human SP-A, as was confirmed by Oosting et al. (1991, 1992). Interestingly, Weber et al. did not see any inhibitory effect of SP-A on the respiratory burst of activated macrophages after treatment of SP-A with collagenase. Wispe et al. (1990) recently demonstrated that tumor necrosis factor alpha, another macrophage-derived enzyme such as collagenase, inhibits surfactant protein (SP-A, SP-B) expression in human pulmonary adenocarcinoma cell lines.

Thus complex interactions between the pulmonary surfactant system and alveolar macrophages occur especially during inflammatory processes in the alveolar space.

Surfactant and Pulmonary Diseases

The classical concept about surfactant and pulmonary diseases is based on the findings of Avery and Mead (1959), who were the first to describe surfactant deficiency as the decisive pathogenetic factor in IRDS. In the meantime several investigations have confirmed that surfactant abnormalities are present in a number of respiratory tract affections such as ARDS (Hallman et al. 1982; Mason 1987), alveolar proteinosis (Honda et al. 1989; Hook et al. 1986), idiopathic pulmonary fibrosis (Honda et al. 1988; Hughes et al. 1989; McCormack et al. 1988; Robinson et al. 1988), sarcoidesis (Baugham et al. 1985; Honda et al. 1988; Sallerin et al. 1984), extrinsic allergic alveolitis (Hughes and Haslam 1990), and others (Hallman et al. 1985). Subject to discussion nowadays is the way in which surfactant alteration and subsequent macrophage function changes are involved in the pathogenesis of pneumonia (Baugham et al. 1984).

The most comprehensive knowledge about pathogenetic effects of surfactant has been gained in regard to IRDS. It is well established that the surfactant deficiency encountered in these preterm infants causes atelectasis and thus life-threatening hypoxemia (Avery and Mead 1959; Robertson 1989c). Multicenter trials conducted to evaluate the benefit of surfactant replacement therapy underlined the efficiency of this therapeutic procedure, although there may still be some controversy about timing, dose, and preparation of the artificial surfactant (Gitlin et al. 1987; Hallman et al. 1989b; Merritt et al. 1989; Robertson 1989a,b,d; Shapiro and Notter 1988; Strayer et al. 1989). Lethality and long-term complications such as bronchopulmonary dysplasia were significantly reduced (Robertson 1989a,b,d). Some concern arose with regard to the immunological implications of surfactant replacement therapy. In 1986 Strayer et al. described circulating immune complexes between surfactant and surfactant antibodies in children with IRDS. In subsequent investigations (Strayer et al. 1991a,b) they assessed the immunogenicity of human and animal surfactant preparations as used in the therapy of the respiratory distress syndrome. They were able to show antibody-related inhibition of in vitro surface activity of human and animal surfactant as assessed by the pulsating bubble surfactometer.

One of the difficulties encountered in the therapy of ARDS that disables simple transcription of IRDS treatment principles is that in ARDS inhibition of surfactant effects seems to be more important than deficiency (Enhorning 1989; Hallman et al. 1989a; Lachmann 1989b; Mason 1987; O'Brodovich et al. 1990). Inhibition occurs due to leakage of plasma proteins into the alveolar space. Thus research is focusing on surfactant preparations less sensitive to functional impairment by fibrinogen degradation products (Seeger et al. 1989). Furthermore, products of activated inflammatory cells recruited into the alveolar space in the course of the ARDS have been thought to participate in surfactant inhibition and degradation (Ryan et al. 1991).

Alveolar proteinosis is characterized by excessive accumulation of surfactant material in the alveolar space (Hook et al. 1986). Similar pathological changes have been found in rats exposed to silica representing an animal model for pneumoconiosis (Heppleston and Young 1972; Heppleston et al. 1972, 1975). The surface activity of surfactant from lungs with proteinosis did not seem to be adversely affected (Heppleston et al. 1975). In terms of pneumoconiosis, increased extracellular surfactant can be seen as a protective device. Surfactant coats the foreign particle thus enhancing its phagocytosis and inhibits the intracellular particle contact with lysosomal enzymes (Schimmelpfeng et al. 1989). On the other hand, overloading of alveolar macrophages with phagocytosed surfactant material may also occur and could impair macrophage activities.

As far as surfactant is concerned the idiopathic pulmonary fibrosis is marked by a reduction in PG and SP-A (Honda et al. 1988; Hughes et al. 1989; McCormack et al. 1988, 1991; Robinson et al. 1988) whereas in the bronchoalveolar lavage fluid (BALF) of sarcoidosis patients PC was reduced (Gitlin et al. 1987).

Characteristic surfactant lipid alterations, i.e., increases in PE levels, have also been encountered in the BALF of patients suffering from extrinsic allergic alveolits (also known as hypersensitivity pneumonitis) (Hughes and Haslam 1990). Interestingly, PE has been shown to induce lymphocyte responses in the peripheral airways, and lung biopsies of patients suffering from extrinsic allergic alveolitis showed increased numbers of lymphocytes in the alveolar walls.

Surfactant and Inhalation Toxicology

Inhaled pollutants penetrating deep into the lung inevitably come into contact with the surfactant layer as it is closest to the intraalveolar space. As mentioned above, surfactant exerts a number of protective effects in this area, and the question arises as to how it is affected by interaction with common environmental pollutants. Such an interaction may take place directly or indirectly by virtue of type II cell damage, recruitment of inflammatory cells with subsequent release of mediators, activation of alveolar macrophages, damage to the alveolocapillary membrane leading to transudation of inhibitory proteins into the alveolar space, and by other mechanisms.

For clinical purposes the pulmonary surfactant system is usually assessed by harvesting BALF and subjecting it to the analytical procedure of interest. As BALF in small laboratory rodents commonly is collected postmortem by rinsing saline solution through the whole lung, instead of a bronchoalveolar segment as in patients, the term bronchoalveolar lavage is subsequently replaced by the more exact term lung lavage.

Evidence has been shown for impairment of the pulmonary surfactant system following exposure to a variety of inhalative pollutants such as O_3, NO_2, diesel exhaust, cigarette smoke, dusts and other substances (Haagsman and van Golde 1985). What is known at present about effects of some important environmental pollutants on the pulmonary surfactant system is discussed in more detail below.

Effects of Inhalative Pollutants on the Pulmonary Surfactant System

Ozone

Ozone is the most important component of photooxidative smog. Photolysis of NO_2 results in the generation of NO and highly reactive oxygen. The latter reacts with oxygen to generate ozone. Ozone is water soluble only to a small extent. It advances easily down to the alveolar region and reacts there with phospholipid components of the cell membranes (Mustafa and Tierney 1978). Alveolar type I cell damage is the characteristic morphologic finding of ozone-induced alveolar lesions (Dungworth 1989). Epidemiologic and experimental evidence has been presented for a variety of detrimental ozone effects on the respiratory tract, including decreased pulmonary function, increased nonspecific airway reacticity, airway inflammation, enhanced lung infectivity, and even impact on carcinogenic processes (Gardner 1984; Lippmann 1989).

Mechanisms of ozone toxicity may include free radical generation as well as lipid peroxidation and sulf-hydryl oxidation. Little information is available about direct toxic effects of ozone on pulmonary surfactant. Ozone-induced effects on phospholipid synthesis have been the subject of a number of animal experiments. Using [$methyl$-^{14}C] choline as a marker, Haagsman et al. (1985) found inhibition of the synthesis of PC, PG, and PE in type II alveolar cells after exposure to ozone. These in vitro studies resulted in the hypothesis that the glycerol-3-phosphate acyltransferase mediated step of the synthesis is inhibited. An ozone-induced decrease in the activity of this enzyme was also found by Peters and Mudd (1982). They exposed a suspension of mitochondria, derived from lung tissue. A decrease in choline phosphotransferase activity after ozone exposure was reported (Haagsman et al. 1985) as well as an increased activity of lysophophatidyl-choline acyltransferase after ozone exposure of type II alveolar cells (0.4 lg/ 18 cm^2 plate) (Ichikawa and Yokoyama 1982) and exposure of rats (1– 5 ppm; 3 h) (Haagsman et al. 1985). However, not only synthesis but also release of surfactant can be affected by ozone exposure. Shimura et al. (1984) reported an increased number and a marked enlargement of lamellar bodies in type II alveolar cells of rats after ozone exposure. Recently ES Wright et al. (1990) also suggested a decreased rate of surfactant secretion in rats subsequent to chronic exposure to ozone (0.12–0.5 ppm). They found a decreased de novo synthesis as assessed by incorporation of ^{14}C and an increased lung tissue phospholipid content without corresponding changes in the phospholipid content in lung lavage fluid (LLF) of exposed animals.

The concentrations of ozone applied by Oosting et al. (1992) (0.4 ppm O_3, 3 and 12 h/day) were similar to those used by Shimura. Oosting et al.

found an inhibition of the surfactant-induced oxidative burst when adding surfactant from ozone-exposed rats to alveolar macrophages from control animals. The surfactant component stimulating the generation of oxygen radicals seems to be the apoprotein SP-A, as traced with SP-A antibody studies. The ozone-induced inhibition of the oxidative burst may therefore be caused by an alteration of this apoprotein. Oosting also reported an enhanced susceptibility of ozone exposed SP-A to proteolysis. Proteolytic enzymes may be liberated in the course of inflammatory processes by leukocytes infiltrating the alveolus. The authors also detected oxidation of methionine and trytptophan residues in ozone exposed canine SP-A. Others findings of these investigations conducted by Oosting et al. (1991, 1992) were functional impairment of SP-A in terms of self-association, lipid vesicle aggregation, mannose-binding capacity, and a decreased ability to enhance the phagocytosis of herpes simplex virus by alveolar macrophages.

The effects of an acute exposure (2–8 h) to ozone in rats on the formation of the intraalveolar surfactant monolayer have been assessed by Balis et al. (1991). The authors found that the unfolding of secreted lamellar bodies and the surfactant reorganization to tubular myelin which represents an intermediate form of surfactant in the alveolar space were inhibited.

Several recent studies deal with oxygen toxicity, which is thought to involve the generation of radicals, as found with ozone. Holm et al. (1985) described a reduced rate of synthesis for PC, a decreased intracellular lipid content, and, as a further parallel to the findings with ozone toxicity, a suppressed activity of the enzyme glycerol-3-phosphate acyltransferase. Enlarged lamellar bodies have also been described (Loo et al. 1989) subsequent to in vitro exposure of rat type II pneumocytes. Nogee et al. found increased apoprotein recovery (SP-A, SP-B, SP-C) in the lung lavage fluid (LLF) of rats following 1–7 days of exposure to an aerosol containing 85% oxygen (Nogee et al. 1991). Interestingly, instillation of exogenous surfactant following experimental hyperoxic injury mitigated the alveolar permeability, improved mechanical lung function, and increased the amount of lavagable phospholipids compared to that in the control group.

These findings underline the importance of the pulmonary surfactant system for the mechanisms of action of lung injury due to oxidant gases. Furthermore, there are theurapeutic implications for the treatment of patients with hyperoxic injury.

NO_2

Nitrogen dioxide originates from NO by oxidation. NO is generated during combustion processes for heat and energy production and is biologically inert. NO_2, however, which is an indoor as well as an outdoor pollutant, may cause alterations in pulmonary function, transient bronchial hyperreactivity, pulmonary edema, impairment of host defense mechanisms, and other effects depending on the exposure characteristics (Gardner 1984; Morrow 1984; Mustafa and Tierney 1978).

Nitrogen dioxide is soluble in tissue fluids to a greater extent than ozone and is thought not to react primarly with the epithelium but the interstitium and endothelium (Mustafa and Tierney 1978). Nevertheless, NO_2 and ozone share similar mechanisms of injury induction, such as initiation of free radical reactions and enzyme inhibition.

A number of in vitro and in vivo studies have been carried out on the effects of NO_2 on pulmonary surfactant. Arner et al. found evidence for impairment of LLF surface activity as well as a reduction in the disaturated PC fraction (DPPC) in rats after exposure to 2.9 ppm NO_2 for 9 months (Arner and Rhoades 1973). Exposure to NO_2 for 1–40 h did not result in a change (Kobayashi et al. 1980; Leung 1983) or increase in synthesis rates of lung phospholipids (Blank et al. 1978, 1982). Blank et al. (1978) found a dose-dependent increase in total lung phospholipids in rats 2–3 days after the end of the NO_2 exposure (40 ppm, 5 h). Exposure to 30 ppm NO_2 for 1 h showed comparable results. Glycerol-3-phosphate acyltransferase and glycerol-3-phosphatidyltransferase activity as well as the total number of type II alveolar cells were increased after in vitro exposure to 40 ppm NO_2 for 5 h.

DNA synthesis in rat lungs and the type II pneumocyte labeling index have been investigated by ES Wright (1986) following exposure to 2 ppm and 7 ppm NO_2 up to 14 days. The most distinct change was found to be the increase in DNA synthesis after 2 days of exposure to 7 ppm NO_2, returning to near control values after 2 weeks. Also the cell labeling index in the 7-ppm NO_2 group showed a significant elevation, returning to the control level within 14 days.

Müller et al. (1989) reported an increase in phospholipid and apoprotein content in lung lavage fluid of rats exposed to 10 ppm NO_2 for 72 h, although the secretion of type II pneumocytes seemed to be affected negatively. They explained the increased lavage content by an influx from the vascular system.

These results suggest a biphasic effect of NO_2 exposure on surfactant synthesis in the lung. An initial stimulation of type II cell proliferation and metabolic activity occurring within hours up to 2–3 days seems to decline gradually and may be followed in the long run by surfactant suppression possibly due to affection of the type II pneumocyte. Furthermore, differences between ozone and NO_2 toxicity, although basically sharing similar injury mechanisms, are likely to exist.

Diesel Exhaust

One of the first studies dealing with exhaust effects on lung phospholipids was performed by Eskelson et al. (1981). An increased phospholipid content was observed in saline wash of tracheobronchial airways after 9 months' exposure to diesel engine emissions containing $750 \, \mu g/m^3$ particles in rats and guinea pigs. Other studies (Chen and Vostal 1983; Strom 1983; E.S. Wright 1986; Wright and Vostal 1983) confirmed the finding of increased lavage content of phospholipids subsequent to diesel exhaust exposure up to 3 months. In addition, an increased phospholipid content in alveolar macrophages and an augmented DNA synthesis in type II cells, indicating proliferation of this cell type, were described (Strom 1983; Wright and Vostal 1983). In the study of E.S. Wright (1986) rats were exposed to diesel engine exhaust containing $6 \, mg/m^3$ soot particles for up to 14 days to evaluate exhaust-related effects on type II cells and phospholipid metabolism. A transient increase in DNA synthesis and type II labeling index was found. Lavage phospholipid content was increased without a corresponding increase in biosynthesis as was investigated by glycerol-3-phosphate acyl-transferase analysis and in vivo incorporation of [^{14}C]palmitic acid. In a further investigation Eskelson et al. (1987) presented evidence for a phospholipidosis in rat lung lavage subsequent to chronic exposure to diesel exhaust containing $750 \, \mu g/m^3$ soot particles. They related the increased pulmonary phospholipid content to proliferation of type II cells, increased de novo phospholipid synthesis, reduced clearance rate, and higher hepatic phospholipogenesis.

Silica

Several authors have reported surfactant accumulation in the lungs of silica-treated animals (Adachi et al. 1989; Gabor et al. 1978; Heppleston et al. 1972, 1974; Kawada et al. 1989; Richards et al. 1983). The reasons for this increase are still subject to discussion. Heppleston et al. (1974) investigated surfactant synthesis and clearance rates and encountered an imbalance. The clearance, although also increased, could not keep pace with the incited biosynthesis. Miller and coworkers (Miller and Hook 1988; Miller et al. 1986, 1987) described hypertrophic and hyperplastic type II cells in the lungs of silica-treated rats as well as increased intracellular SP-A content and synthesis rate (Miller et al. 1990). Augmented activity of enzymes involved in the phospholipid biosynthesis was found by Kawada et al. (1989). It is still unclear in what way the silica particle interacts with the type II cell. Bruch and Schlösser (1989) suggested the alveolar macrophage as the main effector cell of silica, subsequently stimulating the type II pneumocyte by release of mediators. He based his view on investigations performed with polyvinyl-*N*-oxide (PVNO)-coated quartz particles. PVNO inhibited the characteristic silica-induced lesions in the alveolar micromilieu. Obviously, phospholipid and protein biosynthesis are increased after silica exposure almost to the same extent (10- to 12-fold) (Kawada et al. 1989). The phospholipid profile of the surfactant fraction was found to be changed (Adachi et al. 1989;

Kawada et al. 1989). The relative amount of PG was decreased and that of PI increased, leading to a decrease in the PG/PI ratio, otherwise found to be reduced in the lung lavage fluid subsequent to alveolar injury (Sheehan et al. 1986; Thrall et al. 1987).

The changes in the intra- and extracellular surfactant pool seem not to represent simply a nonspecific alveolar reaction but some kind of a defense mechanism. Surfactant may inhibit the cellular toxicity of silica particles by coating their surface, thus preventing a direct contact of the silica surface with cellular and subcellular membranes (Haagsman and van Golde 1985; Schimmelpfeng et al. 1989; Wallace et al. 1988). Retoxification of the particle may occur by gradual degradation of such a phospholipid membrane by phospholipase.

Tobacco Smoke

Compared to environmental pollutants tobacco smoke is inhaled in unusually high concentrations. Its involvement in the pathogenesis of epidemiologically important lung diseases such as chronic bronchitis, emphysema, and lung cancer is well established (Doll and Peto 1976). The question arises as to how the pulmonary surfactant system is affected, and what role such effects may play with regard to lung disease processes.

The findings about surfactant yield in BALF of smokers and smoke-exposed animal species are still somewhat contradictory. Hughes and Haslam (1990) found increased levels of PG, PE, and SPH in the BALF of smokers. Oulton et al. (1991) described a twofold increase in LLF phospholipid content of mice exposed for 30 min to smoke generated from the burning of polyurethane foam. The intracellular phospholipid pool was unchanged, suggesting an impaired alveolar clearance of surfactant rather than an increased de novo synthesis. Other investigators also found increases or no differences in the lavagate phospholipid content harvested from smoke exposure groups compared to the control group (Clements 1972; Hamosh et al. 1979; Hughes and Haslam 1990; Low et al. 1977). In contrast, Finley and Ladman (1972), Le Mesurier et al. (1980, 1981), and recently De Bernardi et al. (1990) reported decreased amounts of surfactant in the lavage fluid of smokers and smoke-exposed animals. Le Mesurier et al. (1981) described ultrastructural changes of hypertrophied type II cells in rats following 25 days of exposure to cigarette smoke. At that time intracellular lamellar bodies were prominent and stained intensively osmiophilic. Further exposure up to 50 days led to the disappearance of the lamellar bodies. A reduced number of lamellar bodies in type II pneumocytes was also mentioned by De Bernardi et al. (1990), who exposed rats to cigarette smoke for 6 months.

Studies dealing with the surface activity of surfactant underlined the detrimental impact of tobacco smoke. Miller and Bondwant (1962) exposed a surfactant layer extracted from rat lungs in vitro to cigarette smoke and found lower surface tension of the expanded monolayer compared to control group samples. Rises in minimum surface tension were also described (Cook and Webb 1966; Higenbottam 1989). In vitro studies with surfactant showed evidence that the particulate constituents of tobacco smoke are responsible for the increase in minimum surface tension (Cook and Webb 1966; Higenbottam 1989). Surface-active substances present in smoke particles, such as sterol and fatty acids, were seen as penetrating into the monolayer and impairing surface activity.

Various Substances with Surfactant Toxicity

In 1985 Haagsman and van Golde published their comprehensive review on surfactant and pulmonary toxicology. They noted a paucity of knowledge on this subject despite its importance for pulmonary well-being. Not much is known about surfactant toxicity attributable to less widespread pollutants. Kynast et al. (1987) reported impairment of the pulmonary surfactant system in rats after exposure to technical aerosols (water-proofing sprays). They found an initial decrease within 2 h after the start of exposure, a reactive increase probably due to shedding out of the cellular phospholipid reservoir within 24 h, and a subsequent decrease until returning to control levels after 2 weeks after treatment.

    In our laboratory evidence was found for impairment of the surfactant system in rats by inhalation of methylene diphenyl diisocyanate (MDI) (Klingebiel et al. 1991; Martin-Carrera et al. 1991). MDI is known to induce affections of the respiratory tract in exposed workers, extending from cough and nasal congestion to acute bronchospasm and allergic asthma. Total phospholipid content as well as the relative PC content in rat LLF were significantly reduced after 4 weeks of exposure to $3.0 \, \text{mg/m}^3$ monomeric MDI. The percentage of all other surfactant phospholipids was significantly increased, with the PS/PI ratio showing the highest level of statistical significance ($p \leq 0.001$). Interestingly, neither dynamic nor quasistatic lung compliance, as assessed by whole-body plethysmography, were altered compared to the control group. In another investigation concerning pollutant surfactant interactions (Klingebiel et al. 1991) we exposed adult male Wistar rats to $1.0 \, \text{mg/m}^3$ monomeric MDI during 18 h/day, 5 days/week for 12 weeks. Total phospholipid content of LLF was significantly reduced whereas the relative PI content increased ($p \leq 0.05$) in the MDI group compared to the clean-air group. The relative PC content was reduced but not significantly ($p = 0.053$). Also in this study there were no statistically significant alterations in terms of lung resistance and compliance in the exposure group. Thus, regarding MDI effects on pulmonary surfactant, the aerosol concentration applied seems to be a more decisive factor for the extent of phospholipid concentration changes in LLF than the duration of exposure.

Narayan et al. (1990) reported effects of intratracheally administered insecticides (DDI, endosulfan) on lipid metabolism of rat lung subcellular fractions. They found an increased phospholipid content in the surfactant system as collected by lung lavage and an enhanced PC/DPPC synthesis via the cytidine diphosphate choline (CDPcholine) pathway.

The impact of exposure to hydrogen sulfide on surface properties of lung surfactant in rats has been recently assessed by Green et al. (1991). Concentrations above and below the threshold concentration for pulmonary edema in rats (200 ppm) were used and surface activity was measured using a so-called captive bubble surface tensiometer. The authors described significant increases in minimum surface tension subsequent to exposure to 300 ppm hydrogen sulfide. They related these changes in surface activity to inhibition of pulmonary surfactant by surfactant inhibitors in the edema fluid as in vitro addition of sodium sulfide (being hydrolysed to hydrogen sulfide) to rat LLF did not result in similar changes as observed in vivo. In contrast, addition of serum proteins to rat LLF in vitro did result in abnormalities of the surface active properties of the samples.

In vitro investigations with cultured rat alveolar type II pneumocytes being exposed to various concentrations of carbon tetrachloride showed a decrease of intracellular ATP content concomitant with inhibition of PC synthesis (Ma et al. 1989). Some reports have been published about experimentally induced respiratory distress syndrome by various noxious agents. Several animal models have been used to elucidate the patho-mechanism and the therapeutic benefit of surfactant replacement in ARDS (Lachmann 1989a,b). Inductive noxae for respiratory distress used in the more recent investigations were N-nitroso-N-methylurethane in dogs (Liau et al. 1987) and rats (Harris et al. 1989), oleic acid in rabbits (Casals et al. 1989), endotoxin in guinea pigs (Tahvanainen and Hattman 1987), and a betaine hydrochloride-pepsin mixture in rabbits (Strohmaier et al. 1990). Reduced recovery and altered composition of phospholipids in lung lavage fluid as well as an increased protein content were common findings.

Bleomycin-induced interstitial pneumonia in rats is used as a model for fibrosing diseases in the human lung (Sulavik and Thrall 1987). There was a reproducible decrease in the PG/PI ratio (Horiuchi et al. 1990; Sulavik and Thrall 1987) as found in patients suffering from idiopathic pulmonary fibrosis (Honda et al. 1988; McCormack et al. 1988).

Effects of Pollutants on the Interaction of Pulmonary Surfactant and Alveolar Macrophages

As mentioned above (see "Nonspecific Local Defense Mechanisms"), the pulmonary surfactant system is able to modulate the pulmonary immune response to inhaled foreign bodies. Especially the stimulation of alveolar macrophages in terms of migration, phagocytosis, and oxygen radical generation (Baughman and Strohofer 1989; Baughman et al. 1987; O'Neill et al. 1984a,b; Van Iwaarden et al. 1990, 1991; Wright and Tenner 1989) must be considered when talking about detrimental impact of pollutants on the surfactant system. Epidemiologic evidence was presented that environmental pollutants may play a role in increasing susceptibility to respiratory infections (Bates and Sitzo 1983, 1986, 1987, 1989). Knowing that the pulmonary surfactant system supports alveolar defense mechanisms, and that it is also sensitive to a variety of inhalative pollutants suggests in vitro investigation of surfactant macrophage interaction subsequent to in vivo pollutant exposure.

To our knowledge only one group of scientists, Oosting and coworkers from the group of van Golde (University of Utrecht, Netherlands) has addressed this intriguing subject up to now (Oosting et al. 1991, 1992). The authors reported an impaired SP-A activity in terms of self-association, lipid aggregation, and mannose-binding capacity, which is thought to represent a putative mechanism for macrophage stimulation (Oosting et al. 1991a). Oosting et al. were able to demonstrate the following effects of in vitro or in vivo exposure of SP-A of different species to ozone: inhibition of SP-A impact on surfactant secretion from the type II pneumocyte, increased susceptibility of (canine) SP-A to proteolysis, decreased ability of (human) SP-A to enhance phagocytosis of herpes simplex virus and to stimulate superoxide anion production by alveolar macrophages. The latter finding was confirmed by investigations with SP-A isolated from the lungs of ozone-exposed rats.

Conclusions and Prospects

Uptake of pulmonary noxae via the inhalation route may result in a variety of disease processes, such as airway hyperreactivity, epithelial damage and alterations of the alveolocapillary membrane, acute and chronic inflammation, and tumor development. What kind of disease process is induced in the lung, if at all, depends among other factors on the physical and chemical properties of the inhaled toxicant, on the local dosimetry, on its deposition and clearance in the airways, and on the metabolic and immunologic status of the lung. For more detailed information about basic principles in inhalation toxicology the reader is referred to other publications (Dungworth 1989).

In terms of surfactant toxicology the terminal airways, i.e., the terminal bronchioli and respiratory bronchioli as well as the alveolar ducts, are of special interest. The type I pneumocyte covering the major surface area of the alveolus reacts sensitively to toxic pollutants, and cell death occurs early. The type II pneumocyte, being a secretory cell, is in general less sensitive to direct acting toxicants (Dungworth 1989) and can proliferate and differentiate into type I cells. The interstitial tissue shows evidence of inflammatory cell influx, fibroblast activity, and plasma extravasation. Cellular and humoral mediators are present here as well as in the alveolar space where desquamized cells and secretory products accumulate.

Chronic exposure to inhaled toxicants represents a permanent stimulus for proliferative repair and cell differentiation. Metaplasia and transdifferentiation of the type II cell may occur (Dungworth 1989). The more sensitive type I cell is increasingly replaced by the secretory type II cell. Particle contact with the alveolar surface seems to exert an inciting effect on cellular metabolism and proliferation. Increases in DNA synthesis and type II cell labeling index were found as well as augmented activity of enzymes involved in the phospholipid biosynthesis (Kawada et al. 1989; E.S. Wright 1986). It has been argued that type II cell stimulation is mediated via the alveolar macrophage (Bruch and Schlösser 1989; Finkelstein 1990), possibly by a macrophage-released growth factor.

On the other hand, extension of the bronchiolar epithelial cells into the alveolar duct ("brochiolarization") may occur, leading to a reduction in alveolar surface area. The bronchiolarization of alveolar ducts is associated with interstitial fibrosis, a characteristic interstitial response in chronic inflammation. Another detrimental effect of prolonged inhalative exposure to air pollutants may be affection of elastic fibers and subsequent pulmonary emphysema, also leading to diminished surface area for alveolar gas exchange.

Whether incited to proliferate and replace the type I pneumocyte, or whether rarefied due to bronchiolarization or emphysema, the type II pneumocyte is of importance in toxicological processes of the lung periphery. As surfactant is a characteristic metabolic product of the type II cell type, its quantitative and qualitative determination should provide valuable information about the cellular integrity and metabolic activity of the alveolar type II cell. Nevertheless, some aspects should be kept in mind when surfactant analysis in LLF has been carried out, and conclusions must be drawn. The extracellular surfactant pool does not necessarily correspond to the intracellular one. An elevated LLF phospholipid concentration could be due to an impaired surfactant clearance from the alveolar space or an increase in the number of type II cells rather than an enhanced de novo synthesis. And a reduced extracellular surfactant content may occur while the intracellular storage granules, the lamellar bodies, have considerably gained volume, suggesting affection of surfactant secretion. To obtain more precise information about changes in surfactant synthesis and/or secretion the use of radioactively labeled precursors were useful.

The pulmonary surfactant system, however, is not only a characteristic metabolic product of a specific cell type but an important functional, biochemical, and immunological factor for the well-being of the respiratory tract. It is indispensable for intact lung mechanics und participates directly and indirectly in the local defense system against inhaled particles, and microorganisms. The results of Oosting et al. (see "Effects of Inhalative Pollutants on the Interaction of Pulmonary Surfactant and Alveolar Macrophages") indicating functional impairment of alveolar macrophages subsequent to ozone exposure mediated by affection of the surfactant-associated protein A (SP-A) underline the need for further research in this area. Also the reports of Schürch, Gehr, and coworkers on surfactant impact on particle deposition in the upper respiratory tract (Gehr et al. 1990a,b; Schürch et al. 1990) deserve further investigation. The mechanisms and the pathophysiological meaning of surfactant changes occurring in the course of pollutant exposure are still not well understood.

Regarding the variety of effects exerted by the pulmonary surfactant system, it is difficult to understand why this system has only rarely been addressed in inhalation toxicity studies. One of the reasons contributing to underestimation of efficacy of surfactant assessment in inhalation toxicology may have been analytical problems. Two-dimensional thin-layer chromatography is still the analytical method of choice in many surfactant laboratories. This method does not require expensive analytical equipment but is time consuming, and satisfactory recovery, especially of the smaller phospholipid fractions (PI, PS, PE), is difficult to achieve. Analysis of surfactant-associated proteins was done by means of sodium dodecyl sulfate–polyacrylamide gel electrophoresis and only those laboratories having SP-A antiserum at their disposal could perform immunoblotting or even establish an immunoassay of their own for quantification. In the meantime several publications about phospholipid analysis in biological matrices by high-performance liquid chromatography have appeared (Becart et al. 1990; Breton et al. 1989; Heinze et al. 1988; Kuhnz et al. 1985; Kynast and Schmitz 1988; Pison et al. 1986; Rimpler et al. 1987; Scarim et al. 1989). In our own laboratory such a method has recently been developed that permits separation and quantification of all surfactant phospholipids (see R. Klingebiel et al., this volume). By now, all three surfactant proteins (SP-A, SP-B, SP-C) have been synthesized by the pharmaceutical industry using gene technological procedures, and some laboratories have established SP-A immunoassays (Akino et al. 1988; Katyal and Singh 1983; Kuroki et al. 1985a,b). At least for the human SP-A an immunoassay will be commercially available in the near future (T. Akino, personal communication).

Numerous publications underline the correlation of pollutant-induced pulmonary affections and concomitant quantitative and qualitative changes of the pulmonary surfactant system. What pathophysiological mechanisms are involved in surfactant toxicology, and whether phospholipid or apoprotein analysis or specific ratios of them are more promising for toxicological purposes is still a matter of discussion. Evidence was also shown that the pulmonary surfactant system extends its influence beyond bronchoalveolar mechanics and affects the local immune response to inhaled foreign material as well as the fate of particles deposited in the upper conducting airways.

Further investigation in this intriguing research area is needed, and the high performance analytical equipment now being disposable will undoubtfully facilitate this work.

Reference

Adachi H, Hayashi H, Sato H, Dempo K, Akino T (1989) Characterization of phospholipids accumulated in pulmonary-surfactant compartments of rats intratracheally exposed to silica. Biochemistry 262:781–786

Akino T, Shimizu H, Mizumoto M, Kuroki Y, Satoh H, Kataoka K, Hagisawa M, Fujimoto S, Hosoda K, Suzuki H (1988) Simplified monoclonal immunoassay for pulmonary surfactant 35-kDa apoprotein in human amniotic fluid. Clin Chem 34/7:1513

Ansfield MJ, Benson BJ (1980) Identification of the immunosuppressove components of canine pulmonary surface active material. J Immunol 125/3:1093–1098

Ansfield MJ, Benfer Kaltreider H, Benson BJ, Caldwell JL (1979) Immunosuppressive activity of canine pulmonary surface active material. J Immunol 122/3:1062–1066

Arner EC, Rhoades RA (1973) Long-term nitrogen dioxide exposure. Arch Environ Health 26:156

Avery ME, Mead J (1959) Surface properties in relation to atelectasis and hyaline membrane disease. Am J Dis Child 97:517–523

Balis JU, Paterson JF, Lundh JM, Haller EM, Shelley SA, Montgomery MR (1991) Ozone stress initiates acute pertubations of secreted surfactant membranes. Am J Pathol 138/4:847–857

Bates DV, Sizto R (1983) Relationship between air pollutant levels and hospital admissions in Southern Ontario. Can J Public Health 74:117–122

Bates DV, Sizto R (1986) A study of hospital admissions and air pollutants in southern Ontario. In: Less SD, Schneider T, Grant LD (eds) Aerosols: research risk assessment and control strategies: proceedings of the second U.S.-Dutch international symposium, May 1985, Williamsburg. Lewis, Chelsea, pp 767–777

Bates DV, Sizto R (1987) Air pollution and hospital admissions in southern Ontario: the acid summer haze effect. Environ Res 43:317–331

Bates DV, Sizto R (1989) The Ontario air pollution study: identification of the causative agent. Environ Health Perspect 79:69–72

Baughman RP, Strohofer S (1989) Lung derived surface active material (SAM) inhibits natural killer cell tumor cytotoxicity. J Clin Lab Immunol 28:51–54

Baughman RP, Mangels DJ, Strohofer S, Corser BC (1987) Enhancement of macrophage and monocyte cytotoxicity by the surface active material of lung lining fluid. J Lab Clin Med 109:692–697

Baughman RP, Stein E, MacGee J, Roshkin M, Sahebjami H (1984) Changes in fatty acids in phospholipids of the bronchoalveolar fluid in bacterial pneumonia and in adult respiratory distress syndrome. Clin Chem 30/4:521–523

Baughman RP, Strohofer S, Dohn M (1985) Decreased phosphatidylcholine in the lung fluid of patients with sarcoidosis. Lipids 20:496–499

Becard J, Chevalier C, Biesse JP (1990) Quantitative analysis of phospholipids by HPLC with a light scattering evaporating detector – application to raw materials for cosmetic use. J High Resolution Chromatogr 13:126–129

Blank ML, Dalbey W, Nettesheim P, Price J, Creasia D, Snyder F (1978) Sequential changes in phospholipid composition and synthesis in lungs exposed to nitrogen dioxide. Am Rev Respir Dis 117:273–280

Blank ML, Dalbey W, Cress EA, Garfinkel S, Snyder T (1982) Pulmonary NO_2-toxicity: phosphatidylcholine levels and incorporation of [^{3}H]thymidine into DNA. Environ Res 27:352–360

Breton L, Serkiz B, Volland J-P (1989) A new rapid method for phospholipid separation by high performance liquid chromatography with light-scattering detection. J Chromatogr 497:243–249

Bruch J, Schlösser W (1989) The therapeutic influence of PVNO on the quartz induced pneumonitis in rat. Eur Respir J 2/8/408:722s (abstr)

Casals C, Herrera L, Miguel E, Garcia-Barreto P, Municio AM (1989) Comparison between intra- and extracellular surfactant in respiratory distress induced by oleic acid. Biochim Biophys Acta 1003:201–203

Catanzaro A, Richman P, Batcher S, Hallman M (1988) Immunomodulation by pulmonary surfactant. J Lab Clin Med 112:727–734

Chen KC, Vostal JJ (1983) Proliferation of pulmonary alveolar type II cells in rats exposed to high concentration of diesel exhaust (DE). Toxicologist 3:9 (abstr)

Clements JA (1972) Smoking and pulmonary surfactant. N Engl J Med 286:261–262

Clements JA, Chambers WH (1957) Surface tension of lung extracts. Proc Soc Exp Biol Med 95:170–172

Cockshutt AM, Weitz J, Possmayer F (1990) Pulmonary surfactant-associated protein A enhances the surface activity of lipid extract surfactant and reverses inhibition by blood proteins in vitro. Biochemistry 29:8424–8429

Cook WD, Webb WR (1966) Surfactant in chronic smokers. Ann Thorac Surg 2:327–333

Coonrod JD (1987) Role of surfactant free fatty acids in antimicrobial defenses. Eur J Respir Dis 71/153:209–214

De Bernardi M, Zanasi A, Feletti F, Ricevuti G, Barni S (1990) Toxicity of cigarette smoke and aerosol therapy: biochemical and ultrastructural findings. Eur J Respir Dis 3 [Suppl 10]:430s (abstr)

Doll R, Peto R (1976) Mortality and relation to smoking; 20 years observation on male British doctors. Br Med J ii:1525

Dungworth DL (1989) Noncarcinogenic responses of the respiratory tract to inhaled toxicants. In: McClellan RO, Henderson RF (eds) Concepts in inhalation toxicology. Hemisphere, New York, pp 273–298

Enhorning G (1989) Surfactant replacement in adult respiratory distress syndrome. Am Rev Respir Dis 140:281–283

Eskelson CD, Strom KA, Vostal JJ, Misiorowski RL, Chvapil M (1981) Lipids in the lung and lung lavage fluid of animals exposed to diesel particulates. Toxicologist 1:74–75 (abstr)

Eskelson CD, Chvapil M, Strom KA, Vostal JJ (1987) Pulmonary phospholipidosis in rats respiring air containing diesel particulates. Environ Res 44:260–271

Finkelstein JN (1990) Physiologic and toxicologic responses of alveolar type II cells. Toxicology 60:41–52

Finley TN, Ladman AJ (1972) Low yield of pulmonary surfactant in cigarette smokers. N Engl J Med 286/5:223–227

Fujiwara T, Chida S, Watabe Y (1980) Artificial surfactant therapy in hyaline-membrane disease. Lancet i:55–59

Gabor S, Zugravu E, Kovats A, Böhm B, Andrasoni D (1978) Effects of quartz on lung surfactant. Environ Res 16:443–448

Gardner DE (1984) Oxidant-induced enhanced sensitivity to infection in animal models and their extrapolation to man. J Toxicol Environ Health 13(2–3):423–439

Gehr P, Schürch S, Geiser M, Im Hof V (1990a) Retention and clearance mechanisms of inhaled particles. J Aerosol Sci 21/1:S491–S496

Gehr P, Schürich S, Berthiaume Y (1990b) Particle retention in airways by surfactant. J Aerosol Med 3/1:27–43

Gitlin JD, Soll RF, Parad RB, Horbar JD, Feldman HA, Lucey JF, Taeusch HW (1987) Randomized controlled trial of exogenous surfactant for the treatment of hyaline membrane disease. Pediatrics 79/1:31–37

Goerke J (1974) Lung surfactant. Biochim Biophys Acta 344:241–261

Green FHY, Schürch S, De Sanctis GT, Wallace JA, Cheng S, Prior M (1991) Effects of hydrogen sulfide exposure on surface properties of lung surfactant. J Appl Physiol 70/5:1943–1949

Haagsman HP, van Golde LMG (1985) Lung surfactant and pulmonary toxicology. Lung 163:275–303

Haagsman HP, Schuurmans EAJM, Alink GM, Batenburg JJ, Van Golde LMG (1985) Effects of ozone on phospholipid synthesis by alveolar type II cells isolated from adult rat lung. Exp Lung Res 9:67–84

Hallman M, Spragg R, Harrell JH, Moser KM (1982) Evidence of lung surfactant abnormality in respiratory failure. Study of broncholalveolar lavage phospholipids, surface activity, phospholipase activity, and plasma myoinositol. J Clin Invest 70:673–683

Hallman M, Arjomaa P, Tahvanainen J, Lachmann B, Spragg R (1985) Endobronchial surface active phospholipids in various pulmonary diseases. Eur J Respir Dis 142S:37–47

Hallman M, Maasilta P, Sipilä I, Tahvanainen J (1989a) Composition and function of pulmonary surfactant in adult respiratory distress syndrome. Eur Respir J 2/3:104s–108s

Hallman M, Pohjavuori M, Järvenpää AL, Bry K, Merritt TA, Pesonen E (1989b) Human surfactant in the treatment of respiratory distress syndrome. A spectrum of clinical responses. Eur Respir J 2/3:77s–80s

Hamosh M, Schlechter Y, Hamosh P (1979) Effect of tobacco smoke on the metabolism of rat lung. Lung Arch Environ Health 34:17–23

Harris JD, Jackson F Jr, Moxley MA (1989) Effect of exogenous surfactant instillation on experimental acute lung injury. J Appl Physiol 66/4:1846–1851

Harwood JL (1987) Lung surfactant. Prog Lipid Res 26:211–256

Harwood JL, Desai R, Hext P (1975) Characterization of pulmonary surfactant from ox, rabbit, rat and sheep. Biochem J 151:707–714

Heinze T, Kynast G, Dudenhausen JW, Schmitz C, Saling E (1988) Quantitative determination of phospholipids in amniotic fluid by high-performance liquid chromatography. Chromatographia 25/6:497–503

Heppleston AG, Young AE (1972) Alveolar lipo-proteinosis: an ultrastructural comparison of the experimental and human forms. J Pathol 107:107–117

Heppleston AG, Fletcher K, Wyatt I (1972) Abnormalities of lung lipids following inhalation of quartz. Experientia 28:938–939

Heppleston AG, Fletcher K, Wyatt I (1974) Changes in the composition of lung lipids and the "turnover" of dipalmitoyl lecithin in experimental alveolar lipoproteinosis induced by inhaled quartz. Br J Exp Pathol 55:384–395

Heppleston AG, McDermott M, Collins MM (1975) The surface properties of the lung in rats with alveolar lipo-proteinosis. Br J Exp Pathol 56:444–453

Higenbottam T (1989) Lung lipids and disease. Respiration 55:14–27

Hildebran JN, Goerke J, Clements JA (1981) Surfactant release in excised rat lung is stimulated by air inflation. J Appl Physiol 51:905–910

Hills BA (1990) The role of lung surfactant. Br J Anaesth 65:13–29

Holm BA, Notter RH, Siegle J, Matalou S (1985) Pulmonary physiological and surfactant changes during injury and recovery from hyperoxia. J Appl Physiol 59/5:1402–1409

Honda Y, Kataoka K, Hayashi H, Takahashi H, Suzuki A, Akino T (1989) Alternations of acidic phospholipids in bronchoalveolar lavage fluids of patients with pulmonary alveolar proteinosis. Clin Chim Acta 181:11-18

Honda Y, Tsunematsu K, Suzuki A, Akino T (1988) Changes in phospholipids in bronchoalveolar lavage fluid of patients with interstitial lung diseases. Lung 166:293-301

Hook GER, Gilmore LB, Talley FA (1986) Dissolution and reassembly of tubular myelin-like multilamellated structures form the lungs of patients with pulmonary alveolar proteinosis. Lab Invest 55/2:194

Horiuchi T, Mason RJ, Kuroki Y, Cherniack RM (1990) Surface and tissue forces, surfactant protein A, and the phospholipid components of pulmonary surfactant in bleomycin-induced pulmonary fibrosis in the rat. Am Rev Respir Dis 141:1006-1013

Hughes DA, Haslam PL, Path MRC (1989) Changes in phosphatidylglycerol in bronchoalveolar lavage fluids from patients with cryptogenic fibrosing alveolitis. Chest 95:82-89

Hughes DA, Haslam PL (1990) Effect of smoking on the lipid composition of lung lining fluid and relationship between immunostimulatory lipids, inflammatory cells and foamy macrophages in extrinsic allergic alveolitis. Eur Respir J 3:1128-1139

Ichikawa I, Yokoyama E (1982) Effect of short-term exposure to ozone on lecithin metabolism of rat lung. J Toxicol Environ Health 10:1005-1015

Jonsson S, Musher DM, Goree A, Lawrence EC (1986) Human alveolar lining material and antibacterial defenses. Am Rev Respir Dis 133:136-140

Juers JA, Rogers RM, McCurdy JB, Cook WW (1976) Enhancement of bacterial capacity of alveolar macrophages by hyman alveolar lining material. J Clin Invest 58:271-275

Kakuta Y, Sasaki H, Takishima T (1991) Effect of artificial surfactant on ciliary beat frequency in guinea pig trachea. Respir Physiol 83/3:313-322

Katyal SL, Singh G (1983) An enzyme-linked immunoassay of surfactant apoproteins. Its application to the study of fetal lung development in the rat. Pediatr Res 17:439-443

Kawada H, Horiuchi T, Shannon JM, Kuroki Y, Voelker DR, Mason RJ (1989) Alveolar type II cells, surfactant protein A (SP-A), and the phospholipid components of surfactant in acute silicosis in the rat. Am Rev Respir Dis 140:460-470

Klingebiel R, Creutzenberg O, Hoymann HG, Dettmer M, Schüler T, Heinrich U (1991) Effects of 12 weeks exposure to a diisocyanate (MDI) on the pulmonary surfactant system and bronchoalveolar cell content in rats. Eur Resp J 4/ 14:352s-353s (abstr)

Kobayashi T, Noguchi T, Kikuno M, Kubota (1980) Effect of acute nitrogen dioxide exposure on the composition of fatty acids in lung and liver phospholipids. Toxicol Lett 6:149-155

Kuhnz W, Zimmermann B, Nau H (1985) Improved separation of phospholipids by high-performance liquid chromatography. J Chromatogr 344:309-312

Kuroki Y, Fukada Y, Takahashi H, Akino T (1985a) Monoclonal antibodies against human pulmonary surfactant apoproteins: Specificity and application in immunoassay. Biochim Biophys Acta 836:201-209

Kuroki Y, Takahashi H, Fukada Y, Mikawa M, Inagawa A, Fujimoto S, Akino T (1985b) Two-site "simultaneous" immunoassay with monoclonal antibodies for the determination of surfactant apoproteins in human amniotic fluid. Pediatr Res 19/10:1017-1020

Kynast G, Schmitz C (1988) Determination of the phospholipid content of human milk, cow's milk and various infant formulas. Z Ernahrungswiss 27:252-265

Kynast G, Schmitz C, Dudenhausen JW, Schnoy N, Wagner M (1987) Investigations on the influence of water-proofing sprays on the phospholipid composition of the lungs. Wiss Umwelt 4:200–205

Lachmann B (1989a) Animal studies of surfactant replacement therapy. Dev Pharmacol Ther 13:164–172

Lachmann B (1989b) Animal models and clinical pilot studies of surfactant replacement in adult respiratory distress syndrome. Eur Respir J 2/3:98s–103s

LaForce FM, Kelly WJ, Huber GL (1973) Inactivation of staphylococci by alveolar macrophages with preliminary observations on the importance of alveolar lining material. Am Rev Respir Dis 108:784–790

Le Mesurier SM, Lykke AWJ, Stewart BW (1980) Reduced yield of pulmonary surfactant: patterns of response following administration of chemicals to rats by inhalation. Toxicol Lett 5:89–93

Le Mesurier SM, Stewart BW, Lykke AWJ (1981) Injury to type II pneumocytes in rats exposed to cigarette smoke. Environ Res 24:207–217

Leung H-W (1983) Effect of nitrogen dioxide exposure on rat lung lipids. Res Commun Chem Pathol Pharmacol 40/3:519–523

Liau DF, Barrett CR, Bell ALL, Ryan SF (1987) Functional abnormalities of lung surfactant in experimental acute alveolar injury in the dog. Am Rev Respir Dis 136:395–401

Lippmann M (1989) Health effects of ozone. A critical review. JAPCA 39/5:672–695

Liu M, Wang L, Li E, Enhorning G (1991) Pulmonary surfactant will secure airflow through a narrow tube. J Appl Physiol 71/2:742–748

Longmuir KJ, Haynes S (1991) Evidence that fatty acid chain length is a type II cell lipid-sorting signal. Am J Physiol (Lung Cell Mol Physiol) 260/4:L44–L51

Loo CKC, Smith GJ, Lykke AWJ (1989) Effects of hyperoxia on surfactant morphology and cell viability in organotypic cultures of fetal rat lung. Exp Lung Res 15:597–617

Low ES, Low RB, Green GM (1977) Correlated effects of cigarette smoke components on alveolar macrophage adenosine triphosphatase activity and phagocytosis. Am Rev Respir Dis 115:963

Ma JVC, LaCagnin LB, Bowman L, Miles PR (1989) Carbon tetrachloride inhibits synthesis of pulmonary surfactant disaturated phosphatidylcholines and ATP production in alveolar type II cells. Biochim Biophys Acta 1003:136–144

Martin-Carrera I, Klingebiel R, Hoymann HG, Heinrich U (1991) Effects of subchronic exposure to a diisoyanate (MDI) on the pulmonary surfactant system and lung function. Aerosol Med 4/1:35 (abstr)

Mason RJ (1987) Surfactant in adult respiratory distress syndrome. Eur J Respir Dis 153:229–236

Mathe AA, Volicer L, Puri SK (1974) Effect of anaphylaxis and histamine, pyrilamine and burimamide on levels of cyclic AMP and cyclic GMP in guinea-pig lung. Res Commun Chem Pathol Pharmacol 8/4:635–651

McCormack FX Jr, Voelker DR, King TE Jr, Mason RJ (1988) Decreased levels of phosphatidylglycerol but not levels of surfactant protein correlate with severity of illness in patients with idiopathic pulmonary fibrosis. Am Rev Respir Dis 137/4:275

McCormack FX, Talmadge EK Jr, Voelker DR, Robinson PC, Mason RJ (1991) Idiopathic pulmonary fibrosis. Abnormalities in the bronchoalveolar lavage content of surfactant protein A. Am Rev Respir Dis 144:160–166

Merritt TA, Hallman M, Spragg R, Heldt GP, Gilliard N (1989) Exogenous surfactant treatments for neonatal respiratory distress syndrome and their potential role in the adult respiratory distress syndrome. Drugs 38/49:591–611

Miller BE, Hook GER (1988) Isolation and characterization of hypertrophic type II cells from the lungs of silica-treated rats. Lab Invest 58/5:565–575

Miller BE, Dethloff LA, Hook GER (1986) Silica-induced hypertrophy of type II cells in the lungs of rats. Lab Invest 55/2:153–163

Miller BE, Dethloff LA, Gladen BC, Hook GER (1987) Progression of type II cell hypertrophy and hyperplasia during silica-induced pulmonary inflammation. Lab Invest 57/5:546–554

Miller BE, Bakewell WE, Katyal SL, Singh G, Hook GER (1990) Induction of surfactant protein (SP-A) biosynthesis and SP-A mRNA in activated type II cells during acute silicosis in rats. Am J Respir Cell Mol Biol 3:217–226

Miller D, Bondurant S (1962) Effects of cigarette smoke on the surface characteristics of lung extracts. Am Rev Respir Dis 85:692–696

Morgenroth K (1986) Das Surfactantsystem der Lunge. de Gruyter, Berlin, pp 1–110

Morgenroth K, Newhouse M (1988) The surfactant system of the lungs. de Gruyter, Berlin

Morrow P (1984) Toxicoplogical data on NO_x: an overview. J Toxicol Environ Health 13:205–227

Mustafa MG, Tierney DF (1978) Biochemical and metabolic changes in the lung with oxygen, ozone, and nitrogen dioxide toxicity. Am Rev Respir Dis 118:1061–1090

Müller B (1989) Increased phospholipid synthesis in diseased lungs. Floating congress on the River Rhine, 11–17 Nov 1989 (abstr)

Narayan S, Dani HM, Misra UK (1990) Lung subcellular fractions and surfactant lipid metabolism of rats exposed with DDT or endosulfan intratracheally. J Environ Sci Health B25/2:259–272

Nicholas TE, Power JHT, Barr HA (1982) The pulmonary consequences of a deep breath. Respir Physiol 49:315–324

Nogee LM, Wispe JR, Clark JC (1991) Increased expression of pulmonary surfactant proteins in oxygen-exposed rats. Am J Respir Cell Mol Biol 4:102–107

O'Brodovich HM, Weitz JI, Possmayer F (1990) Effect of fibrinogen degradation products and lung ground substance on surfactant function. Biol Neonate 57:325–333

O'Neill SJ, Lesperance E, Klass DJ (1984a) Rat lung lavage surfactant enhances bacterial phagocytosis and intracellular killing by alveolar macrophages. Am Rev Respir Dis 130:225–230

O'Neill SJ, Lesperance E, Klass DJ (1984b) Human lung lavage surfactant enhances staphylococcal phagocytosis by alveolar macrophages. Am Rev Respir Dis 130:1177–1179

Oosterlaken-Dijksterhuis MA, van Eijk M, van Buel BLM (1991) Surfactant protein composition of lamellar bodies isolated from rat lung. Biochem J 274:115–119

Oosting RS, van Greevenbroek MMJ, Verhoef J, van Golde LMG, Haagsman HP (1991) Structural and functional changes of surfactant protein A induced by ozone. Am J Physiol (Lung Cell Mol Physiol) 261/5:L77–L83

Oosting RS, van Iwaarden JF, van Bree L, Verhoef J, van Golde LMG, Haagsman HP (1992) Exposure of surfactant protein A to ozone in vitro and in vivo impairs its interactions with alveolar cells. Am J Physiol (Lung Cell Mol Physiol) 262:L63–L68

Oulton M, Moores HK, Scott JE (1991) Effects of smoke inhalation on surfactant phospholipids and phospholipase A_2 activity in the mouse lung. Am J Pathol 138:195–202

Pattle RE (1955) Properties, function and origin of the alveolar lining layer. Nature 175/4469:1125–1126

Persson A, Chang D, Rust K, Moxley M, Longmore W, Crouch E (1989) Purification and biochemical characterization of CP4 (SP-D), a collagenous surfactant-associated protein. Biochemistry 28:6361–6367

Persson A, Chang D, Crouch E (1990) Surfactant protein D is a divalent cation-dependent carbohydrate-binding protein. J Biol Chem 265/10:5755–5760

Peters RE, Mudd JB (1982) Inhibition by ozone of the acylation of glycerol 3-phosphate in mitochondria and microsomes from rat lung. Arch Biochem Biophys 216/1:34–41

Pison U, Gono E, Joka T, Obertake U, Obladen M (1986) High-performance liquid chromatography of adult human bronchoalveolar lavage: assay for phospholipid lung profile. J Chromatogr 377:79–89

Possmayer F (1990) The role of surfactant-associated proteins. Am Rev Respir Dis 142:749–752

Rice WR, Sarin VK, Fox JL, Baatz J, Wert S, Whitsett JA (1989) Surfacant peptides stimulate uptake of phophatidylcholine by isolated cells. Biochim Biophys Acta 1006:237–245

Rich EA (1990) Pulmonary surfactant as a physiologic immunosuppressive agent. J Lab Clin Med 116/1:4–5

Richards R, Hunt J, George G (1983) Pulmonary surfactant and mineral-induced diseases. In: Cosmi EV, Scarpelli EM (eds) Pulmonary surfactant system. Elsevier, Amsterdam, pp 287–296

Rimpler M, Gerull A, Dörwald ML, Zaremba W, Degen E (1987) Quantitative determination of phospholipids in biological samples by high-performance liquid chromatography (abstract). Fresenius Z Anal Chem 327:37

Robertson B (1989a) Background to neonatal respiratory distress syndrome and treatment with exogenous surfactant. Dev Pharmacol Ther 13:159–163

Robertson B (1989b) European multicenter trials of Curosurf for treatment of neonatal respiratory distress syndrome (RDS). Eur Resp J 2/S8/598:763s

Robertson B (1989c) The evolution of neonatal respiratory distress syndrome into chronic lung disease. Eur Respir J 2/3:33s–37s

Robertson B (1989d) Neonatal respiratory distress syndrome and surfactant therapy; a brief review. Eur Respir J 2/3:73s–76s

Robinson PC, Watters LC, King TE, Mason RJ (1988) Idiopathic pulmonary fibrosis. Abnormalities in bronchoalveolar lavage fluid phospholipids. Am Rev Respir Dis 137:585–591

Rooney SA (1985) The surfactant system of the lung. In: Witschi HP, Brain JD (eds) Toxicology of inhaled materials. Springer, Berlin Heidelberg New York, pp. 471–502

Rooney SA (1987) The surfactant system and lung phospholipid biochemistry. Am Rev Respir Dis 131:439–460

Ryan SF, Ghassibi Y, Liau DF (1991) Effects of activated polymorphonuclear leucocytes upon pulmonary surfactant in vitro. Am J Respir Cell Mol Biol 4:33–41

Sallerin F, Prevost MC, De Graeve P (1984) Etude cytologique et phospholipidique du liquide de lavage broncho-alveolaire au cours des pneumopathies interstitielles diffuses et des sarcoidoses. Rev Mal Respir 1:181–185

Scarim J, Ghanbari H, Taylor V, Menon G (1989) Determination of phosphatidylcholine and disaturated phosphatidylcholine content in lung surfactant by high performance liquid chromatography. J Lipid Res 30:607–611

Schimmelpfeng J, Pätzold S, Seidel A (1989) Studies on the protective action of surfactant components on quartz and chrysotile asbestos toxicity. Eur Resp J 2/S8/411:722s (abstr)

Schlepper-Schäfer J, Wintergerst E, Plattner H, Manz-Keinke H (1989) SP-A interacts with macrophages and monocytes in a mannose dependent manner (abstract). Floating congress on the River Rhine, 11–17 Nov 1989 (abstr)

Schürch S, Gehr P, Im Hof V, Geiser M, Green F, (1990) Surfactant displaces particles toward the epithelium in airways and alveoli. Respir Physiol 80:17–32

Schürch S, Gehr P, Im Hof V, Geiser M, Green F (1990) Surfactant displaces particles to the epithelium in airways and alveoli. Respir Physiol 80:17–32

Seeger W, Günther A, Thede C (1989) Differential sensitivity to fibrinogen-inhibition of SP-C- versus SP-B-based surfactants. Floating congress on the River Rhine, 11–17 Nov 1989 (abstr)

Shapiro DL, Notter RH (1988) Controversies regarding surfactant replacement therapy. Clin Perinatol 1514:891–903

Sheehan PM, Stokes OC, Yeh Y-Y, Hughes WT (1986) Surfactant phospholipids and lavage phospholipase A_2 in experimental pneumocystis carinii pneumonia. Am Rev Respir Dis 134:526–531

Shimura S, Maeda S, Takismima T (1984) Giant lamellar bodies in alveolar type II cells of rats exposed to a low concentration of ozone. Respiration 46:303–309

Singh G, Katyal SL, Brown WE, Kennedy AL, Wong-Chong M-L, Gottron SA (1991) Identification, isolation, and partial characterization of a 7.5-kDa surfactant-associated protein. Exp Lung Res 17:559–567

Strayer DS, Merritt TA, Lwebuga-Mukasa J, Hallman M (1986) Surfactant-anti-surfactant immune complexes in infants with respiratory distress syndrome. Am J Pathol 122:353

Strayer DS, Merritt TA, Hallman M (1989) Surfactant replacement: immunological considerations. Eur Respir J 2/3:91s–96s

Strayer DS, Hallman M, Merritt TA (1991a) Immunogenicity of surfactant: I. Human alveolar surfactant. Clin Exp Immunol 83:35–40

Strayer DS, Hallman M, Merritt TA (1991b) Immunogenicity of surfactant: II. Porcine and bovine surfactants. Clin Exp Immunol 83:41–46

Strohmaier W, Redl H, Schlag G (1990) Studies of the potential role of a semisynthetic surfactant preparation in an experimental aspiration trauma in rabbits. Exp Lung Res 16:101–110

Strom KA (1983) Increase in lipid contents of alveolar macrophages from diesel particulates exposed rats. Toxicologist 3:8 (abstr)

Sulavik SB, Thrall RS (1987) Surfactant and physiologic alternations in an animal model of adult human lung disease. Respiration 51/1:10–14

Tahvanainen J, Hallman M (1987) Surfactant abnormality after endotoxin-induced lung injury in guinea-pigs. Eur J Respir Dis 71:250–258

Tenner AJ, Robinson SL, Borchelt J, Wright JR (1989) Human pulmonary surfactant protein (SP-A), a protein structurally homologous to C1q, can enhance FcR- and CR1-mediated phagocytosis. J Biol Chem 264/23:13923–13928

Thrall RS, Swendsen CL, Shannon TH, Kennedy CA, Frederick DS, Grunze MF, Sulavik SB (1987) Correlation of changes in pulmonary surfactant phospholipids with compliance in bleomycin-induced pulmonary fibrosis in the rat. Am Rev Respir Dis 136:113–118

Tierney DF (1989) Lung surfactant: some historical perspectives leading to its cellular and molecular biology. Am J Physiol 257:L1–L12

Van Golde LMG (1985) Synthesis of surfactant lipids in the adult and fetal lung: pathways and regulatory aspects. Eur J Respir Dis 142:19–24

Van Golde LMG, Batenburg JJ, Robertson B (1988) The pulmonary surfactant system: biochemical aspects and functional significance. Physiol Rev 68/2:374–455

Van Iwaarden F, Welmers B, Verhoef J (1990) Pulmonary surfactant protein A enhances the host-defense mechanism of rat alveolar macrophages. Am J Respir Cell Mol Biol 2:91–98

Van Iwaarden JF, van Strijp JAG, Ebskamp MJM, Welmers AC, Verhoef J, van Golde, LMG (1991) Surfactant protein A is opsonin in phagocytosis of herpes simplex virus type 1 by rat alveolar macrophages. Am J Physiol (Lung Cell Mol Physiol) 261/5:L204–209

Venkitaraman AR, Hall SB, Whitsett JA, Notter RH (1990) Enhancement of biophysical activity of lung surfactant extracts and phospholipid-apoprotein mixtures by surfactant protein A. Chem Phys Lipids 56:185–194

von Neergard K, (1929) Neue Auffassungen über einen Begriff der Atemmechanik. Die Retraktionskraft der Lunge, abhängig von der Oberflächenspannung in den Alveolen. Z Gesamte Exp Med 66:373–381

Wallace WE, Keane MJ, Vallythan V (1988) Suppression of inhaled particle cytotoxicity by pulmonary surfactant and re-toxification by phospholipase: distinguishing properties of quartz and kaolin. Ann Occup Hyg 32:291–298

Webb DSA, Jeska EL (1986) Enhanced luminol-dependent chemiluminescence of stimulated rat alveolar macrophages by pretreatment with alveolar lining material. J Leukoc Biol 40:55–64

Weber H, Heilmann P, Meyer B, Maier KL (1990) Effect of canine surfactant protein (SP-A) on the respiratory burst of phagocytic cells. FEBS Lett 270(1,2):90–94

Wilsher ML, Hughes DA, Haslam PL (1988a) Immunomodulatory effects of pulmonary surfactant on lymphocyte mediated cytotoxicity. Am Rev Respir Dis 137/4:52

Wilsher ML, Hughes DA, Haslam PL (1988b) Immunoregulatory properties of pulmonary surfactant: influence of variations in the phospholipid profile. Clin Exp Immunol 73:117–122

Wilsher ML, Hughes DA, Haslam PL (1988c) Immunomodulatory effects of pulmonary surfactant on natural killer cell and antibody-dependent cytotoxicity. Clin Exp Immunol 74:465–470

Wispe JR, Clark JC, Warner BB, Fajardo D, Hull WE, Holtzman RB, Whitsett JA (1990) Tumor necrosis factor-alpha inhibits expression of pulmonary surfactant protein. J Clin Invest 86:1954–1960

Wright ES (1986) Effects of short-term exposure to diesel exhaust on lung cell proliferation and phospholipid metabolism. Exp Lung Res 10:39–55

Wright ES, Vostal JJ (1983) Changes in lung cell population and phospholipid (PL) metabolism during inhalation exposure of rats to diesel exhaust. Toxicologist 3:8 (abstr)

Wright ES, White DM, Smiler KL (1990) Effects of chronic exposure to ozone on pulmonary lipids in rats. Toxicology 64:313–324

Wright JR (1990) Clearance and recycling of pulmonary surfactant. Lung Cell Mol Physiol 259/3:L1–L12

Wright JR, Tenner AJ (1989) Metabolism of lung surfactant components: could SP-A be a mediator of both surfactant metabolism and immune function? Floating congress on the River Rhine, 11–17 Nov 1989 (abstr)

New Approaches to Evaluating the Pulmonary Effects of Controlled Inhalation Exposures in Human Volunteers

P.A. Bromberg

University of North Carolina, Center for Environmental Medicine and Lung Biology, Medical Research Building C, Chapel Hill, NC 27599-7310, USA

Introduction

The respiratory tract serves as a passive portal of entry for various inhaled gases (e.g., CO) and vapors (e.g., benzene, toluene, methanol) as well as a target organ for the toxicologic effects of certain reactive gases (e.g., O_3) and inhaled particulate matter. I will limit my remarks to the latter class of air pollutants and discuss only effects on the respiratory system. Nevertheless, we should bear in mind the possibility that systemic as well as localized respiratory tract effects may be attributable to inhaled toxicants. My remarks will deal with some issues in experimental protocol development, with newer experimental techniques suitable for use in human subjects, and with the promise and pitfalls of in vitro toxicologic study of human cells. Most of my illustrations will come from ozone toxicology with which I have the greatest familiarity, but which I hope will be generalizable.

Experimental Protocols

Subject Selection

The use of human volunteers for experimental inhalation exposures is of course limited by ethical imperatives. In addition, the great interindividual diversity of healthy and diseased humankind poses problems as well as opportunities for the clinical investigator.

Normals

"Healthy" human subjects are usually characterized in terms of age, size, and sex. But even when an apparently homogeneous group of non-smoking, nonatopic, young, male, Caucasian subjects was subjected to an identical ozone exposure protocol, a wide range of spirometric response was observed

U. Mohr et al. (Eds.)
Advances in Controlled Clinical
Inhalation Studies
© Springer-Verlag Berlin Heidelberg 1993

(McDonnell et al. 1983). Interestingly, individual subjects display much more predictable responses when retested (Gliner et al. 1983; McDonnell et al. 1985a). This suggests that genetic factors may play a significant role in modulating this particular response. The role of genetic factors in determining biological response in man can be evaluated by studying identical (monozygotic) twins. Powerful methods for data analysis have been developed to allow reduction in size of the study population (DeFries and Fulker 1985).

Although it is currently not possible to predict the spirometric response of an untested subject to O_3 exposure, the reproducibility of an established response pattern allows preselection of subjects as "responders" or "nonresponders". One may then advantageously study these preselected groups further. For example, the role of nociceptive sensory nerve stimulation in determining the degree of ozone-induced decrement of inspiratory capacity (Hazucha et al. 1989) could be explored pharmacologically using an opioid receptor agonist in "responders" and an antagonist in "nonresponders". Alternatively, an attempt to define a "no-effect threshold" for ozone might be pursued in a group of "responders".

In pursuing subject preselection to reduce biologic variability and increase sensitivity in controlled exposure studies, one must bear in mind the implications for risk assessment. Extremely rigorous criteria for subject selection will reduce the extrapolated size of the at-risk population and may therefore diminish the weight given to that study in the development of environmental air quality criteria and policy. Indeed, one may question to what extent study volunteers recruited from the general population are truly representative of that population for the purpose of risk assessment.

An extension of this preselection procedure to the realm of epidemiology might involve identifying individuals in field studies who exhibit the largest responses to spontaneously occurring air pollution and then inviting them (and suitable controls) to participate in controlled exposure studies. Furthermore, an analysis of the characteristics of "responders" in field studies may provide guidance in defining subject selection criteria for controlled exposure studies.

Environmental factors that may affect response must also be considered in defining a study population. Thus, the spirometric response to ozone is influenced by cigarette smoking, recent prior exposure to ozone, and administration of antiinflammatory drugs such as indomethacin (Schelegle et al. 1987) or ibuprofen (Hazucha et al. 1991). Studies of monozygotic twins may be useful in uncovering such factors, since discrepant responses to an identical exposure implies that environmental (rather than genetic) factors are modulating the response (Webster et al. 1979).

Diseased

When a study population is selected for the presence of a particular disease that may confer unusual sensitivity to a certain toxicant, the elicited responses can again be very heterogeneous. This is the case, for example, with the bronchoconstrictive response of asthmatic subjects to brief exercise in atmospheres containing SO_2 (Horstman et al. 1986). Indeed, when examined closely, patients characterized as having a particular disease may constitute a quite heterogeneous group. "Asthma" is such a disease. It exhibits a broad spectrum of clinical severity and overlaps with chronic bronchitis. It is found in all age groups and has a variety of etiologies and special features. The use of clinically indicated treatment (medications) may interfere with the experimental study design.

The study of diseased subjects can also impose experimental limitations. Thus, individuals with chronic obstructive lung disease are unable to perform strenuous exercise. This may account for the fact that such subjects have not been found to be particularly susceptible to controlled ozone exposures (Kehrl et al. 1985), although one might expect such individuals to be at particularly high risk upon exposure to inhaled toxicants. Prolonged exposures at tolerated levels of exercise and repeated daily exposures may be worth considering when rethinking such experiments.

Age

Age is an important variable in designing toxicologic studies. Children are of particular concern because their lungs are still developing and may therefore be at greater risk for irreversible injury. Epidemiologic studies of respiratory health in a number of communities in the USA indicate that children residing in regions with higher levels of respirable particulate matter may be at risk for developing "bronchitis".

Acute studies of children exposed to ozone in outdoor play situations (Avol et al. 1985; Avol et al. 1987; Spektor et al. 1988; Higgins et al. 1990) and in controlled exposure experiments (McDonnell et al. 1985b; Koenig et al. 1988) suggest that children over 8 years old are about as susceptible as young adults to the effects of ozone on lung function.

Cross-sectional studies of the spirometric response to controlled exposures indicate that in adults ozone reactivity diminishes with increasing age (Drechsler-Parks et al. 1987; McDonnell et al. 1993). Whether the same can be said for the inflammatory response to ozone is not known. In any event, an age-related decrease of spirometric reactivity to ozone may offer another explanation for the previously noted insensitivity of patients with chronic obstructive pulmonary disease (COPD).

Exposure Conditions

The addition of exercise to controlled exposure protocols was essential to the demonstration of effects of ozone and of SO_2 exposure at "relevant" concentrations (less than 0.3 ppm for ozone and less than 1 ppm for SO_2, the latter in asthmatic subjects). Exposure protocols now almost invariably include exercise. This is not unreasonable given the nature of outdoor activities but would be less relevant to indoor air studies.

It is often recommended that controlled exposures should mimic "real-life" exposures. This implies not only that the concentration, duration, and subject activity level be realistic for a given pollutant, but also that mixtures of pollutants be studied. A recent example of controlled exposure protocol development driven by atmospheric monitoring data and field studies is the work of Horstman et al. (1990) and McDonnell et al. (1991) on prolonged exposures to very low concentrations of ozone. These studies demonstrated significant spirometric decrements developing several hours into 6.6-h exposures to 0.10 and 0.08 ppm O_3 in healthy young adults. Furthermore, analysis of bronchoalveolar lavage (BAL) fluid obtained 16 h after exposure in a subset of these subjects showed a significant inflammatory response (Devlin et al. 1991a). These data lend substantial additional weight to the argument (Rombout et al. 1986) that the U.S. National Ambient Air Quality Standard for ozone needs revision.

One of the unresolved issues in air pollution research is a certain lack of coherence between the serious health effects observed during so-called air pollution "disasters" and the modest effects of controlled exposures to low levels of SO_2 and acid sulfate aerosols, even in asthmatic patients. There is increasing evidence from cross-sectional epidemiologic studies of urban populations in the United States that even very low levels of particulate exposure cause significant health effects such as bronchitis in children and exacerbations of lung disease in adults. We have not yet devised the proper controlled exposure protocol to shed light on this problem. Whether the difficulty is in subject selection, exposure conditions, duration, or the health effect parameters selected for measurement is unclear.

Controlled exposures to pollutant *mixtures* are easy to recommend but difficult to organize in the absence of good clues from field studies. Even for only 2 pollutant species, the selection of concentration ranges and of exposure sequences and duration greatly complicates the task of the experimentalist. The interaction of pollutant exposure with the response of allergic individuals to antigen challenge will be of particular interest (Bascom et al. 1990; Molfino et al. 1991). The possible role of pollutant exposure in the genesis of undesirable immunologic sensitization to inhaled substances also needs study.

Measurement Selection

Not too surprisingly, experimentalists tend to measure effects that are known to occur from previous studies and are safe and relatively easy to measure. These constraints result in a great deal of descriptive data which are nevertheless useful in risk assessment and standard setting.

A more mechanistic approach to measurement selection is driven by the desire to explain the genesis of previously observed effects and to provide a firm basis for extrapolation and interpretation of limited experimental data. Thus, an attempt to correlate apparently separate effects such as increased prostaglandin (PGE_2) content in BAL liquid and spirometric decrements after ozone exposure stimulated me and my colleagues to study the effects of pretreatment with cyclooxygenase inhibitors on these variables (Hazucha et al. 1991). Basic principles of cell biology can also direct experimental design. For example, the respiratory tract polymorphonuclear cell influx following O_3 exposure (Seltzer et al. 1986; Koren et al. 1989) suggests the presence of some chemoattractant. Agents like leukotrienes (LTB_4) and complement-derived moieties do not appear to be involved (Seltzer et al. 1986; Koren et al. 1989). However, interleukin (IL-8) (S. Becker, personal communication) and platelet-activating factor (PAF) (J. Samet and M. Friedman, personal communication) are under study as candidate chemoattractants.

Another example of the use of a mechanistic approach to experimental design derives from the recognition that ozone can attack unsaturated lipids in aqueous media to form aldehydes and H_2O_2 (Pryor et al. 1991), both of which are toxic species. This finding suggests the utility of a search for these chemical species in vivo following ozone exposure. In addition, it focuses attention on the possible role of components of respiratory tract surface liquid in mediating the effects of O_3 exposure on the underlying tissue structures.

Techniques

It is a truism that new techniques resolve old questions and unveil new problems, while new concepts drive technical innovation. Early controlled exposure studies in clinical respiratory toxicology applied established techniques of pulmonary physiology to explore effects on respiratory mechanics, gas exchange, and respiratory control. These approaches have yielded important information and continue to be very useful.

Imaging

Newer physiologic techniques like the inhalation of isotopically labelled soluble substances and insoluble particles to measure deposition and clearance of probes deposited on the respiratory surfaces have been applied to studies of O_3 aerosols using the gamma-camera (Gerrity et al. 1991; Kehrl et al. 1987). Other imaging techniques when combined with suitable probes may provide new means of noninvasively exploring the pulmonary and bronchial microvasculature.

Microprobes

Microprobes of airway surfaces could produce valuable information. For example, measurement of *surface liquid pH* would be very useful in SO_2 and acid aerosol investigations, *surface temperature* could be applied to measurement of mucosal blood flow in airways, and *transepithelial electrical potential difference* has been applied to the in vivo study of effects of ozone inhalation in airways epithelial ion transport (Bromberg et al. 1991).

Dosimetry

Analyzers of pollutant gases with response time constants less than 250 ms would provide invaluable data on the dose of pollutant delivered to different levels along the airways. Progress in building such devices for ozone and in applying them to toxicologic studies has been reported (Gerrity et al. 1988; Ben-Jebria et al. 1989, 1990). Solid data from such experiments would allow more rigorous testing of the models that currently dominate our thinking about regional dosimetry in the human respiratory tract (Hu et al. 1992).

Other approaches to dosimetry involve the use of nonradioactive, isotopically labelled pollutants. For example, $^{18}O_2$ (nonradioactive) can be transformed into $^{18}O_3$ for inhalation studies. Postexposure samples are analyzed for their $^{18}O/^{16}O$ ratio by mass spectrometry. Since the natural abundance of ^{18}O (i.e., background) is about 2% of total oxygen atoms, extremely precise analytical techniques are needed to detect excess ^{18}O atoms. Nevertheless, analysis of the cellular and fluid phases of BAL liquid following exposure of human volunteers to 0.4 ppm $^{18}O_3$ appears to indicate that most of the isotope is in the fluid phase rather than the cellular fraction (G. Hatch, personal communication).

In my opinion, it is essential to pursue the issue of dosimetry in order to understand the pathogenesis of pollutant effects, to devise relevant in vitro exposure systems, and to compare animal with human exposures. Naturally, the relation between local tissue dose and the conventional exposure conditions (ambient concentration, ventilation, duration, etc.) will need to be explored and defined as well. Such information may also help us understand some of the intersubject response variability that has previously been discussed.

Small Airways Dysfunction

The development or application of methods designed to evaluate pollutant effects on small airways function deserves emphasis, given the importance of this region of the lung as a site for occult damage. In addition to more conventional techniques, such methods include the measurement of peripheral resistance with the wedged bronchoscope technique (Menkes and Traystman 1977), first described in humans by Bartels (1972), and the further application of the "bolus" dispersion technique (Heyder et al. 1988; McCawley and Lippmann 1988). The latter technique has recently been applied to the study of ozone effects (Keefe et al. 1991).

Cellular and Molecular Biology

Moving away from applied physiology and toward cellular/molecular biology, the development of techniques to explore the upper and lower airways and lung in human subjects have revolutionized our thinking.

Bronchoalveolar Lavage (BAL)

The application of transbronchoscopic BAL has defined the inflammatory response to O_3 inhalation in man and established that it develops within 1–2 h of the termination of a 2-h exposure to 0.4 ppm O_3 and evolves over a time course of more than 18 h (Seltzer et al. 1986; Koren et al. 1989, and in press). The initial neutrophil response as well as sharply increased levels of soluble mediators like IL-6 and PGE_2 decrease over the first 18 h following exposure, total protein remains about constant, but fibronectin increases (Koren et al. 1991). The pathogenesis and the health implications of these findings and their relation to the spirometric decrements observed after exposure to similar levels of ozone (McDonnell et al. 1983) and to the phenomenon of postozone bronchial hyperreactivity (Seltzer et al. 1986) are under active study.

It should be noted that the BAL procedure samples the airways and lung only beyond the point of wedging of the bronchoscope tip. This is generally in the middle lobe (right) or lingular (left) bronchus. There are further limitations in this type of sampling. One is that there is no distinction between airways and parenchyma; a second is that the surface liquid components are diluted to an unknown extent by the lavage procedure; a third is that the cellular fraction of the lavage is not necessarily representative of the cellular composition of the subadjacent tissues.

Rennard et al. (1990) pointed out the usefulness of an initial "small volume" (20 ml) lavage. By use of markers specific for airway secretions this fraction was shown to reflect preferentially airways surface liquid. Schelegle et al. (1991) used this technique to show selective neutrophilia in the airways only 1 h after a 1-h exposure to 0.3 ppm O_3. Others have developed specialized catheters with balloons that can be temporarily inflated to isolate briefly a portion of the left main stem bronchus for the purpose of a localized lavage or a localized instillation of antigen in a large airway.

The dilutional problem remains unresolved despite the interesting proposal by Rennard et al. (1986) to use endogenous urea as a marker for the original volume of surface liquid. Urea in the surface liquid is reasonably assumed to be in thermodynamic equilibrium with the extracellular fluid and blood plasma at the start of the lavage. The problem is that additional urea diffuses into the lavage liquid during the course of procedure, resulting in some overestimate of the original surface liquid volume.

Biopsy

The limited sampling achieved by lavage has been addressed by adding biopsy procedures. Atraumatic curette-scrape biopsy of the respiratory epithelium lining the surface of the inferior nasal turbinate provides about 10^5 epithelial cells per scrape. Brushing of lower airways provides $0.5-2.5 \times 10^5$ viable cells per brush. The brushings can be obtained at multiple levels along the airway to look for regional effects, including the trachea and main bronchi which are excluded by conventional BAL. In addition, trans-bronchoscopic endobronchial biopsy under direct vision is an extremely safe procedure. It provides small samples of intact mucosal tissue suitable for histologic examination, for immunohistochemistry, and for in situ hybridization.

Most of the cells ordinarily recovered from BAL are alveolar macrophages. These can be cultured and their functional properties assessed. Most of the cells recovered from nasal curette or airways brush biopsies are epithelial. These cells can be cultured on suitable supports and culture media. Even with as few as several thousand cells, specific mRNA levels can be assessed by first producing complementary DNA with reverse transcriptase and then amplifying specific cDNA regions using the polymerase chain reaction (PCR) with suitable primers. If precautions are observed, the resultant specific cDNA levels can be interpreted quantitatively in terms of the original level of mRNA.

Using such techniques, key questions related to the response of respiratory epithelium to toxicant exposure can be addressed. For example, are airways epithelial cells a source of the increased levels of IL-6 and IL-8 observed in BAL after ozone exposure? Are these changes present in selected regions only, and do these regions conform to the pattern of tissue uptake of the toxicant?

In Vitro Toxicology

Progress in cell biology has made it possible to use normal human respiratory cells in primary culture or immortalized human bronchial epithelial cell or monocytic lines in culture to study the effects of in vitro exposure to gases and particles. The advantages of such procedures include: the ability to study substances to which human subjects cannot ethically be exposed; studying human cells without being dependent on costly subject recruitment and controlled exposure procedures; the ability to control more rigorously the experimental conditions, e.g., composition of the extracellular medium, nature of the substrate supporting the cell layer, etc.; the ability to sample the basal as well as the apical side of the cell layer in the case of epithelial cells; and the ability to test specific mechanistic hypotheses.

For example, a serum-sensitive clone of a human bronchial epithelial cell line (BEAS-2B/S6), originally derived in the laboratory of Lechner and Harris at the National Institutes of Health (NIH) by infection with an adenovirus 12-SV40 (simian virus) hybrid (Reddel et al. 1988; Ke et al. 1988), has been extensively studied at the Environmental Protection Agency (USEPA) Clinical Research Branch and University of North Carolina (UNC) Center for Environmental Medicine in Chapel Hill. The culture conditions have been standardized, and a number of properties of these cells have been found to be comparable with those of primary airways epithelial cell cultures. Following brief apical side exposures to as little as $0.1\,ppm\ O_3$ in the absence of apical surface liquid, the cells remain viable and attached but show increased release of arachidonate metabolities, PAF, and cytokines (Devlin et al. 1991b; Samet et al. 1991). These findings suggest a proinflammatory function for epithelial cells.

Primary cultures of human respiratory epithelium as well as BEAS-2B/S6 cells have allowed the development of an in vitro model of infectivity (Becker et al. 1991a). Respiratory syncytial virus (RSV) can infect these cells and cause plaque formation in the cell layer, accompanied by the production of viral proteins. The development of this model will allow exploration of the interaction of experimental RSV infection with exposure to relevant toxicants, as well as other studies of the biology of human RSV infections.

Of course, cultured cell systems do not perfectly reflect in vivo conditions. Thus, the relevant toxicant dose range for cells that normally are found deep within the lung is not yet clear, the cultured cells are not rigorously identical to their counterparts in vivo, and the milieu of the cultured cells is far from representing reality. For example, Devlin and Koren (1990) described extensive changes in protein synthesis in alveolar macrophages obtained by BAL following an in vivo ozone exposure and cultured briefly in the presence of [^{35}S]methionine. However, when alveolar macrophages were exposed to ozone ex vivo, these changes were not reproduced (Becker et al. 1991b). It appears that the in vivo milieu is essential for these particular ozone-induced changes to occur. The creation of interactive, multicellular, in vitro systems requires another level of experimental complexity.

Conclusion

It is clear that our ability to study the effect of inhaled toxicants on the human respiratory system is far from being exhausted. The design of controlled chamber exposures of human subjects will need closer coordination with epidemiologists. More attention needs to be paid to dosimetry and to the mechanisms underlying the phenomenology of observed responses. The development of new physiologic and biologic tools will allow this goal to be pursued vigorously. The use of cultured human cells opens the way to studies of agents and of interactions that would otherwise not be possible. It will be important to document the quantitative relevance of in vitro to in vivo toxicology, and ozone is a toxicant that is well suited for such comparisons.

References

Avol EL, Linn WS, Shamoo DA, Valencia LM, Anzar UT, Hackney JD (1985) Respiratory effects of photochemical oxidant air pollution in exercising adolescents. Am Rev Respir Dis 132:619–622

Avol EL, Linn WS, Shamoo DA, Valencia LM, Venet TG, Trim SC, Hackney JD (1987) Short-term respiratory effects of photochemical oxidant exposure in exercising children. J Air Pollut Control Assoc 37:158–162

Bartels M (1972) Collaterale Ventilation beim Menschen. Thesis, Tübingen University

Bascom R, Naclerio RM, Fitzgerald TK, Kagey-Sobotka A, Proud D (1990) Effect of ozone inhalation on the response to nasal challenge with antigen of allergic subjects. Am Rev Respir Dis 142:594–601

Becker S, Soukup J, Yankaskas JR (1991a) Respiratory syncytial virus infection of human primary nasal and bronchial epithelial cell cultures and bronchoalveolar macrophages. Am J Respir Cell Mol Biol (in press)

Becker S, Madden M, Newman SL, Devlin RB, Koren HS (1991b) Modulation of human alveolar macrophage properties by ozone exposure in vitro. Toxicol Appl Pharmacol (in press)

Ben-Jebria A, Ultman JS (1989) Fast-responding chemiluminescent ozone analyzer for respiratory applications. Rev Sci Instrum 60:3004–3011

Ben-Jebria A, Hu S-C, Ultman JS (1990) Improvements in a chemiluminescent analyzer for respiratory applications. Rev Sci Instrum 61:3435–3439

Bromberg PA, Ranga V, Stutts MJ (1991) Effects of ozone on airways epithelial permeability and ion transport. Research report 48, Health Effects Institute, Cambridge, MA, pp 1–21

DeFries JC, Fulker DW (1985) Multiple regression analysis of twin data. Behav Genet 15:467–473

Devlin RB, Koren HS (1990) The use of two-dimensional gel electrophoresis to analyze changes in alveolar macrophage proteins in humans exposed to ozone. Am J Respir Cell Mol Biol 2:281–288

Devlin RB, McDonnell WF, Mann R, Becker S, House DE, Schreinemachers D, Koren HS (1991a) Exposure of humans to ambient levels of ozone for 6.6 hours causes cellular and biochemical changes in the lung. Am J Respir Cell Mol Biol 4:72–81

Devlin, RB, Noah T, McKinnon KP, Koren HS (1991b) The use of a cell line as a model system to study the interaction of environmental toxicants with human airway epithelial cells. Toxicologist 11:851

Drechsler-Parks DM, Bedi JF, Horvath SM (1987) Pulmonary function response of older men and women to ozone exposure. Exp Gerontol 22:91–101

Gerrity TR, Weaver RA, Berntsen J, House DE, O'Neil JJ (1988) Extrathoracic and intrathoracic removal of ozone in tidal-breathing humans. J Appl Physiol 65:393–400

Gerrity TR, Bennett WD, Keefe M, DeWitt P, Chapman W (1991) The response of tracheobronchial clearance of inhaled particles to acute ozone exposure in healthy humans. Am Rev Respir Dis 143:A91

Gliner JA, Horvath SM, Folinsbee LJ (1983) Pre-exposure to low ozone concentrations does not diminish the pulmonary function response on exposure to higher ozone concentration. Am Rev Respir Dis 127:51–55

Hazucha MJ, Bates DV, Bromberg PA (1989) Mechanism of action of ozone on the human lung. J Appl Physiol 67:1535–1541

Hazucha MJ, Pape G, Madden M, Koren H, Kehrl H, Bromberg P (1991) Effects of cyclooxygenase inhibition on ozone-induced respiratory inflammation and lung function changes. Am Rev Respir Dis 143:A701

Heyder J, Blanchard JD, Feldman HA, Brain JD (1988) Convective mixing in human respiratory tract: estimates with aerosol boli. J Appl Physiol 64:1273–1278

Higgins ITT, D'Arcy JB, Gibbons DI, Avol EL, Gross KB (1990) Effect of exposures to ambient ozone on ventilatory lung function in children. Am Rev Respir Dis 141:1136–1146

Horstman D, Roger LJ, Kehrl H, Hazucha MJ (1986) Airway sensitivity of asthmatics to sulfur dioxide. Toxicol Ind Health 2:289–298

Horstman DH, Folinsbee LJ, Ives PJ, Abdul-Salaam S, McDonnell WF (1990) Ozone concentration and pulmonary response relationships for 6.6-hour exposures with five hours of moderate exercise. Am Rev Respir Dis 142:1158–1163

Hu S-C, Ben-Jebria A, Ultman JS (1992) Longitudinal distribution of ozone absorption in the lung: quiet respiration in healthy subjects. J Appl Physiol 73:1655–1661

Ke Y, Reddel RR, Gerwin BI, Miyashita M, McMenamin M, Lechner JF, Harris CC (1988) Human bronchial epithelial cells with integrated SV40 virus T antigen genes retain the ability to undergo squamous differentiation. Differentiation 38:60–66

Keefe MJ, Bennett WD, DeWitt P, Seal E, Strong AA, Gerrity TR (1991) The effect of ozone exposure on the dispersion of inhaled aerosol boluses in healthy human subjects. Am Rev Respir Dis 144:23–30

Kehrl HR, Hazucha MJ, Solic JJ, Bromberg PA (1985) Responses of subjects with chronic obstructive pulmonary disease after exposure to 0.3 ppm ozone. Am Rev Respir Dis 131:719–724

Kehrl HR, Vincent LM, Kowalsky RJ, Horstman DH, O'Neil JJ, McCartney WH, Bromberg PA (1987) Ozone exposure increases respiratory epithelial permeability in man. Am Rev Respir Dis 135:1124–1128

Koenig JQ, Covert DS, Smith MS, Van Belle G, Pierson WE (1988) The pulmonary effects of O_3 and NO_2 alone and combined in healthy and asthmatic adolescent subjects. Toxicol Ind Health 4:521–532

Koren HS, Devlin RB, Graham DE, Mann R, McGee MP, Horstman DH, Kozumbo WJ, Becker S, House DE, McDonnell WF, Bromberg PA (1989) Ozone-induced inflammation in the lower airways of human subjects. Am Rev Respir Dis 139:407–415

Koren HS, Devlin RB, Becker S, Perez R, McDonnell WF (1991) Time-dependent changes of markers associated with inflammation in the lungs of humans exposed to ozone. Toxicol Pathol 19:406–411

McCawley M, Lippmann M (1988) Development of an aerosol dispersion test to detect early changes in lung function. Am Ind Hyg Assoc J 49:357–366

McDonnell WF, Horstman DH, Hazucha MJ, Seal E Jr, Haak ED, Salaam SA, House DE (1983) Pulmonary effects of ozone exposure during exercise: dose-response characteristics. J Appl Physiol 54:1345–1352

McDonnell WF, Horstman DH, Salaam SA, House DE (1985a) Reproducibility of individual responses to ozone exposure. Am Rev Respir Dis 131:36–40

McDonnell WF, Chapman RS, Leigh MW, Strope GL, Collier AM (1985b) Respiratory response of vigorously exercising children to 0.12 ppm ozone exposure. Am Rev Respir Dis 132:875–879

McDonnell WF, Kehrl HR, Abdul-Salaam S, Ives PJ, Folinsbee LJ, Devlin RB, O'Neil JJ, Horstman DH (1991) Respiratory responses of humans exposed to low levels of ozone for 6.6 hours. Arch Environ Health 46:145–150

McDonnell WF, Muller KE, Bromberg PA, Shy CM (1993) Predictors of individual differences in acute response to ozone exposure. Am Rev Respir Dis 147: xxx–xxx (in press)

Menkes HA, Traystman RJ (1977) Collateral ventilation. Am Rev Respir Dis 116:287–309

Molfino NA, Wright SC, Katz I, Tarlo S, Silverman F, McClean PA, Szalai JP, Raizenne M, Slutsky AS, Zamel N (1991) Effect of low concentrations of ozone on inhaled allergen responses in asthmatic subjects. Lancet 338:199–203

Pryor WA, Das B, Church DF (1991) The ozonation of unsaturated fatty acids: aldehydes and hydrogen peroxide as products and possible mediators of ozone toxicity. Chem Res Toxicol 4:341–348

Reddel RR, Ke Y, Gerwin BI, McMenamin MG, Lechner JF, Su RT, Brash DE, Park J-B, Rhim JS, Harris CC (1988) Transformation of human bronchial epithelial cells by infection with SV40 or adenovirus-12 SV40 hybrid virus, or transfection via strontium phosphate coprecipitation with a plasmid containing SV40 early region genes. Cancer Res 48:1904–1909

Rennard SI, Basset G, Lecossier D, O'Donnell K, Martin P, Crystal RG (1986) Estimation of volume of epithelial lining fluid recovered by lavage using urea as a marker of dilution. J Appl Physiol 60:532–538

Rennard SI, Ghafouri M, Thompson AB, Linder J, Vaughan W, Jones K, Ertl RF, Christensen K, Prince A, Stahl MG, Robbins RA (1990) Fractional processing of sequential bronchoalveolar lavage to separate bronchial and alveolar samples. Am Rev Respir Dis 141:208–217

Rombout P, Lioy PJ, Goldstein BD (1986) Rationale for an eight-hour ozone standard. J Air Pollut Control Assoc 36:913–917

Samet JM, Noah T, McKinnon K, Devlin RB, Friedman M (1991) Effect of ozone on platelet activating factor (PAF) synthesis in human bronchial epithelial cells. FASEB J 5:A484

Schelegle ES, Adams WC, Siefkin AD (1987) Indomethacin pretreatment reduces ozone-induced pulmonary function decrements in human subjects. Am Rev Respir Dis 136:1350–1354

Schelegle ES, Siefkin AD, McDonald RJ (1991) Time course of ozone-induced neutrophilia in normal humans. Am Rev Respir Dis 143:1353–1358

Seltzer J, Bigby BG, Stulbarg M, Holtzman MJ, Nadel JA, Ueki IF, Leikauf GD, Goetzl EJ, Boushey HA (1986) Ozone-induced change in bronchial reactivity to methacholine and airway inflammation in humans. J Appl Physiol 60:1321–1326

Spektor DM, Lippmann M, Lioy PJ, Thurston GD, Citak K, James DJ, Bock N, Speizer FE, Hayes C (1988) Effects of ambient ozone on respiratory function in active, normal children. Am Rev Respir Dis 137:313–320

Webster PM, Lorimer EG, Paul SF, Woolf CR, Zamel N (1979) Pulmonary function in identical twins: comparison of non-smokers and smokers. Am Rev Respir Dis 119:223–228

Section 6. Clinical Data and Regulatory Decisions

Meta-analysis and "Effective Dose" Revisited

M.J. Hazucha

University of North Carolina, Center for Environmental Medicine and Lung Biology, Chapel Hill, NC 27599–7310, USA

Introduction

Quantitative reanalyses of data from various laboratories have been done for more than 30 years. However, the development of more formal rules for combining the results of controlled trials, the adaptation of existing statistical techniques to this type of data, and the development of new methods to advance such secondary analyses have taken place only over the past decade. Although the process of combining and synthesizing the results from separate but similar experiments – called meta-analysis – is still controversial, it is steadily gaining ground. In the area of health effects of ozone on pulmonary function, the objective of meta-analyses has been to characterize the ozone dose-effect relationship from diverse studies. Attempts have also been made to test the validity of the previously advanced notion of "effective dose," the product of ozone concentration, minute ventilation, and duration of exposure (Silverman et al. 1976). One study of pooled data found that a linear regression model expressed the best dose-effect association; the author also concluded that the "effective dose" concept is valid (Colucci 1983). However, a later study based on a larger data set reported a quadratic function as the best-fitting model and implicitly demonstrated that in its present mathematical form, "effective dose" might be invalid (Hazucha 1987). Subsequent studies appear to support the conclusions of the latter study.

Although the number of studies available for meta-analysis is still quite small compared with the numbers in other fields of research, the small reported data sample variances partially compensate for the lack of numbers. It is this tightness of data which permits us to go beyond simple pooling of results to clarify inconsistencies, to answer the controversial questions of interest, or to explore new associations. In the meta-analysis reported here, the ozone dose-response relationship and the influence of additional determinants on its form were reevaluated, the validity of the "effective" dose concept retested, and the existence of an ozone threshold as well as a temporal pattern of adaptation to ozone reexamined.

U. Mohr et al. (Eds.)
Advances in Controlled Clinical
Inhalation Studies
© Springer-Verlag Berlin Heidelberg 1993

Meta-analysis

General Methodology

Clearly, the traditional methods such as a literature review or identification of key studies are inadequate to unify the sometimes conflicting results such as those mentioned earlier. Meta-analyses, however, can be used to discern which factors have influenced the regression equations even when those factors are not obvious. The general goals of meta-analysis are the following:

1. To evaluate objectively and synthesize findings from different experimental studies
2. To increase the utilization of available experimental data and, in particular, (a) to improve estimates of effect size, (b) to enhance statistical power for key variables of interest, and (c) to identify and evaluate the strength of the associations between variables of interest
3. To resolve uncertainties and controversies among the findings of different studies
4. To identify the inadequacies of past experimental work
5. To answer more general questions which are not answerable by individual or even multiple experimental trials (Sacks et al. 1987)
6. To develop new hypotheses and ideas for future research (Jenicek 1989)

At present, there are no criteria for when meta-analysis should be performed; however, methodological approaches and, in particular, the general rules for selection of studies have been well established.

As with any research endeavor, the first step in meta-analysis is assessment of the problem(s) and definition of an objective(s). Subsequent steps in a well-organized analysis include a critical review of the literature and selection of pertinent studies, identification of and selection of common endpoints, a definition of analytical strategies with model identification, and finally, synthesis of the results and their interpretation (Laird and Mosteller 1990).

Concentration-Response Relationship in Healthy Populations

Since the publication in 1987 of a quantitative analysis of the relationship between ozone concentration and spirometric response (Hazucha 1987), the number of new studies reporting ozone-induced effects has been substantial. Therefore, the primary goals of the current analysis were to incorporate these studies into the original database and then to update and expand the application of regression models in order to evaluate the influence of key parameters on the magnitude of the response.

The criteria for inclusion were the same as those previously reported (Hazucha 1987). Data from 20 new technical and research publications augmented the total number of studies to 49. To facilitate comparisons between the previous and current meta-analyses, the data were grouped by minute ventilation into four sets: light exercise set, $\dot{V}_E \leq 23\,l/min$; moderate exercise set, $\dot{V}_E = 24-43\,l/min$; heavy exercise set, $\dot{V}_E = 44-63\,l/min$; and very heavy exercise set, $\dot{V}_E \geq 64\,l/min$. Within each ventilation (exercise) group, data were subdivided by duration of exposure into two subgroups: 1-h and 2-h ozone exposure sets. These two subgroups were further subdivided by the activity pattern utilized during exposure trials into rest, intermittent, and continuous exercise data sets. Subsets with less than 6 data points from at least three different studies were excluded from the analysis. The reported primary test for the assessment of exposure effects was invariably spirometry, and the forced expiratory volume in 1 S (FEV_1) was selected as the key spirometric variable of interest. In the exploratory phase of the analysis, several second-order regression models, weighted by a number of subjects per study cohort, were tested. Although several models performed well, the pure quadratic function with restricted intercept for a dependent variable to 100 was the simplest and one of the best-fitting. Mathematically, the function has the form $PCT = 100 - A * CONC^2$ (a parabola with its vertex at a 100% value), where PCT is a selected spirometric variable expressed in percentage change from control, A is a quadratic coefficient, and CONC is ozone concentration in ppm.

The largest subgroup of studies used 2-h exposure with moderate intermittent exercise. The scatter plot of 143 points from 18 studies, the mean +/- standard deviation by ozone concentration, and the 95% confidence intervals for mean and predicted values for this subgroup are shown in Fig. 1. The regression function in this plot was not restricted by the intercept = 100. A similar distribution of data points was observed in other subgroups regardless of category. Fig. 2 shows the regression curves for the rest (no exercise) subgroup and the 2-h intermittent exercise subgroups. The pattern of response and the quadratic coefficients were very close to those reported previously (Hazucha 1987).

Regression curves for 1-h continuous exercise at three different ventilation levels, as well as a regression curve obtained with 1-h rest (no exercise) data, are shown in Fig. 3. All regression curve parameter estimates were based on 23-33 data points (4-5 studies). Insufficient data for the light exercise group prevented any meaningful analysis. The correlation coefficients from moderate to the highest exercise load were 0.710, 0.795, and 0.985, respectively. At a moderate exercise load, the quadratic coefficient was found to be lower for continuous than for intermittent exercise; for heavy and very heavy exercise regressions, the coefficients were higher for continuous than for intermittent exercise. This indicates that at higher exercise loads the same ozone concentration will elicit a greater spirometric response following continuous exercise than following intermittent exercise.

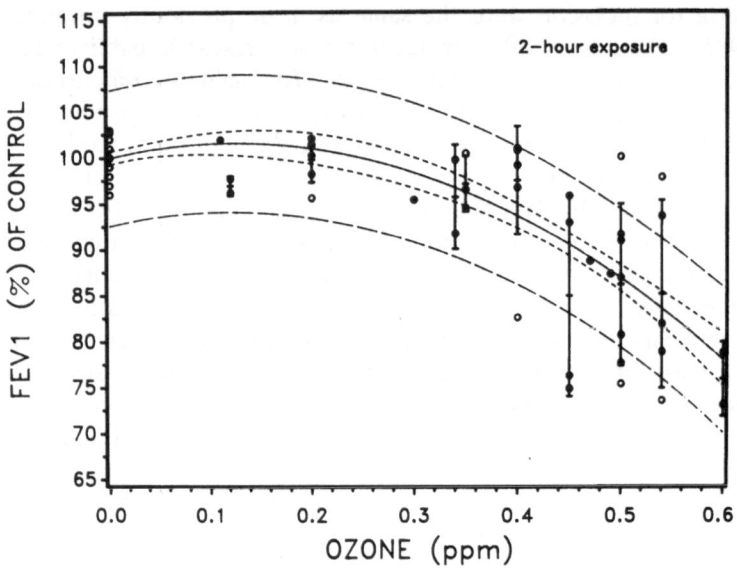

Fig. 1. Scatter plot of ozone concentration vs. mean decrements in FEV_1, following 2 h of exposure with intermittent moderate exercise. *Vertical bars* indicate mean +/− SD at a particular ozone concentration. Regression line (*solid line*) is bracketed by an upper and a lower 95% confidence interval for the expected mean of the dependent variable (*inner dashed lines*) and by an upper and a lower 95% confidence interval for individual predictions (*outer dashed lines*)

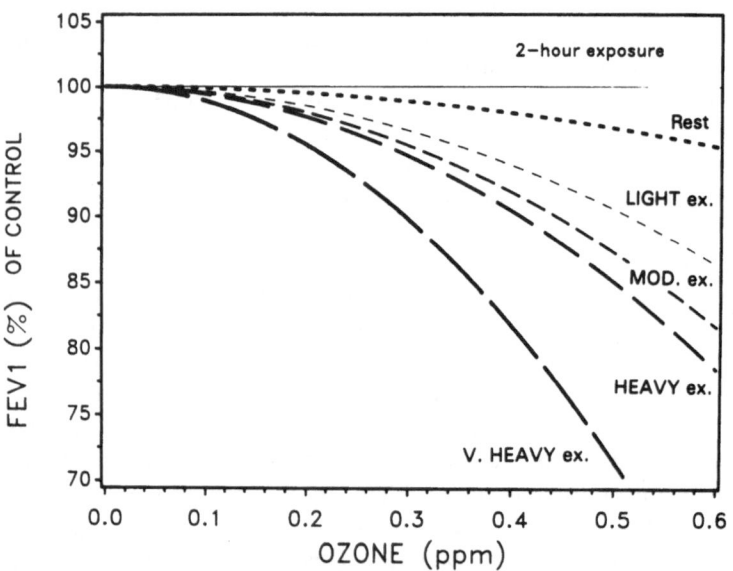

Fig. 2. Effects of minute ventilation, expressed in terms of intermittent exercise intensity, on FEV_1-ozone concentration regression (2-h exposures)

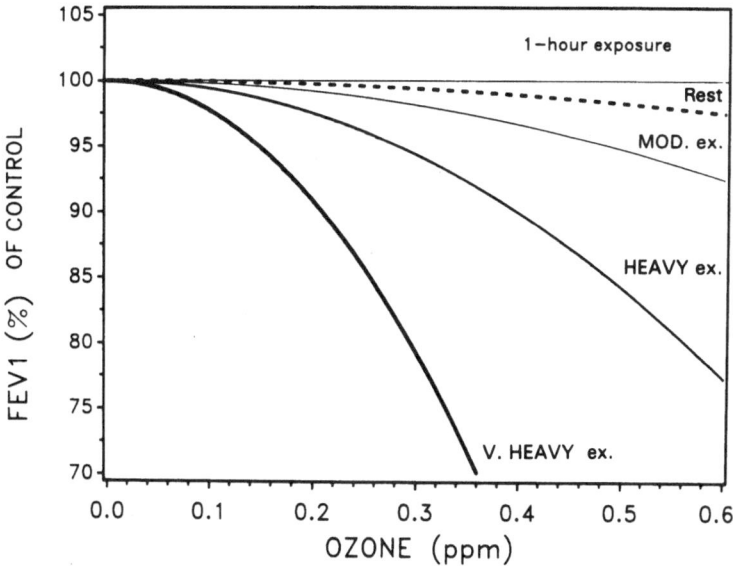

Fig. 3. Effects of minute ventilation, expressed in terms of continuous exercise load, on FEV_1-ozone concentration regression (1-h exposures)

The effect of ventilation and the exercise activity mode on lung function response during exposure is more apparent when the continuous and intermittent exercise regression curves, stratified by level of exercise, are combined (Fig. 4). Despite different exposure times (1 h for continuous and 2 h for intermittent exercise), the cumulative ventilation for each study at a corresponding exercise level was about the same. Since the ozone doses within the subgroups were more or less equivalent, intuitively they were expected to elicit an equal response. Indeed, some investigators have reported that regardless of exercise continuity, spirometric responses to a comparable dose of ozone are in "relatively close agreement" (Adams et al. 1981; Colucci 1983). The current analysis, however, shows that only the heavy exercise group regressions support this paradigm (Fig. 4).

The most convenient explanation for such "inconsistency" of response is imbalance in the number of trials per subgroup used in multiregression analysis; the ratios of the number of trials used in the intermittent exercise group to the number used in continuous exercise sets were approximately 3, 1, and 1, from the moderate to the intense exercise set. Although this factor might influence the regression, it is more likely that the "numerically equivalent dose" does not necessarily mean an "equal effect dose". Indeed, findings from several studies imply that under otherwise comparable conditions, "equivalent doses" induced a spectrum of responses. More systematic evaluation of "equivalent dose" effects strongly suggests that the concept might not be valid (Silverman et al. 1976, 1977).

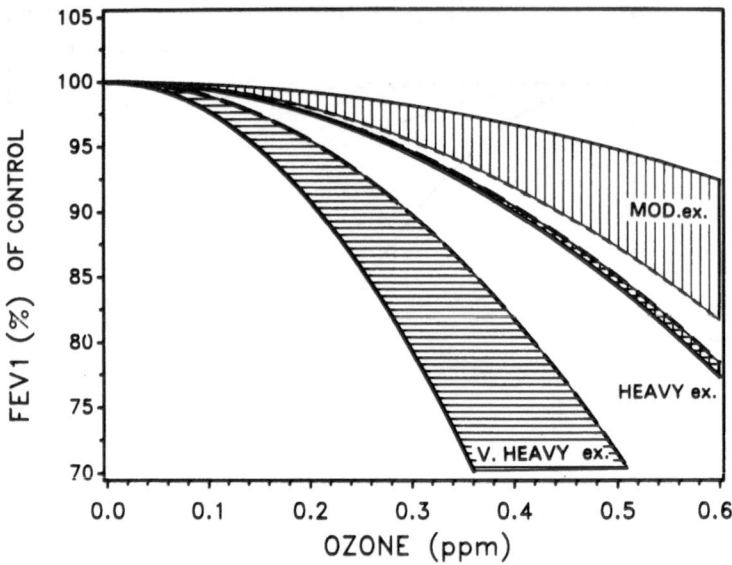

Fig. 4. Regression curves of FEV_1 vs. ozone concentration for 1-h exposures with continuous exercise (*solid lines*) and comparable 2-h exposures with intermittent exercise (*dashed lines*), *Shaded areas* represent differences between pairs of curves at equivalent workloads; *vertical lines*, moderate exercise; *crosshatched*, heavy exercise; *horizontal lines*, very heavy exercise pair of regression curves

Ozone Response of Sensitive Populations

The paucity of studies reporting ozone effects on populations at risk prevents any exploration of the dose-effect relationship. Minimally acceptable meta-analysis would require at least twice as many studies as are currently available. The findings of existing studies, however, can still be meaningfully compared with a prediction range for a healthy population. Although more specific tests have shown that some of the potentially susceptible groups might be, on average, more responsive to ozone than normal subjects, the results of routine spirometry, a test used invariably in the assessment of the effects of ozone in healthy populations, have been equivocal. Fig. 5 graphically illustrates postexposure changes in FEV_1, obtained from the available studies and plotted over the 95% confidence range for a healthy population intermittently exercising in ozone under a moderate workload for 2 h. The scatter plot does not suggest that these groups considered to be at risk are indeed at greater risk to ozone than is the general population.

Similarly, because of the insufficient number of laboratory trials on cohorts of females, smokers, and older individuals, no quantitative integration and analysis of these populations is possible at present.

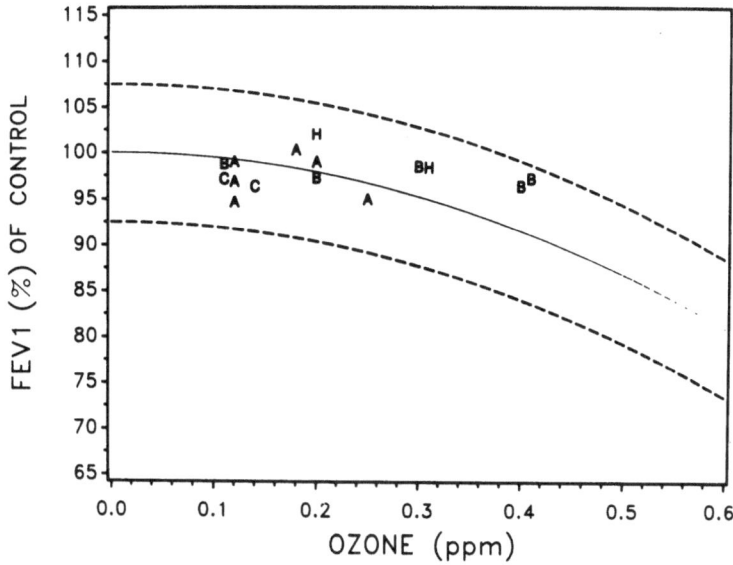

Fig. 5. Average FEV_1 responses of groups of individuals considered to be at risk following 2-h exposures to ozone with moderate intermittent exercise; *A*, asthmatics; *B*, chronic bronchitics; *C*, children; *H*, patients with coronary heart disease. Data are superimposed over a regression curve (*solid line*) and upper and lower 95% confidence limits (*dashed lines*) for predicted values; the curves were derived from 2-h exposures of healthy subjects, intermittently exercising at moderate loads

Effective Dose

As demonstrated in Fig. 4 and briefly discussed in an earlier section, the available literature clearly indicates that the "equivalent" ventilation paradigm might at best be valid only within narrowly defined exposure conditions. The reported observations also suggest that the extension of the "equivalent" ventilation model by including exposure duration as a codeterminant of the "effective" dose (ozone concentraion × minute ventilation × exposure duration) does not generalize the application; even this model appears to be valid only under restricted conditions. To date, the most convincing evidence that the same "effective" dose does not induce the same magnitude of effects has come from our laboratory (Hazucha et al. 1990). Twenty-four young, healthy nonsmokers were randomly exposed to clean air, steady-state 0.12 ppm ozone, and a variable concentration rising steadily from 0 to 0.24 ppm ozone over a 4-h period, and then regressing back to 0 over the subsequent 4-h period. Three of the subjects were exposed to air and 0.12 ppm ozone for up to 10 h. During the exposure, subjects alternately exercised at a moderate load (38 l/min) and rested for 30 min. Both ozone exposures induced subjective symptoms and significantly

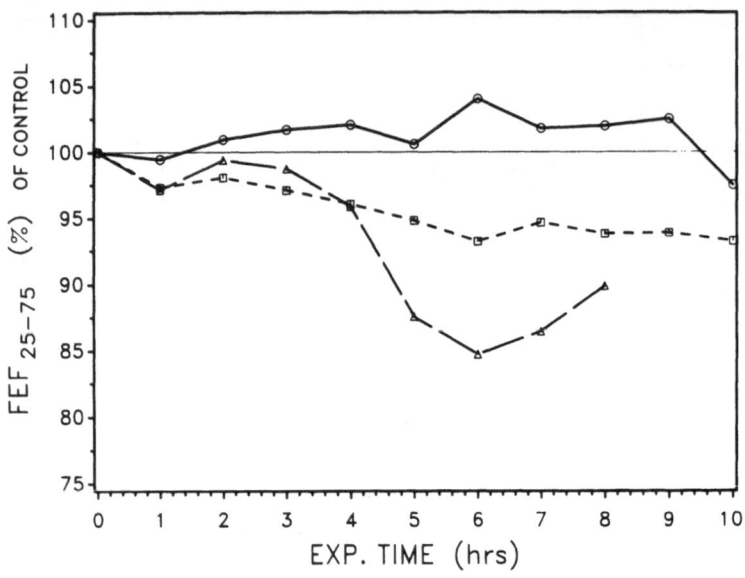

Fig. 6. Plot of average changes in forced expiratory flow (FEF_{25-75}) vs. 10-h exposure to air (*circles, solid line*), steady-state 0.12 ppm ozone (*squares, dashed line*), and transient concentration of ozone (*triangles, broken line*); $n = 24$ except for 9th and 10th h wherre $n = 3$

decreased lung function. The elicited effects of two equivalent "effective" doses (4th and 8th h) were not of the same magnitude (Fig. 6). Midway through the exposure the variable concentration profile induced smaller effects, and at the end of the 8-h exposure, significantly greater effects than constant exposure. These results confirm that the "effective" dose is not a sufficient index of exposure; ozone concentration must be weighted more heavily in the "effective" dose product.

Adaptation to Ozone

Many laboratories have studied the effects on pulmonary function of repeated daily exposures over a range of ozone concentrations. In general, it has been found that the mean decrement in key spirometric variables was largest on the 1st or 2nd day of exposure. The decrement in response to ozone on the 3rd day was less than on a previous day; subsequent daily exposures attenuated the response further. Several authors have suggested that adaptation will develop only above "threshold" ($\geqslant 0.2$ ppm) ozone concentrations, and that above this level, regardless of concentration, adaptation is more or less complete within 3 days following the maximum effect day. Our most recent findings, however, indicate that adaptation can develop even at a low ozone concentration (Hazucha et al. 1990). In 8-h

CONSECUTIVE DAILY EXPOSURES to OZONE

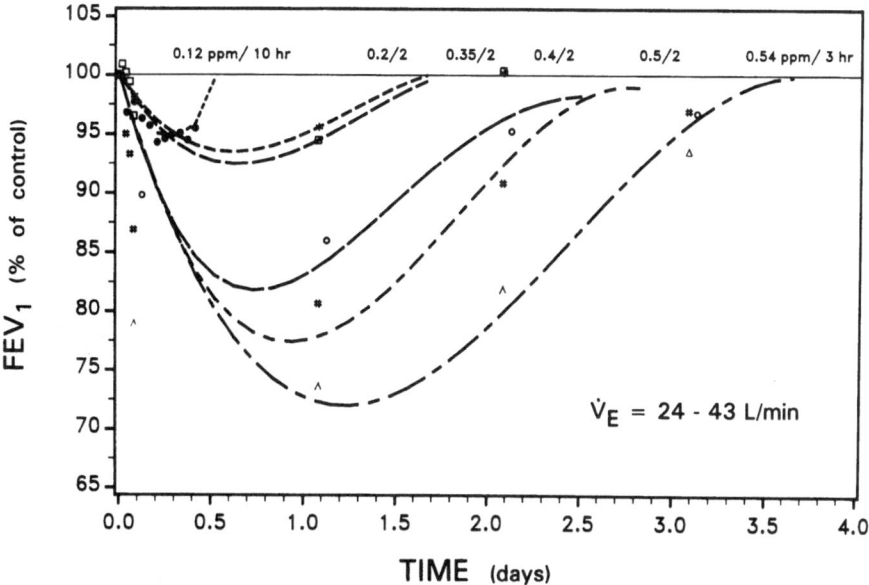

Fig. 7. A set of regression curves fitted to day by day postexposure values in FEV_1 obtained following repeated daily acute exposures to ozone for 2–4 h (adaptation studies). Each curve and associated symbol represent one study at an indicated ozone exposure concentration (ppm)

exposures to 0.12 ppm ozone with moderate intermittent exercise, we observed that the effects assessed by spirometry leveled off after the 6th h of exposure (Fig. 6). Some individuals even showed improvement of lung function while the exposure continued. Three additional subjects exposed for 10 h to 0.12 ppm ozone showed a similar pattern of response (Fig. 6). These observations strongly suggest that adaptation to ozone might not only develop at lower concentrations, but it might develop during actual exposure. The limited number of published studies on ozone adaptation curtails rigorous analysis; however, a simple pooling of the results reveals some relationships between spirometric decrements, ozone concentration, and a daily reexposure sequence which are not apparent by evaluating individual studies. Study by study regression curves (Fig. 7) suggest that adaptation occurs at any concentration of ozone and that the time required for adaptation to develop is directly related to the concentration of ozone.

References

Adams WC, Savin WM, Christo AE (1981) Detection of ozone toxicity during continuous exercise via the effective dose concept. J Appl Physiol 51:415–422

Colucci AV (1983) Pulmonary dose/effect relationships in ozone exposure. In: Lee SD, Mustafa MG, Mehlman MA (eds) International symposium on the biochemical effects of ozone and related photochemical oxidants. Princeton Science, Princeton, pp 21–44 (Advances in modern environmental toxicology, vol 5)

Hazucha MJ (1987) Relationship between ozone exposure and pulmonary function changes. J Appl Pysiol 62:1671–1680

Hazucha MJ, Seal E, Folinsbee LJ (1990) Effects of steady-state and variable ozone concentration profiles on pulmonary function of man. Am Rev Resp Dis 141:A71

Jenicek M (1989) Meta-analysis in medicine, where we are and where we want to go. J Clin Epidemiol 42:35–44

Laird NM, Mosteller F (1990) Some statistical methods for combining experimental results. International Journal of Technology Assessment in Health Care 6:5–30

Sacks HS, Bernier J, Reitman D, Ancona-Berk VA, Chalmers TC (1987) Meta-analyses of randomized controlled trials. N Engl J Med 316:450–455

Silverman F, Folinsbee LJ, Barnard J, Shephard RJ (1976) Pulmonary function changes in ozone – interaction of concentration and ventilation. J Appl Physiol 41:859–864

Silverman F, Shephard RJ, Folinsbee LJ (1977) Effects of physical activity on lung responses to acute ozone exposure. In: Kasuga S, Suzuki N, Yamada T, Kimura G, Imagaki K, Onoi M (eds) Proceedings of the 4th International Clean Air Congress, Tokyo, pp 15–19

Regulating Indoor Air[*]

B. Seifert

Institut für Wasser-, Boden- und Lufthygiene des Bundesgesundheitsamtes,
Corrensplatz 1, 1000 Berlin 33, FRG

Introduction

To reduce air pollution, many countries have regulations which limit emissions of air pollutants into outdoor air. These regulations include ambient air quality standards valid for both the short term and the long term. Generally, such standards are the result of a compromise between scientific knowledge and political will.

Like outdoor air, the air quality of industrial workplaces is subject to regulations. Limit values have been set by the various bodies responsible for the protection of the working population. Averages over one shift of several hours and short-term exposure limits have been defined.

As to the nonindustrial indoor environment, potential exposure to air pollutants has also been subject to certain regulations for many years. In many countries, building codes contain proscriptions which have an influence on the design of indoor spaces. In addition, research related to human comfort has been carried out with the aim of defining the acceptable indoor climate (cf. Pettenkofer 1858; Fanger 1970; McIntyre 1980). National and international bodies have issued recommendations (e.g., ASHRAE 1981; ISO 1984). However, the presence of chemical and microbiological pollutants in the air of private spaces, schools, offices, transportation systems, etc. has only become a matter of greater concern since the mid-1970s and has only been the subject of regulations to a very limited extent.

The major difficulty that one faces in dealing with indoor air regulation is that this topic is not under the responsibility of one single department or ministry and that no special law comprehensively addressing the subject exists in any country.

In the absence of clearly defined responsibilities, regulations are not easily established. As a result, private litigation becomes important in protecting individuals against damage such as that caused by environmental

---

[*] This article expresses the personal views of the author and does not necessarily reflect the position of the Federal Health Office (Bundesgesundheitsamt).

U. Mohr et al. (Eds.)
Advances in Controlled Clinical
Inhalation Studies
© Springer-Verlag Berlin Heidelberg 1993

impact (Ricci et al. 1989). But not only is such private litigation costly, it also lays the interpretation of scientific findings into the hands of non-scientists, namely judges. Even if a judge calls on experts for assistance, a court can never assemble and evaluate the full body of scientific knowledge, especially if questions are to be answered for which there is no agreement among scientists.

Therefore, to create a system of legal guaranty is one of the most important rationales for establishing regulations, especially in the environmental field. However, regulations should not be too tight in the case of the indoor environment. Rather, the avenue indicated by O'Riordan (1989) should be followed: "Anticipatory environmental policy should seek to establish the right mix of regulations and incentives – to coordinate planning, fiscal and economical instruments with regulatory measures . . .".

This article discusses the different regulatory options that are available to guarantee satisfactory indoor air quality. In the course of the text, "to regulate" is used in the more general sense of "to adjust by rule, method, or established mode" which goes beyond the more restricted meaning of "to bring under the control of law or constituted authority".

The Possibilities to Reduce Indoor Air Pollution

The fundamental equation which governs indoor air pollution is the following:

$$dc_i/dt = Q/V + n \cdot c_a - A \cdot c_i - n \cdot c_i \qquad (1)$$

with c_i = concentration of compound i in indoor air $(mg \cdot m^{-3})$
  Q = emission rate $(mg \cdot h^{-1})$
  V = volume of the indoor space (m^3)
  n = ventilation rate (h^{-1})
  c_a = concentration of compound i in outdoor air $(mg \cdot m^{-3})$
  A = decay factor (h^{-1})

This equation applies to static conditions – more complex equations are needed to describe dynamic situations (cf. Wadden and Scheff 1983 or other textbooks) – and shows that the concentration of a pollutant in indoor air can be expressed by a source part and a sink part. The source part takes into consideration the emission of a compound into the air, while the sink part comprehends removal precesses.

For various reasons the most trivial way of reducing indoor air pollution, namely obtaining zero emission by avoiding the source completely, is only possible in a limited number of cases. Generally, following Eqn. 1 there are two choices to reduce indoor air pollution: one is to prevent the generation of pollutants (e.g., by controlling the source), while the other is to remove the pollutants (e.g., by ventilating or using an air-cleaning device). Both source control and removal processes are valid approaches to reduce indoor air pollution. However, they do not indicate the level to which this reduction should be conducted. This level must be defined by setting appropriate limit values.

The Source Control Approach

According to Eqn. 1 the rate at which a pollutant is emitted from a product determines the final concentration of this pollutant in indoor air. Thus, setting an emission standard is one means of source control; others include voluntary agreements not to produce and/or use a product or imposing a prohibitive ban on a product.

Emission Standards

One possibility to develop an emission standard is to start from a tolerable indoor concentration level, e.g., a guideline value. With a number of assumptions regarding the average conditions under which the product is used in practice (temperature, relative humidity, air exchange rate, loading factor, etc.), the desired emission factor of a compound can be calculated.

Such a procedure is more easily described than achieved in practice for a number of reasons. For example, one difficulty is that more than one product may emit the compound under consideration. Assuming that the apportionment, although difficult, is possible for continuously emitting surface materials, a simple equation can be used to approximate the emission factor E_i $(mg \cdot m^{-2} \cdot h^{-1})$ for compound i in such material:

$$E_i = (c_i \cdot n)/L \tag{2}$$

with c_i = concentration of compound i in the air $(mg \cdot m^{-3})$
n = air exchange rate (h^{-1})
L = loading factor (m^{-1})

More complex equations are used to take into account the influence of parameters such as the variation of the emission factor with time, the effects of removal processes other than ventilation, the temperature, or the relative humidity. An important example for the influence of the last two parameters is formaldehyde, for which special equations have been established describing this influence (e.g., Andersen et al. 1975). Generally, emission factors are obtained from test chamber measurements under well-defined conditions. Recent guidelines published in Europe (COST 613 1989) and in the USA (ASTM 1989) demonstrate that these conditions have to be described precisely and maintained very carefully during the experiment to obtain comparable data. Many difficulties still need to be solved in the testing of emission factors, especially if intermittent rather than continuous sources are being considered.

However, despite all the difficulties, source control is a very, if not the most, appropriate way of reducing indoor air pollution. As a first practical step towards this goal, the Council of the European Communities has issued a Council Directive on construction products (European Communities 1989). The Directive, among other requirements, states that

Construction work must be designed and built in such a way that it will not be a threat to the hygiene or health of the occupants or neighbours, in particular as a result of any of the following:

– the giving off of toxic gas,
– the presence of dangerous particles or gases in the air,
– the emission of dangerous radiation,
– pollution or poisoning of the water or soil,
– faulty elimination of waste water, smoke, solid or liquid wastes,
– the presence of damp in parts of the works or on surfaces within the works.

The Directive does not specify details but leaves the implementation of these requirements to the European standards organizations which have to establish harmonized standards for products. Much work remains to be done to make such standards available. They are urgently needed in view of the Single European Market to come into force in 1993.

Voluntary Agreements

Fortunately enough, concentration levels of most air pollutants are below what may cause immediate adverse health effects. On the other hand, the available knowledge of potential adverse health effects of chronic exposure of humans to contaminants at low concentration levels is inadequate, especially if mixtures are being considered. Thus, the scientific proof of a need to lower the actually encountered exposure levels may be difficult and action only possible on the basis of "prevention is better than cure." In such situations, a reduction of indoor air pollution can only be based on a consensus reached by all parties of the society.

To achieve such a consensus, the dissemination of information beyond scientific circles is urgently needed. The difficulties which scientists and governmental institutions are facing in communicating environmental risks to the public are well recognized (Covello et al. 1987; Covello 1989; Renn 1989), and faulty behaviour of industrial and perhaps also governmental representatives may have contributed to creating some of these difficulties in the past. As has been pointed out recently by Fülgraff (1989), "scientists tend to neglect that they may be experts for risk assessment, but not at all experts for acceptability, adequacy, reasonability, justifiability, etc."

If it comes to voluntary agreements, special incentives may induce a kind of self-regulation of the market. Although the system is far from being perfect, positive experience has been made in the FRG with an environmental label, the so-called "Blue Angel". Under certain conditions, this label can be assigned to products representing a lower burden to the environment than others.

Ranking is in fact an excellent way of driving market forces. However, a sound evaluation system is needed to establish the ranking order. In the case of many consumer products, (governmental) text institutes use such systems to evaluate the technical performance of the product. Only to a very limited extent do these systems take into account a potential negative environmental impact of the product. What is generally not part of the final evaluation at all is the existence or the danger of any adverse health effect due to the emission of air pollutants.

The difficulties encountered in establishing a ranking system for health-related material and product evaluation cannot be underestimated. However, a first step towards developing such system has been made recently (Seifert 1990) in that important criteria to be used to develop a ranking index were defined. The index would take into account the chronic and acute toxicological properties of the material or product as well as the material's influence on the human sensory system. A proposal based on a similar approach has been published recently by Dieter et al. (1990) for the setting of priorities in the clean-up of chemically contaminated sites.

Bans

The most categoric decision which can be taken with regard to an anthropogenic pollutant is to prohibit its production and/or use. Generally, one would expect the decision for a complete ban to be preceded by qualitative and quantitative proof of the detrimental effect of this pollutant. In practice, however, in the few cases in which substances have been banned from the indoor environment, the decision was not based on definite proof but rather on apparent evidence, to some extent perhaps even on public pressure.

A good example is environmental tobacco smoke (ETS). The qualitative evidence of the unhealthy properties of ETS and the results of the majority of the known epidemiological studies on passive smoking have led to a ban on smoking in many places, although no individual case of lung cancer has up to now been and most probably never will be, traced back to the influence of ETS exposure. There can be no doubt that prevention is the driving force in the development of regulations creating smoke-free atmospheres.

The difficulty that generally comes along with the ban of a substance or product is the lack of sufficient knowledge of the properties of potential substitution products. Although science tries hard to forecast any negative properties of a substitution product, the pathways and cross-connections from the first step in the manufacturing of a product to its ultimate disposal are mostly so complex that they are not all well understood.

Despite these difficulties inherent in substitution, it seems as if the development of mankind has been nothing but a continuous series of substitution processes, which from early days on was mostly driven by the desire to make life more comfortable but tends more and more also to take into account the aspect of guaranteeing a healthy environment for all. The question is whether the struggle between these two sides of the coin can ever be solved.

The Dilution Approach

There are cases of indoor pollution in which the emissions of the source(s) cannot be avoided. One of the best examples is the emission caused by the occupants of a room themselves, which includes carbon dioxide and body odours. While the former is even toxic at elevated levels, the other can be highly annoying. Another frequent example is the situation in a room where an already present material or product is only recognized later as being harmful. In both cases, ventilation and air cleaning offer the possibility to reduce the pollution level.

Ventilation Standards

Equation 1 defines the relationship which exists between the emitted amount of a pollutant and its final concentration in indoor air. To lower this concentration, one can either diminish the source strength or use ventilation. In fact, ventilation has been and will continue to be one major option to reduce pollutant concentrations indoors. However, the need for saving energy calls for as low a ventilation rate as possible. This has led to the specification of minimum ventilation rates which provide acceptable indoor air quality (IEA 1987).

The recently published ASHRAE Standard 62-1989 (ASHRAE 1989) describes a ventilation rate procedure which specifies the outdoor air requirements for ventilation and is thought "to provide acceptable indoor air quality, ipso facto". Although not legally binding, ASHRAE 62-1989 reflects the state-of-the-art engineering knowledge and forms the basis of the lay-out of ventilation systems not only in the USA.

Air-Cleaning Devices

Sometimes indoor air pollution problems can be traced back to the presence of special materials and products. Examples include the use of formaldehyde-emitting particle board for construction and the application onto wooden panels of preservatives such as pentachlorophenol. As in such cases the removal of the source is not easy, air-cleaning devices may offer a possibility to lower the level of pollutants. However, the efficiency of some of these devices has sometimes to be questioned even if so claimed by the manufacturer.

Limit Values for Indoor Air Pollutants

It goes without saying that we face many limits in daily life, some of them being more stringent, others less. The same applies in the field of air pollution. Some limit values have a more binding character than others: While the first ones are called "standards," the others are "guideline values".

Standards for Indoor Air Quality

Many countries have set standards for outdoor (ambient) air pollutants. However, worldwide there are no standards for indoor air pollutants. Although there can be no doubt that standards contribute to establishing legal guaranties, two major criticisms can be brought forward against the setting of standards for chemicals (and microorganisms) in indoor air:

1. The existence of a standard favors the impression of having a limit below which there is no reason for concern.
2. The full enforcement of a standard is virtually impossible due to the large number of indoor spaces which would need to be checked.

In addition, the large variety of conditions encountered inside buildings makes it difficult to define the boundary conditions to be associated with the standard. One compound for which these difficulties apply is formaldehyde. The formaldehyde concentration in the air of a room depends critically on temperature and relative humidity. An increase or decrease of the room temperature of only 1°C changes the formaldehyde concentration by roughly 10%. Thus, one and the same room may fulfil the requirements of a standard at 20°C but not at 23°C. However, both temperatures being within the accepted range of thermal comfort, an individual cannot be obliged to live at 20°C simply because at this temperature the standard – if defined for 20°C – would be respected.

Due to the absence of standardized ventilation requirements for naturally ventilated buildings, which show a wide variety of ventilation rates, similar difficulties would arise in practice if standards were defined for a specific ventilation rate.

Guideline Values for Indoor Air Quality

As the word "guideline" indicates, such a value should provide guidance and, thus, is much weaker than a standard. In contrast to a standard, a guideline value generally will not take into account socioeconomic or political aspects. As has been pointed out by the World Health Organization (1987), "inhalation of an air pollutant in concentrations and for exposure times below a guideline value will not have adverse effects on health". However, since by nature the guideline value does not define a sharp borderline and generally does not take synergisms into account, compliance with these values "does not guarantee the absolute exclusion of effects at levels below such values". Consequently, a strategy including two values may be adopted under some circumstances. While the first value would define an action level, the second would indicate a target level to be reached in the future.

Larger sets of air quality guideline values for individual substances (either applicable to or expressively developed for indoor air) have been published by the World Health Organization (1987), Canada (Health and Welfare Canada 1987), and Norway (Helsedirektoratet 1990). In addition to these, guideline values for a few selected substances have been published in some countries. In the case of formaldehyde, a concentration of 0.1 ppm has been adopted in the majority of West European countries, a few of them having set higher levels (up to 0.4 ppm under certain circumstances) (COST 613 1990).

The existing guideline values have been derived on the basis of available knowledge of direct or indirect health effects of individual substances. Besides the fact that such a substance-by-substance approach is very time-consuming, it does not take synergistic effects into account, which are likely to be especially important with mixtures of volatile organic compounds.

Besides indicating the level of concern with regard to an indoor air pollutant, guideline values can serve the very important purpose of setting emission standards.

A Practical Example: Tetrachloroethene

The various possibilities that exist to regulate indoor air can be used to complement each other. This approach has been chosen recently in the FRG to reduce the concentration of tetrachloroethene (TCE) in rooms adjacent to dry-cleaning shops and is described in the following. For easy reference, the different keywords relating to what has been explained in the text are given in italics.

Following complaints of the population living in the vicinity of dry-cleaning shops, measurements were made which showed TCE concentrations of up to several mg/m^3 (1-week average). These levels were elevated by far above the median of $0.015\,mg/m^3$ which had been observed in about 500 randomly distributed German homes (Krause et al. 1987). In an expert hearing (cf. Anonymous 1988), a *guideline value* of $5\,mg/m^3$ was derived from toxicological considerations which could be used as an *action level* demanding immediate countermeasures. Below this level, no immediate action was considered to be necessary. However, control measures were recommended to lower the TCE concentration.

As it seemed very likely that technical changes on the dry-cleaning machines (*source control*) would permit the achievement of an indoor TCE concentration of $0.1\,mg/m^3$, this value was recommended as the *target level*. Following these recommendations an ordinance was issued in December 1990 in which an emission standard of $20\,mg\ TCE/m^3$ was defined for dry-cleaning machines (Anonymous 1990). The ordinance also specifies that the TCE concentration in the air of rooms adjacent to dry-cleaning shops should not exceed $0.1\,mg/m^3$ (7-day average). If this level is found to be exceeded, measures should be taken within 6 months to lower the concentration. Existing installations were given a 2-year period to fulfill the requirements.

Recently, a report was issued containing the results of repetitive TCE measurements which were taken 18 months after the first measurements, during which time control measures had been carried out (Hauptgesundheitsamt Bremen 1990). The percentage of rooms in which the target level had been reached was small; in some cases the authors observed even higher TCE concentrations than during the first campaign. It is not clear to what extent the analytical procedure and/or the sampling strategy contributed to these findings. However, these results do not exclude the possibility for a need to completely *ban* dry-cleaning machines from apartment houses in the future if no other technical means arises to exclude an exposure of the population.

References

Anderson I, Lundqvist GR, Mølhave L (1975) Indoor air pollution due to chipboard used as a construction material. Atmos Environ 9:1121–1127

Anonymous (1988) Empfehlung des Bundesgesundheitsamtes zu Tetrachlorethen in der Inneraumluft (Recommendation of the Federal Health Office concerning tetrachloroethene in indoor air). Bundesgesundheitsbl 31:99–101

Anonymous (1990) Verordnung zur Emissionsbegrenzung von leichtflüchtigen Halogenkohlenwasserstoffen (2. BImSchV) (Ordinance on the limitation of emissions of halogenated hydrocarbons). Bundes-Gesetz-Blatt I (10 Dec 1990):2694–2700

ASHRAE (American Society of Heating, Refrigerating and Air-Conditioning Engineers) (1981) Thermal environmental conditions for human occupancy. ASHRAE Standard 55-1981, Atlanta

ASHRAE (American Society of Heating, Refrigerating and Air-Conditioning Engineers) (1989) Ventilation for acceptable indoor air quality. ASHRAE Standard 62-1989, Atlanta

ASTM (American Society for Testing Materials) (1989) Standard guide for small-scale environmental determinations of organic emissions from indoor materials/products. Draft, Subcommittee D 22.05 on Indoor Air

COST 613 (1989) Formaldehyde emission from wood based materials: guideline for the determination of steady state concentrations in test chambers. European Concerted Action "Indoor air quality and its impact on man", report no. 2. Office for Publication of the EC, Luxembourg (EUR 12196 EN)

COST 613 (1990) Indoor air pollution by formaldehyde in European countries. European Concerted Action "Indoor air quality and its impact on man", report no. 7. Office for Publication of the EC, Luxembourg (EUR 12219 EN)

Covello VT, Slovic P, von Winterfeldt D (1987) Risk communication: a review of the literature. National Academy of Sciences, Washington

Covello VT (1989) Communicating right-to-know information on chemical risks. Environ Sci Technol 23:1444–1449

Dieter HH, Kaiser U, Kerndorff H (1990) Proposal on a standardized toxicological evaluation of chemicals from contaminated sites. Chemosphere 20(1–2):75–90

European Communities (1989) Council directive on the approximation of laws, regulations and administrative provisions of the member states relating to construction products. Official J EC L 40/12, 11 Feb 1989

Fanger PO (1970) Thermal comfort. Danish Technical Press, Copenhagen

Fülgraff G (1989) Akzeptanz von Umweltrisiken (Acceptance of environmental risks). Lecture 25th Anniversary Länderausschuß für Immissionsschutz (German Interstate Committee for the Protection of Ambient Air), Düsseldorf, 11 April 1989

Hauptgesundheitsamt Bremen (1990) Bericht über die TCE-Belastung bei Anwohnern chemischer Reinigungen (Report on the TCE exposure of persons living close to dry-cleaning shops)

Health and Welfare Canada (1987) Exposure guidelines for residential indoor air quality. Department of National Health and Welfare, Ottawa

Helsedirektoratet (1990) Retningslinjer for inneluft-kvalitet (Guidelines for indoor air quality). Helsedirketoratets utredningsserie 6–90. Norwegian Health Directorate

IEA (International Energy Agency) (1987) Energy conservation in buildings and community systems programme, annex IX: minimum ventilation rates. Final report of phases I and II

ISO (International Organization for Standardization) (1984) Moderate thermal environments – determination of the PMV and PPD indices and specification of the conditions for thermal comfort. ISO Standard 7730, Geneva

Krause C, Mailahn W, Nagel R, Schulz C, Seifert B (1987) Occurence of volatile organic substances in the air of 500 homes in the Federal Republic of Germany. In: Seifert B et al. (eds) Indoor Air '87 – Proceedings of the 4th International Conference on Indoor Air Quality and Climate, Berlin (West), 17–21 Aug 1987, vol 1. Institute for Water, Soil and Air Hygiene, Berlin, pp 102–106

McIntyre DA (1980) Indoor climate. Applied Science, London

O'Riordan T (1989) Anticipatory environmental policy – impediments and opportunities. Environ Monit Assess 12:115–125

Pettenkofer M (1858) Über den Luftwechsel in Wohngebäuden (On the air exchange in apartment buildings). Cotta, Müchen

Renn O (1989) Risk communication at the Community level: European lessons from the Seveso Directive. J Air Pollut Control Assoc 39:1301–1308

Ricci PF, Cox LA, Dwyer JP (1989) Acceptable cancer risks: probabilities and beyond. J Air Pollut Control Assoc 39(8):1046–1053

Seifert B (1990) Guidelines for material and product evaluation. Indoor air pollution: characterization of sources and acute effects on health and comfort meeting. Pierce Foundation, New Haven, 22–24 Oct 1990

Wadden RA, Scheff PA (1983) Indoor air pollution. Wiley, New York

World Health Organization (1987) Air quality guidelines for Europe. WHO Regional Publ, European series no. 23, Copenhagen

Perspective on the Regulator's Need for Future Clinical Studies

D.J. McKee

Office of Air Quality Planning and Standards, US Environmental Protection Agency, Mail Drop 12, Research Triangle Park, NC 27711, USA

Introduction

Clinical inhalation studies have been pivotal to making regulatory decisions concerning national ambient air quality standards (NAAQS) since they were first set in 1971. This has been due in part to the fact that interpretation of clinical studies is not limited by many of the uncertainties associated with epidemiology or field studies such as pollutant exposure (i.e., concentration and duration) or coexposure to other pollutants. Because the experimental subjects are human, the development of dosimetry models or consideration of species sensitivity differences has not been necessary in order to use the data quantitatively in setting NAAQS levels or averaging times.

Limitations of clinical research, however, have become more apparent over the past 2 decades of standard setting. For many of the criteria pollutants (i.e., NAAQS pollutants), the most serious health effects of exposure are not the acute ones typically measured in short-term clinical studies but rather the chronic ones resulting from exposures ranging from months to years typically investigated in animal toxicology studies.

Due to difficulties of generating complex mixtures of pollutants, clinical studies have tended to focus on individual pollutant exposures and may underestimate the full health impact of breathing polluted ambient air. Also, for obvious ethical reasons, most invasive techniques cannot be used on human subjects, thus limiting the extent to which morphometric, morphological, and biochemical information can be obtained. Finally, health assessment of highly toxic or carcinogenic substances will continue to be unacceptable using normal clinical inhalation procedures and will necessitate further development of new techniques to address adequately future regulatory needs for the hazardous and highly toxic pollutants. The focus of this discussion is primarily on the criteria pollutants due to legal and ethical constraints of conducting clinical inhalation studies of toxic chemicals. It should be emphasized that the following reflects my review of information and does not necessarily represent EPA policy.

U. Mohr et al. (Eds.)
Advances in Controlled Clinical
Inhalation Studies
© Springer-Verlag Berlin Heidelberg 1993

Background

The Clean Air Act (CAA) provides authority and guidance to regulate ambient air pollutants which are both ubiquitous and endanger public health and/or welfare. The CAA further requires that primary (i.e., health-based) NAAQS be based on health effects criteria and provide an adequate margin of safety to ensure protection of the public.

On 30 April 1971, the EPA promulgated in the *Federal Register* (36 FR 8186) primary (i.e., health-based) NAAQS for carbon monoxide (CO), hydrocarbons, nitrogen dioxide (NO_2), photochemical oxidants, total suspended particulate (TSP), and sulfur dioxide (SO_2). Lead (Pb) was added to the list of criteria pollutants on 5 October 1978 (43 FR 46246) based on evidence that young children developed deficits in IQ, school performance, and social behavior when exposed to excessive lead. This occurred after EPA was sued to list Pb under section 108 of the Clean Air Act. The NAAQS for hydrocarbons was revoked on 5 January 1983 (48 FR 628) due to a lack of evidence showing effects at ambient levels. Revision of the 0.08 ppm photochemical oxidants NAAQS to the 0.12 ppm ozone (O_3) NAAQS on 8 February 1979 (44 FR 8202) was based on compelling evidence that: (1) only O_3 of all photochemical oxidants existed at sufficient concentrations in the ambient air to produce adverse health effects and (2) limited evidence of acute health effects at lower O_3 exposures.

Decisions were published to retain the NO_2 NAAQS on 19 June 1985 (50 FR 25532) and not to revise the CO NAAQS on 13 September 1985 (50 FR 37484). Action was also taken to modify the particulate matter standard in order to place substantially greater emphasis on controlling smaller particles which deposit in the respiratory tract. A size-specific indicator that includes particles less than or equal to 10 μm (PM_{10}) was promulgated on 1 July 1987 (52 FR 24634).

Table 1 is a summary of the current NAAQS. Each of these is currently at some stage in the review process. Clinical inhalation studies have played an important role in making regulatory decisions for these standards in the past and will continue to play a key role in the future. Ethical considerations for human exposure to highly toxic chemicals have restricted the extent to which clinical studies of toxic agents have been possible in the past. However, promising new techniques such as bronchoalveolar lavage (BAL) in combination with in vitro procedures to evaluate recovered cells and other material may permit a better understanding of health effects of noncriteria pollutants in the future.

Regulatory Process and Use of Clinical Inhalation Studies

Prior to using clinical studies in making regulatory decisions the Environmental Criteria and Assessment Office (ECAO) of the EPA conducts a

Table 1. National ambient air quality standards

Pollutant	Primary standards	Averaging time	Secondary standards
Carbon monoxide	9 ppm ($10\,mg/m^3$) 35 ppm ($40\,mg/m^3$)	8 h[a] 1 h[a]	None
Lead	$1.5\,\mu g/m^3$	Quarterly average	Same as primary
Nitrogen dioxide	0.053 ppm ($100\,\mu g/m^3$)	Annual (arithmetic mean)	Same as primary
Particulate matter (PM_{10})	$50\,\mu g/m^3$ $150\,\mu g/m^3$	Annual (arithmetic mean)[b] 24 h[c]	Same as primary
Ozone	0.12 ppm ($235\,\mu g/m^3$)	1 h[d]	Same as primary
Sulfur oxides (SO_2)	0.03 ppm ($80\,\mu g/m^3$) 0.14 ppm ($365\,\mu g/m^3$)	Annual (arithmetic mean) 24 h[a] 3 h[a]	– – 0.5 ppm ($1300\,\mu g/m^3$)

[a] Not to be exceeded more than once per year.
[b] The standard is attained when the expected annual arithmetic mean concentration is less than or equal to $50\,\mu g/m^3$, as determined in accordance with Appendix K.
[c] The standard is attained when the expected number of days per calendar year with a 24-h average concentration above $150\,\mu g/m^3$ is equal to or less than 1, as determined in accordance with Appendix K.
[d] The standard is attained when the expected number of days per calendar year with maximum hourly average concentrations above 0.12 ppm is equal to or less than 1, as determined in accordance with Appendix H.

thorough literature review for purposes of developing a Criteria Document, which serves as the basis for NAAQS for pollutants such as CO and O_3. This review is intended to identify all research which may be potentially pertinent to a final regulatory decision. Papers which have been peer reviewed and published in scientific journals are included initially; however, as the review progresses, other studies which are pertinent, publicly available, and scientifically credible may be added.

Scientists familiar with the literature base carefully analyze the information with particular criteria in mind. Specifically, pollutant exposures used in each study should approximate levels which might be expected in ambient air. While there are no guidelines which clearly define unacceptably high levels of clinical exposure, exposures which are substantially higher than those found in the ambient environment generally are not seen as providing useful information for setting levels for the NAAQS or other standards. Occasionally, some studies are excluded due to methodological problems, but this is unusual and is often explained within the text of the regulatory document. Foreign literature is considered for inclusion in EPA documents as far as possible, but limited resources for translation often restrict the focus of most literature searches to publications written in English. The probability of inclusion of any study, however, is increased by presentation of results at scientific meetings and publication of at least an abstract in English.

After a regulatory document is available as an external review draft, it is reviewed by the Clean Air Scientific Advisory Committee (CASAC), and a public meeting is held to discuss the scientific content of the document and to accept public comment. At this point the CASAC may accept the document with minor modifications or request that a second draft be prepared for review at a subsequent meeting. Concurrently, an OAQPS Staff Paper is prepared based on scientific review conducted in the Criteria Document but also contains staff recommendations. This also reviewed by the CASAC and public. Once closure is reached on these documents, the regulatory review which ensues can be quite complicated, lengthy, and at times litigious. Figure 1 summarizes this process. Thorough discussions of this process have been published (Padgett and Richmond 1983; Lippmann 1987).

Regulatory Need for Clinical Studies

As existing standards continue to be reviewed and new air pollutants are identified for possible regulation, identification of research needs to

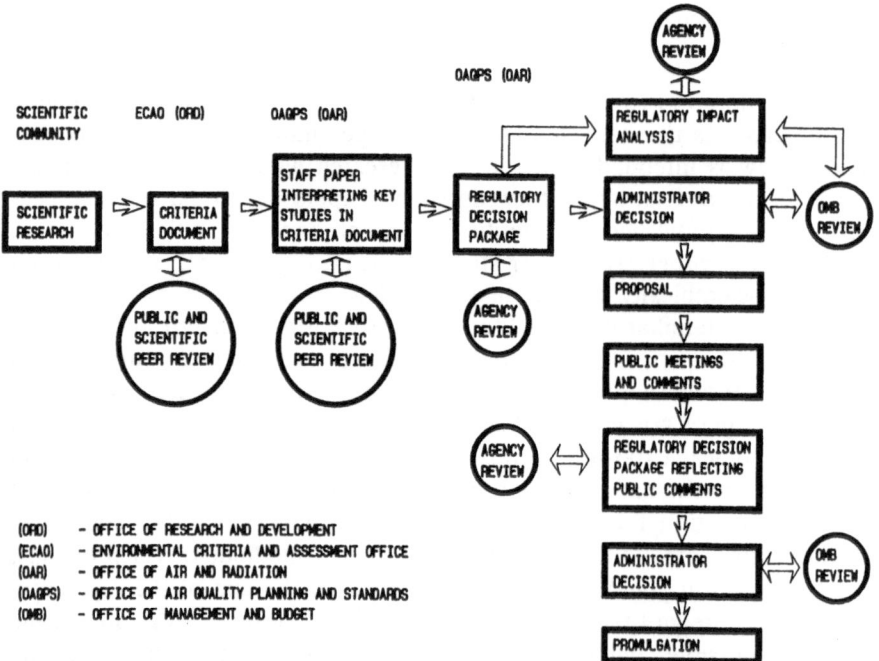

Fig. 1. NAAQS process flow chart

improve understanding of the relationship between pollutant exposure and health effects response has become an integral part of the review process. As the current scientific database is examined in air quality criteria and health assessment documents, gaps in knowledge about exposure-response relationships are uncovered and provided for discussion in criteria documents and at CASAC review meetings. These meetings offer an opportunity for public input and generally result in a "Report of the CASAC" which presents recommendations for future research on a particular pollutant or pollutants. These reports are released subsequent to closure on regulatory documents and have been used by the EPA Air and Radiation Research Committee (ARRC) as an important element in discussing and proposing air health research to be supported by the EPA. EPA research priorities are discussed in ARRC meetings and establish the basis for air research to be recommended. This process continues to change over time but is closely associated with the regulatory review process and research gaps identified during review.

The following sections provide specific examples of clinical studies used in making prior regulatory decisions. Although clearly not comprehensive, significant uncertainties about health effects of air pollution are also discussed which may be resolved by future clinical research.

Carbon Monoxide

The original CO NAAQS (9 ppm/8 h; 35 ppm/1 h) were promulgated based in part on clinical inhalation studies of behavioral impairment associated with small doses of CO (Beard and Wertheim 1967). Clinical CO exposure studies of time to onset of angina for exercising angina patients (Anderson et al. 1973) and of work time to exhaustion of healthy men (Horvath et al. 1975) helped to provide the basis for a decision not to revise the standards in 1985. Many of the key studies conducted since final action was taken on the standards in 1985 have also been clinical inhalation studies of exercising angina patients (Kleinman et al. 1989; Allred et al. 1989a,b; Adams et al. 1988; Sheps et al. 1987). Although the criteria document for the current NAAQS review is nearing completion, future clinical research needs have continued to be identified.

Clinical studies of individuals with preexisting coronary artery disease remain the highest priority for CO. In the USA alone, there are more than one million heart attacks each year resulting in about half a million deaths. Of the half a million survivors, about 10% are asymptomatic, and about 20% of all myocardial infarctions are silent. This suggests that many more individuals may be at risk upon CO exposure than are aware of their risk, particularly the approximately 50 000 survivors of hospital-treated myocardial infarction who are asymptomatic but have signs of ischemia. While it has been clearly shown that CO lowers the blood's oxygen carrying capacity, it appears also to interfere with different vasomotor-active substances and induces vasoconstriction or prevents vasodilation in coronary arteries, thus producing ischemia which is likely to be silent. Clinical studies have not been conducted which address the effects of CO on silent ischemic subjects. These studies are needed to assess the impact of ambient CO levels on this high-risk group.

Other population groups which appear to be at particular risk to CO exposure include individuals with congestive heart failure, peripheral vascular and cerebrovascular disease, anemia and other hematologic disorders, and obstructive lung disease. Those persons with combined exposure to CO and other chemicals (e.g., alcohol, cardiovascular drugs, methylene chloride) as well as those visiting high altitudes may also be at greater risk with regard to cardiovascular effects as well as neurobehavioral effects from elevated ambient CO exposures. In general, more information on the health effects of ambient CO on high-risk groups will provide a better basis for making future regulatory decisions on the CO NAAQS.

Lead

Lead (Pb) levels in the ambient air have been declining in the USA since the Pb primary NAAQS ($1.5\,\mu g/m^3$, quarterly average) was set in 1978, based on preventing most (99.5%) children in the USA from exceeding levels of $30\,\mu g\,Pb/dl$ whole blood. However, while exposure has been reduced, evidence of what constitutes a safe level of exposure suggests reason for concern at lower levels than indicated previously. Essentially all of this evidence is derived from animal and epidemiological studies. Currently, exposure considerations have taken precedence in light of the numerous sources of Pb exposure identified during the past decade.

Due to the highly toxic nature of Pb, clinical inhalation studies cannot be recommended. However, prospective studies of previously exposed subjects to assess the adverse effects on the neurobehavioral development of young children should be considered. More information also is needed to understand the full impact of fetal Pb exposures on fetal and early postnatal development. Prospective studies could also help establish the relationship between blood Pb levels and blood pressure in adults with respect to the incidence of hypertension. Finally, there is a need for a better understanding of the mobilization and deposition of various Pb species in the body, especially among pregnant and postmenopausal women. This research should emphasize the toxic effects of increased bone Pb mobilization during pregnancy and after menopause as well as the toxic effects of low-level Pb exposures over a period of many years or even a lifetime. Since it appears that no threshold may exist for certain Pb-induced neurological effects, every effort should be made to reduce human exposure.

Nitrogen Dioxide

The annual standard for NO_2 (0.053 ppm) originally was based largely on a community epidemiology study (Shy et al. 1970a,b) suggesting respiratory effects in children exposed to long-term, low level NO_2 concentrations. The standard was retained in 1985 on the basis of a significant association between a history of respiratory symptoms/illness in children and exposure to NO_2 emitted from gas stoves (Speizer et al. 1980; Melia et al. 1977, 1979; Florey et al. 1979; Goldstein et al. 1979). Effects reported could not be linked to a particular acute exposure and did not provide a basis for a short-term standard.

Clinical inhalation studies (Orehek et al. 1976; Kerr et al. 1979; von Nieding et al. 1973) were cited in the 1985 decision on the NAAQS as providing limited support for short-term (1–2 h) health effects in asthmatic and chronic bronchitic sufferers exposed to NO_2 at or below 0.5 ppm. At this time, there remains much uncertainty about the extent to which acute, low level exposures to NO_2 affect airway responsiveness in sensitive individuals, particularly when preexposed to an allergen or to another pollutant such as O_3. Another area of concern is its relationship to respiratory infection. A carefully designed clinical inhalation study of the effects of acute NO_2 exposure on upper and lower respiratory tract infection could help to clarify many unanswered questions about averaging times associated with the response in the gas stove studies and the significance of the animal mortality studies for human health effects. New endpoints are now available through BAL, which may provide information that could support the findings of increased respiratory infection from epidemiology studies, i.e., decreased immune response or increased epithelial permeability.

Ozone

The original NAAQS for total oxidants (0.08 ppm) was based largely on an association of increased risk of asthma attacks and ambient oxidant levels reported in an epidemiology study (Schoettlin and Landau 1961). Subsequent clinical inhalation studies (Folinsbee et al. 1978; Horvath et al. 1979; von Nieding et al. 1979) of resting subjects exposed to O_3 reported a relatively minimal effect for exposures at or below 0.25 ppm O_3, and the O_3 NAAQS was revised to 0.12 ppm in 1979. During the 1980s numerous clinical studies (McDonnell et al. 1983; Avol et al. 1984; Kulle et al. 1985; Folinsbee and Horvath 1986) provided evidence of symptoms (e.g., cough, chest pain) and lung function decrements in heavily exercising subjects exposed to levels as low as 0.12 ppm. The severity of the effects was highly variable, with some subjects showing no effects at lower O_3 levels and others showing significant decrements. Studies of respiratory effects in children at summer camps (Lioy et al. 1985; Spektor et al. 1988a,b) suggested a greater respiratory response for prolonged exposures (6–8 h) to ambient O_3 levels than had been demonstrated in clinical studies of 1–2 h duration. This led to a series of clinical studies which reported statistically significant changes in pulmonary function and airway responsiveness in moderately exercising healthy individuals exposed for 6.6 h to O_3 levels in the range of 0.08–0.12 ppm (Horstman et al. 1988, 1989; Folinsbee and Hazucha 1989; Folinsbee et al. 1988). BAL techniques were used following similar exposures to assess O_3-induced inflammation in the lower airways, thought to be a precursor of chronic lung damage (Koren et al. 1989a,b).

From a regulatory perspective, the highest priority need for clinical research is a confirmation of pulmonary effects found in moderately exercising subjects following prolonged exposures (6–8 h) to low levels (0.08–0.12 ppm) of O_3. Of particular interest are investigations of the inflammatory response, as measured by cellular and biochemical markers, which will help to develop a better understanding of the relationship between repeated acute exposures to O_3 and chronic lung damage. Also of significant regulatory value would be acute O_3 inhalation studies which reduce the large uncertainties currently existing between O_3 exposure and increased risk of respiratory infection. The relationship between increased asthma attack rate and O_3 exposure should be explored in clinical studies to help establish whether O_3 is a causative agent or may be sensitizing the respiratory tract for other agents.

Particulate Matter

Although the 1971 *Federal Register* notice did not provide a detailed rationale for the particulate matter (PM) NAAQS ($75 \mu g/m^3$, annual mean; $200 \mu g/m^3$, max 24-h average, measured as TSP), it was generally based on evidence of increased morbidity and mortality reported in the communities of Donora, Pennsylvania, and London, UK (Lawther et al. 1970). As information began to emerge about PM deposition, it became clear that particles of 10 μm and smaller were most likely to enter and deposit in the respiratory tract (Miller et al. 1979, 1984). This led to revision of the health NAAQS for PM on 1 July 1987, which replaced (1) total suspended particulate matter (TSP) with a new indicator which includes particles with a diameter of 10 μm or less (PM_{10}), (2) the 24-h TSP NAAQS with a 24-h PM_{10} NAAQS of $150 \mu g/m^3$, and (3) the annual TSP NAAQS with a PM_{10} NAAQS of $50 \mu g/m^3$.

Although very little clinical inhalation research has been used to establish PM NAAQS thus far, several areas of research could provide useful information in making future regulatory decisions. Studies of regional deposition in both sedentary and exercising individuals will help to determine effective doses for given exposures and to relate such doses and responses to the potential for health effects. Research is needed to define the effects of exercise on particle retention and the influence of oronasal breathing on regional deposition. Data must characterize the extent to which individuals with narrowed airways (e.g., persons with asthma or chronic obstructive pulmonary disease) have enhanced tracheobronchial deposition and identify which factors have the greatest influence in causing the enhancement. Emphasis should be placed on the study of acid aerosols, particularly with regard to effects on respiratory function, airway hyperreactivity, and mucociliary clearance, and on combined effects of O_3 and acid aerosols on tissue injury, altered defenses, inflammation, and epithelial permeability.

Sulfur Dioxide

When the SO_2 primary NAAQS were set in 1971 at 0.14 ppm SO_2 (24-h average) and 0.03 ppm (annual arithmetic mean), they were based primarily on epidemiological studies conducted in London. Peak pollution (>0.38 ppm SO_2, 24-h average) episodes were associated with clear increases in daily mortality during the winters of 1958–1959 (Martin and Bradley 1960; Martin 1964), although subsequent analysis (Mazumdar et al. 1981) of these and other studies suggested that only smoke particles were influential in causing mortality. Lower SO_2 peaks (0.19–0.23 ppm, 24-h average) were associated with daily worsening of health status in bronchitis sufferers during the winters of 1954–1968 (Lawther et al. 1970). Numerous clinical inhalation studies have subsequently shown that asthmatic and, to a lesser extent, atopic subjects appear to be significantly more sensitive than normal subjects to bronchoconstriction induced by SO_2 exposure. Short-duration (5–60 min) exposures of SO_2 can induce changes in airway resistance of: (1) 100%–600% at 1–2 ppm (Schacter et al. 1984; Roger et al. 1985; Horstman et al. 1986), (2) 120%–260% at 0.60–75 ppm (Linn et al. 1983a,b; Hackney et al. 1984), and (3) 50%–100% at 0.50 ppm only when moderately exercising (Bethel et al. 1983a,b; Roger et al. 1985). These and other recent studies have created concern about the possible need for an additional short-term standard, and this alternative is currently being considered.

There continues to be a need for clinical inhalation studies of the effects of SO_2 on asthmatics, particularly at lower levels (0.25–0.50 ppm SO_2) and with more sensitive subjects. Studies are needed on the effects of SO_2 in combination with and following other atmospheric factors such as cold/dry air or other pollutants (e.g., O_3 or NO_2). Clinical inhalation studies of subjects with acute respiratory infection could help establish the impact of SO_2 on the duration or severity of infection and help to identify potential groups of sensitive individuals other than asthmatics (e.g., children, elderly people, those with chronic bronchitis). Finally, using BAL techniques it is possible to study mechanisms of action linking SO_2 exposure with pulmonary tissue response in humans (e.g., stimulation of smooth muscle activity via the autonomic nervous system and via the cell-mediated release of inflammatory agents such as histamine).

Pollutants Associated with Alternative Fuels

The development of various alternatives to conventional gasoline and diesel fuels has gained increasing interest in recent years for various reasons, including economic and environmental concerns. Although some of these "new" chemicals, e.g., methanol, ethanol, and compressed natural gas, have a substantial history of use in modern society, our experience with their application as fuels for motor vehicles is not as extensive. Other compounds, such as methyl-*tert*-butyl ether (MTBE), are less familiar but are already being used in reformulated gasolines in many areas. The growing number of these chemicals and their blends with conventional fuels presents a tremendous challenge for environmental risk assessment. A comprehensive presentation of this problem may be found in the EPA's draft "Alternative fuels research strategy".

Among the many questions that arise with the introduction of alternative fuels are their potential health risks and benefits for human populations. Their net health effects will depend not only on the fuels themselves but on their evaporative and combustion emissions and the by-products of these emissions after chemical transformation in the atmosphere. Much remains to be done to characterize all of these emission products and their potential for human exposure, but certain compounds seem to be likely prospects for investigation. For example, aldehydes such as formaldehyde and acetaldehyde have been identified in relation to methanol and ethanol fuels, respectively. The complexity of potential exposure is further multiplied by the routes of possible human contact, but the fundamental need is for much more information on the effects of exposure via inhalation.

Apart from acute poisoning by ingestion, very little clinical research has been devoted to inhaled methanol vapor, and essentially no such information exists on blends of methanol and gasoline. Unpublished work by Cook et al. (1990) examined visual and other neurobehavioral and cognitive functions in 12 young adult males exposed to $250 \, mg/m^3$ methanol vapor for 75-min periods. Although no clearly adverse effects were detected, a cluster of variables related to cognitive function showed marginally significant effects, thus suggesting the need for a larger study with greater statistical power to detect subtle effects. Nevertheless, much remains to be learned about reproductive and developmental effects in humans exposed to methanol. In addition, some basic metabolic parameters, such as V_{max} and the Michaelis constant, have not been reported for humans.

Ethanol presents the same paradox as methanol in even greater extremes. Only a tiny fraction of the vast information on ethanol pertains to exposure by inhalation. Given this situation, the greatest need is to develop adequate pharmacokinetic and dosimetric data to support the use of data based on oral and nonhuman exposures to ethanol. Blends of ethanol and gasoline are widely used as fuels but have not been the subject of clinical study.

The health effects of inhaled aldehydes have been studied primarily from the standpoint of cancer. However, the irritative and sensitizing effects of aldehydes on the respiratory system warrant attention as well. Moreover, the need for more clinical effects data on these toxic agents exists independently of their relationship to alternative fuels.

Beyond these basic research needs, clinical studies of mixtures of fuels and fuel-related compounds will clearly be required for a comprehensive assessment of the risks and benefits of alternative fuels. Before these studies can be designed, however, more emissions characterization and atmospheric transformation work is necessary to determine exactly which compounds should be included.

Conclusion

In retrospect, it is clear that clinical inhalation research has provided substantial information for making regulatory decisions. It is also apparent, however, that significant questions remain in understanding the full health impact of human exposure to air pollution. Inferences should be based upon data from not only clinical but also epidemiological, in vitro, and animal toxicology studies as well. It is essential that all of these disciplines be used in assessing effects information which is needed to make appropriate regulatory decisions. Under many circumstances, the data generated in each discipline are complementary, and simultaneous assessment of information allows unsolved questions to be answered and consistency of findings among different disciplines to be examined. To the extent feasible this should be attempted. However, only through the careful design and conduct of clinical inhalation studies and development of new techniques such as BAL will many of these problems be resolved adequately.

References

Adams KF, Koch G, Chatterjee B, Goldstein GM, O'Neil JJ, Bromberg PA, Sheps DS, McAllister S, Price CJ, Bissette J (1988) Acute elevation of blood carboxyhemoglobin to 6% impairs exercise performance and aggravates symptoms in patients with ischemic heart disease. J Am Coll Cardiol 12:900–909

Allred EN, Bleecker ER, Chaitman BR, Dahms TE, Gottlieb SO, Hackney JD, Pagano M, Selvester RH, Walden SM, Warren J (1989a) Short-term effects of carbon monoxide exposure on the exercise performance of subjects with coronary artery disease. N Engl J Med 321:1426–1432

Allred EN, Bleecker ER, Chaitman BR, Dahms TE, Gottlieb SO, Hackney JD, Hayes D, Pagano M, Selvester RH, Walden SM, Warren J (1989b) Acute effects of carbon monoxide exposure on individuals with coronary artery disease. Research report no. 25. Health Effects Institute, Cambridge, MA

Anderson EW, Andelman RJ, Strauch JM, Fortuin NJ, Knelson JH (1973) Effect of low-level carbon monoxide exposure on onset and duration of angina pectoris: a study in ten patients with ischemic heart disease. Ann Intern Med 79:46–50

Avol EL, Linn WS, Venet TG, Shamoo DA, Hackney JD (1984) Comparative respiratory effects of ozone and ambient oxidant pollution exposure during heavy exercise. J Air Pollut Control Assoc 34:804–809

Beard RR, Wertheim GA (1967) Behavioral impairment associated with small doses of carbon monoxide. Am J Public Health 57:2012–2022

Bethel RA, Epstein J, Sheppard D, Nadel JA, Boushey HA (1983a) Sulfur dioxide-induced bronchoconstriction in freely breathing, exercising, asthmatic subjects. Am Rev Respir Dis 129:987–990

Bethel RA, Erle DJ, Epstein J, Sheppard D, Nadel JA, Boushey HA (1983b) Effect of exercise rate and route of inhalation on sulfur-dioxide-induced bronchoconstriction in asthmatic subjects. Am Rev Respir Dis 128:592–596

Florey C, Melia RJW, Chinn S, Goldstein BD, Brooks AGF, John HH, Craighead IB, Webster X (1979) The relation between respiratory illness in primary school children and the use of gas for cooking: III Nitrogen dioxide, respiratory illness and lung infection. Int J Epidemiol 8:347

Folinsbee LJ, Hazucha MJ (1989) Persistence of ozoneinduced changes in lung function and airway responsiveness. In: Schneider T, Lee SD, Wolters GJR, Grant LD (eds) Atmospheric ozone research and its policy implications. Proceedings of the 3rd US-Dutch international symposium, May 1988, Nijmegen. Elsevier, Amsterdam, pp 483–492 (Studies in environmental science, vol 35)

Folinsbee LJ, Horvath SM (1986) Persistence of the acute effects of ozone exposure. Aviat Space Environ Med 57:1136–1143

Folinsbee LJ, Drinkwater BL, Bedi JF, Horvath SM (1978) The influence of exercise on the pulmonary changes due to exposure to low concentrations of ozone. In: Folinsbee LJ, Wagner JA, Borgia JF, Drinkwater BL, Gliner JA, Bedi JF (eds) Environmental stress: individual human adaptations. Academic, New York, pp 125–145

Folinsbee LJ, McDonnell WF, Horstman DH (1988) Pulmonary function and symptom responses after 6.6-hour exposure to 0.12 ppm ozone with moderate exercise. J Air Pollut Control Assoc 38:28–35

Goldstein BD, Melia RJW, Chinn S, Florey C, Clark D, John HH (1979) The relation between respiratory illness in primary schoolchildren and the use of gas for cooking: II Factors affecting nitrogen dioxide levels in the home. Int J Epidemiol 8:339

Hackney JD, Linn WS, Bailey RM, Spier CE, Valencia LM (1984) Time course of exercise-induced bronchoconstriction in asthmatics exposed to sulfur dioxide. Environ Res 34:321–327

Horstman DH, Roger LJ, Kehrl HR, Hazucha MJ (1986) Airway sensitivity of asthmatics to sulfur dioxide. Toxicol Ind Health 2:289–298

Horstman D, McDonnell W, Folinsbee L, Abdul-Salaam S, Ives P (1988) Changes in pulmonary function and airway reactivity due to prolonged exposure to typical ambient ozone (O_3) levels. EPA report no. EPA-600/D-88-103. US Environmental Protection Agency, Health Effects Research Laboratory, Research Triangle Park, NC. Available from: NTIS, Springfield, VA; PB88-211891.

Horstman D, McDonnell W, Folinsbee L, Abdul-Salaam S, Ives P (1989) Changes in pulmonary function and airway reactivity due to prolonged exposure to typical ambient ozone (O_3) levels. In: Schneider T, Lee SD, Wolters GJR, Grant LD (eds) Atmospheric ozone research and its policy implications. Proceedings of the 3rd US-Dutch international symposium, May 1988, Nijmegen. Elsevier, Amsterdam, pp 755–762 (Studies in environmental science, vol 35)

Horvath SM, Ravan PB, Dahms TE, Gray DJ (1975) Maximal aerobic capacity at different levels of carboxyhemoglobin. J Appl Physiol 38:300–303

Horvath SM, Gliner JA, Matsen-Twisdale JA (1979) Pulmonary function and maximum exercise responses following acute ozone exposure. Aviat Space Environ Med 50:901–905

Kerr HD, Kulle TJ, McIlhany ML, Swidersky P (1979) Effect of nitrogen dioxide on pulmonary function in human subjects: an environmental chamber study. Environ Res 19:392–404

Kleinman MT, Davidson DM, Vandagriff RB, Caiozzo VJ, Whittenberger JL (1989) Effects of short-term exposure to carbon monoxide in subjects with coronary artery disease. Arch Environ Health 44:361–369

Koren HS, Devlin RB, Graham DE, Mann R, McDonnell WF (1989a) The inflammatory response in human lung exposed to ambient levels of ozone. In: Schneider T, Lee SD, Wolters GJR, Grant LD (eds) Atmospheric ozone research and its policy implications. Proceedings of the 3rd US-Dutch international symposium, May 1988, Nijmegen. Elsevier, Amsterdam, pp 745–753 (Studies in environmental science, vol 35)

Koren HS, Devlin RB, Graham DE, Mann R, McGee MP, Horstman DH, Kozumbo WJ, Becker S, House DE, McDonnell WF, Bromberg PA (1989b) Ozone-induced inflammation in the lower airways of human subjects. Am Rev Respir Dis 139:407–415

Kulle TJ, Sauder LR, Hebel JR, Chatham MD (1985) Ozone response relationships in healthy nonsmokers. Am Rev Respir Dis 132:36–41

Lioy PJ, Vollmuth TA, Lippmann M (1985) Persistence of peak flow decrement in children following ozone exposures exceeding the National Ambient Air Quality Standard. J Air Pollut Control Assoc 35:1068–1071

Lippmann M (1987) Role of science advisory groups in establishing standards for ambient air pollutants. Aerosol Sci Technol 6:93–114

Lawther PJ, Waller RE, Henderson M (1970) Air pollution and exacerbations of bronchitis. Thorax 25:525–539

Martin AE (1964) Mortality and morbidity statistics and air pollution. Proc R Soc Med 57:969–975

Martin AE, Bradley WH (1960) Mortality, fog and atmospheric pollution – an investigation during the winter of 1958–59. Monthly Bulletin Ministry Health Laboratory Services 19:56–72

Mazumdar S, Schimmel H, Higgins I (1981) Daily mortality, smoke and SO_2 in London, England 1959–1972. Proceedings of the proposed SO_x and particulate standard specialty conference. Air Pollution Control Association, Atlanta, Georgia, pp 219–239

McDonnell WF, Horstmann DH, Hazucha MJ, Seal E Jr, Haak ED, Salaam S, House DE (1983) Pulmonary effects of ozone exposure during exercise: dose-response characteristics. J Appl Physiol Respir Environ Exercise Physiol 54:1345–1352

Miller FJ, Gardner DE, Graham JA, Lee RE, Wilson WE Jr, Bachmann JD (1979) Size considerations for establishing a standard for inhalable particles. J Air Pollut Control Assoc 29:610–615

Miller FJ, Grady MA, Martonen TB (1984) Coarse mode aerosol behavior in man: theory and experiment. In: Liu BYH, Piu DYH, Fissan H (eds) Aerosols: science, technology, and industrial applications of airborne particles. New York, Elsevier, pp 999–1002

Melia RJW, Florey C, Altman DS, Swan AV (1977) Association between gas cooling and respiratory disease in children. Br Med J 2:149–152

Melia RJW, Florey C, Chinn S (1979) The relation between respiratory illness in primary schoolchildren and the use of gas for cooking: I Results from a national survey. Int J Epidemiol 8:333

Orehek J, Massari JP, Gayrard P, Grimaud C, Charpin J (1976) Effect of short-term, low-level nitrogen dioxide exposure on bronchial sensitivity of asthmatic patients. J Clin Invest 57:301–307

Padgett J, Richmond H (1983) The process of establishing and revising national ambient air quality standards. J Air Pollut Control Assoc 33/1: 13–16

Roger LJ, Kehrl HR, Hazucha M, Horstman DH (1985) Bronchocon-striction in asthmatics exposed to sulfur dioxide during repeated exercise. J Appl Physiol 59:784–791

Schachter EN, Witek TJ Jr, Beck GJ, Hosein HR, Colice G, Leaderer BP, Cain W (1984) Airway effects of low concentrations of sulfur dioxide: dose-response characteristics. Arch Environ Health 39:34–42

Schoettlin CE, Landau E (1961) Air pollution and asthmatic attacks in the Los Angeles area. Public Health Rep 76:545–548

Sheps DS, Adams KF, Bromberg PA, Goldstein GM, O'Neil JJ, Horstman D, Koch G (1987) Lack of effect of low levels of carboxy hemoglobin on cardiovascular function in patients with ischemic heart disease. Arch Environ Health 42:108–116

Shy CM, Creason JP, Pearlman ME, McClain KE, Benson FB, Young MM (1970a) The Chattanooga school children study: effects of community exposure of nitrogen dioxide: I. Methods, description of pollutant exposure and results of ventilatory function testing. J Air Pollut Control Assoc 20/8:539–545

Shy CM, Creason JP, Pearlman ME, McClain KE, Benson FB, Young MM (1970b) The Chattanooga school study: effects of community exposure to nitrogen dioxide: II. Incidence of acute respiratory illness. J Air Pollut Control Assoc 20/9:582–588

Speizer FE, Ferris BG Jr, Bishop YMM, Spengler J (1980) Respiratory disease rates and pulmonary function in children associated with NO_2 exposure. Am Rev Respir Dis 121:3–10

Spektor DM, Lippmann M, Lioy PJ, Thurston GD, Citak K, James DJ, Bock N, Speizer FE, Hayes C (1988a) Effects of ambient ozone on respiratory function in active normal children. Am Rev Respir Dis 137:313–320

Spektor SM, Lippmann M, Thurston GD, Lioy PJ, Stecko J, O'Connor G, Garshick E, Speizer FE, Hayes C (1988b) Effects of ambient ozone on respiratory function in healthy adults exercising outdoors. Am Rev Respir Dis 138:821–828

Von Nieding G, Krekeler H, Fuchs R, Wagner HM, Koppenhagen K (1973) Studies of the acute effect of NO_2 on lung function: influence on diffusion, perfusion and ventilation in the lungs. Int Arch Arbeitsmed 31:61–72

Von Nieding G, Wagner HM, Krekeler H, Lollgen H, Fries W, Beuthan A (1979) Controlled studies of human exposure to single and combined action of NO_2, O_3, and SO_2. Int Arch Occup Environ Health 43:195–210

Part II
Poster Presentations

Part 4
Future Perspectives

Use of Questionnaires for Assessment of Exposure to Airborne Pollutants

N.C.G. Freeman and P.J. Lioy

Robert Wood Johnson Medical School, Univ. of Med. & Dentistry of New Jersey, Dept. of Environmental and Community Med., 675 Hoes Lane, Piscataway, NJ 08854-5635, USA

Introduction

Accurate estimates of exposure to air pollutants are necessary for interpreting the causes of health outcomes and for the development of meaningful risk assessments. Numerous studies have shown that the levels of certain air pollutants, including respirable particles, volatile organic compounds, and polycyclic aromatic hydrocarbons, may be greater within than outside the home (Dockery and Spengler 1981; Wallace et al. 1985, 1987; Wallace 1987; Sexton et al. 1984; Silverman et al. 1982; Lioy et al. 1988a, 1990; Waldman et al. 1990). In addition, the typical American spends 60%–70% of each day in the home environment (Dockery and Spengler 1981; Chapin 1984; Robinson 1977) and therefore may be exposed to substantially higher levels of certain pollutants than would be estimated using fixed outdoor air samplers. At the same time, for some pollutants which do not have clearly defined indoor sources outdoor ambient concentrations may be the dominant influence on indoor levels (Lioy et al. 1988a, 1990; Waldman et al. 1990; Buckley et al. 1991). Thus it is important to understand the influence of household and life-style activities on both the sources of pollution and the routes of exposure.

Questionnaires can provide information about sources of pollution and routes of exposure (Lebowitz et al. 1989; Quackenboss et al. 1982). Questionnaires help refine indirect estimates of exposure by providing information about the time spent by individuals in specific microenvironments. This information, together with pollution levels obtained from fixed microenvironmental samplers, provides a time-weighted estimate of exposure. In addition, questionnaire data can be used as surrogates for measurements of specific sources by providing information about the presence or absence of those sources (environmental tobacco smoke, ETS; coal-burning stoves; site contamination) and estimates of exposure through the amount of time spent near these sources or the duration of use of these sources (Freeman et al. 1991).

U. Mohr et al. (Eds.)
Advances in Controlled Clinical
Inhalation Studies
© Springer-Verlag Berlin Heidelberg 1993

Exposure questionnaires can focus on either the household or the individual. Household questionnaires are typically surveys completed by one member of the home and may include estimates of activities for all members of the house. Personal exposure questionnaires may be survey instruments based on estimates, or real time or 24-h recall activity diaries and logs.

Methods

Study Designs

The effectiveness of questionnaire use is illustrated in two studies assessing (a) residential and personal exposure to ambient levels of benzo(a)pyrene (BaP), the Total Human Environmental Exposure Study (THEES), and (b) residential exposure to chromium from industrial waste deposits, the Hudson County Chromium Exposure Study (HCCES).

THEES was designed to examine and characterize household and individual daily exposure to BaP from multimedia sources. BaP is a ubiquitous combustion product and potential carcinogen, with less than 10% of the particles greater than 1 μm in diameter (Miguel and Friedlander 1978). Fourteen volunteers from eight households in a small industrial community in northwestern New Jersey participated in a 3-year study. The community had been identified as having the highest ambient levels of BaP of 27 sites analyzed in New Jersey (Lioy et al. 1988b; Waldman et al. 1990).

HCCES was designed to assess household levels of chromium (Cr) in areas in which chromium slag had been used extensively as apparently clean fill. Analysis of residential soil samples from areas where the chromium containing slag was used as fill found total Cr levels as high as 46 000 ppm at a depth of 2–4 ft and as high as 3580 ppm on the surface. These samples contained varying amounts of hexavalent Cr, the carcinogenic and irritant form of Cr. Eighteen households from four residential areas in Hudson County, New Jersey, identified by the New Jersey Department of Environmental Protection as having high Cr levels in soil or having contaminated buildings in the area, have been studied. Because there are a variety of sources of Cr exposure other than the contaminated sites, the study was designed to identify other sources and determine each pathway of possible contact.

Sampling Methodology

The sampling protocols for the two studies are shown on Table 1.

Air Samples. All air samples were based on the PM-10 fraction, which is that portion of airborne particles which can be deposited in the tracheo-

Table 1. Comparison of THEES and HCCES study protocols

	THEES			HCCES
	Phase 1	Phase 2	Phase 3	
Date	2/1987	1/1988	9/1988	5–6/1990
Period	14 days	14 days	14 days	7 days
No. participants	14	14	14	54
No. households	10	8	8	18
Samples				
Air				
Indoor	Daily	Daily	Daily	Weekly
Outdoor	Daily	Daily	Daily	Weekly
Personal	ND	Daily	Daily	ND
Diet	Daily	Daily	Daily	
Dust				
Wipe	ND	ND	ND	(Bi-)weekly
Vacuum	ND	ND	ND	(Bi-)weekly
Household survey	+	+	+	+
Daily diary	H	P	P	H
Biomonitoring interview	ND	ND	ND	P
Biological samples				
Urine	ND	Daily	Daily	Once
Blood	ND	Once	Once	ND

H, household; P, personal; ND, not determined.

bronchial and gas exchange regions of the lungs. Indoor and outdoor samplers were run simultaneously. Household monitors (indoor air sampling impactors) run at 10 l/min were placed in the main living areas of each house (Lioy et al. 1988a, 1990; Waldman et al. 1990). Outdoor samplers were sited at three locations within the community in THEES and in each study neighborhood in HCCES. THEES personal monitors, which employed a Marple PM-10 impactor attached to a lapel clip, were worn by each participant for 14 days and collected 24-h samples (Buckley et al. 1991).

Dietary Samples. Both BaP and Cr are contained in foods. BaP occurs in food products predominantly through the cooking process, especially through the smoking and broiling of fatty meats. Cr is a natural trace element found in a wide variety of fruits, vegetables, and shell fish. Daily food samples were collected for BaP analysis in THEES. Information about consumption of Cr containing foods was gathered in HCCES, but no food samples were collected.

Biomonitoring. Urine samples were collected from participants in both studies in order to assess the body burden of the contaminants being studied. Daily urine samples were collected from participants in THEES and analyzed for BaP metabolites and creatinine. One urine sample was collected from each participant in HCCES and analyzed for Cr and creatinine.

Questionnaires. Questionnaires used in THEES and HCCES were designed to provide time/activity information used to identify routes of exposure and high-risk behaviors. Content of the questions was pollutant specific. The questionnaires were pretested for comprehension and content with a computer diagnostic program (Right Writer 2.1, Right Soft, Sarasota, FL). The questionnaires were designed to be read and understood by an average American 11-year-old (5th grade level). Household time/activity survey instruments were used in both studies. The survey characterized the house construction, household activities, and estimates of the participants' use of five environmental compartments: outdoors, home, work, indoors other than home or work, and travel. Self-administered daily activity diaries were used to follow individuals in THEES and household activities in HCCES. HCCES participants were interviewed using a 48-h recall questionnaire and the data composited to provide total household information.

Information Retrieval

In THEES, survey instruments were filled out for each house during each phase of THEES. Household and personal activity 24-h recall diaries were collected from 95% of the homes and participants. Diary completion rates were 100%, that is, if a participant started to fill out a diary, it was filled out completely.

In HCCES, survey instruments were filled out for all 18 households. Self-administered daily household activity logs were filled out by 61% of the homes. Compliance was poorest at site 100 with only two of six logs completed. One household from each of the other sites did not complete the activity log. Compliance seemed to be associated with both literacy and motivation. Individuals who were semiliterate or for whom English was a second language and was not used in the home did not complete the diary. These represented 85% of the noncompliance cases.

Results

THEES

The mean concentrations of PM10 and BaP over the last two phases of THEES are shown in Table 2. Both BaP and PM10 concentrations outdoors and in the home were higher in the winter than in the early fall. Since none of the participants or their family smoked, the primary influence on indoor PM10 and BaP levels in the winter were the outdoor levels. Using total number of person days in a stepwise regression model, several indoor

Table 2. THEES phases 2 and 3 – air sampling measurements by phase: means (SD)

	BaP (ng/m³)		PM10 (μg/m³)	
	Phase 2	Phase 3	Phase 2	Phase 3
n^a	158	201	159	192
Personal	1.87 (8.32)	0.18 (0.20)	82.86 (83.20)	102.52 (190.90)
Home	1.10 (0.93)	0.16 (0.20)	52.93 (30.23)	37.93 (14.13)
Outdoor	1.05 (0.88)	0.14 (0.12)	55.90 (37.03)	30.19 (10.62)

[a] Number of person-days with complete information.

sources were found to have modest influences on winter indoor PM10 and BaP levels. These include use of supplemental heating sources and house-keeping activities.

Personal exposure levels of PM10 and BaP in THEES 2 and THEES 3 were similar to or highter than indoor and outdoor concentrations (Table 2). Stepwise regression analysis identified several variables contributing to personal exposure including use of supplementary heat sources, appliance use, and ETS exposure during THEES 2 (Table 3). Inclusion of time-weighted

Table 3. THEES phase 2 – proportion of variation (R^2) explained by diary variables, and by ambient air levels and diary variable for personal exposure (170 person days; 13 subjects, 14 days; outliers removed)

Intercept	Independent variable	β	Total R^2
BaP			
0.78	ETS	0.365***	
	Coal stove use	0.230***	0.18
0.07	Ambient BaP	0.706***	
	ETS	0.286***	
	Range cooking	0.104*	
	Unvented space heater	0.089	
	Coal stove use	0.079	0.63
PM-10			
54.5	Coal stove use	0.296***	
	Appliance use	0.277***	
	Unvented space heater	0.186**	
	Range cooking	0.189**	
	ETS	0.171*	0.22
18.9	Ambient PM-10	0.487***	
	Coal stove use	0.244***	
	Appliance use	0.241***	
	Range cooking	0.196**	
	Unvented space heater	0.169**	
	ETS	0.094	0.44

$^*p \le 0.05$; $^{**} p \le 0.01$; $^{***} p \le 0.001$; otherwise, $p = 0.05–0.10$.

ambient air levels in the models substantially improved the estimates of personal exposure. Analysis of THEES 3 based on person-days did not identify any significant influences of household or personal activities on either indoor or personal levels of BaP or PM10.

The availability of 14 daily measures on each household during THEES 2 and 3 allowed analysis of BaP and PM10 by household and participant. Looked at in this way, several idiosyncratic influences on personal exposure could be identified, including arc welding, cooking activities, and ETS in THEES 2, and housecleaning, cooking activities, ETS, and working with combustion engines in THEES 3.

HCCES

The focus of HCCES was on the household rather than the individual. Statistical analysis was carried out using each of the questionnaires. The three questionnaires produced similar models for indoor PM10 and Cr. Analyses have shown significant differences between the residential sites in both PM10 and Cr air concentrations (Table 4). Evaluation of indoor/outdoor PM10 and Cr ratios by site suggested that sites 100 and 400 had indoor pollutant sources. Further, the differences between sites was confounded by the fact that most of the smokers were at site 100, and that there

Table 4. HCCES – air sampling measurements by site: means (SD)

Site	n^a	PM10 (μg/m^3)		Cr (ng/m^3)	
		Outdoor	Indoor	Outdoor	Indoor
100	7	46.9	157.7 (128.5)	7	9.1 (5.2)
Smokers	4		237.5 (113.4)		11.5 (4.9)
Nonsmokers	3		51.3 (23.2)		6.0 (4.4)
200	8	25.5 (3.5)	21.8 (8.7)	6	2.4 (1.2)
300	3	32.5 (21.9)	28.0 (6.0)	4.0 (1.4)	4.0 (1.8)
400	10	31.0 (2.1)	40.8 (9.8)	6.0 (1.9)	4.9 (1.2)
Smokers	2		58.0 (4.2)		4.0 (1.4)
Nonsmokers	8		36.5 (4.0)		4.8 (1.1)

[a] Number of samples.
Statistical comparison of indoor air PM10 and Cr between sites (Kruskal-Wallis nonparametric analysis of variance):
  Indoor PM10   K-W 19.97, $p = 0.001$, df $= 3$, site 100 > 400 > 300, 200
  Indoor Air Cr K-W 14.81, $p = 0.002$, df $= 3$, site 100 > 400, 300 > 200

Statistical comparison – nonsmoker houses only:
  Indoor PM10   K-W 14.00, $p = 0.003$, df $= 3$, site 100, 400 > 300, 200
  Indoor Air Cr K-W 10.86, $p = 0.013$, df $= 3$, site 100, 400, 300 > 200

Table 5. HCCES – comparison of exposure sources by questionnaire type (sites 100, 200, 300, 400)

Dependent variable	n^a	Independent variables	β	R^2	p
Preliminary survey					
PM-10 (μg/m^3)	18	Cigarettes smoked (Σ all smokers in house)	0.819	0.672	<0.001
Air Cr (ng/m^3)	17	Cigarettes smoked (Σ all smokers in house)	0.926	0.857	<0.001
Wipe Cr (ng/cm^2)	18	Floor washing	0.405	0.164	0.096
Daily activity diary					
PM-10 (μg/m^3)	13	Smoke hours in home	0.978	0.956	<0.001
Air Cr (ng/m^3)	13	Smoke hours in home	0.965	0.836	<0.001
		Windows open	0.305	0.920	0.003
		Vacuum	0.200	0.954	0.023
Wipe Cr (ng/cm^2)	13	Frequency front door open	0.442	0.195	0.130
Biosurvey variables combined for households					
PM-10 (μg/m^3)	17	Cigarettes smoked	0.787	0.620	<0.001
Air Cr (ng/m^3)	17	Cigarettes smoked	0.632	0.399	0.031
Wipe Cr (ng/cm^2)	17	Sweeping	0.425	0.181	0.089

[a] Number of households.

were no smokers at sites 200 or 300. Smoking in the home was found to be the primary contributor to both indoor PM10 and Cr models (Table 5).

The discrepancy between models associated with the influence of smoking on Cr concentrations in air may be due to several factors. (a) The samples used in the biosurvey and activity log do not reflect the total sample for which surveys were completed. (b) The biosurvey reflects the responses only of those who participated in the biomonitoring study. Two known smokers did not participate in this aspect of the study. (c) The way in which the questions on smoking were phrased was different for each questionnaire. The biomonitoring questionnaire asked for the number of cigarettes smoked within a specific 36-h period. The survey smoking questions dealt with typical smoking habits, and the activity log asked for the actual number of cigarettes smoked by each household member day by day.

Dust samples obtained in HCCES were also analyzed for Cr (Table 6). There was enormous variability within homes and between homes in the amount of Cr on the wipes. Site 400 had significantly less Cr in dust samples than did the other three sites. Wipe sample levels of Cr were found to be related to the frequency of housecleaning activities (sweeping and floor washing), although these were weaker associations than those to smoking habits and air levels and were not consistent across diary analyses.

Survey information on house dimensions was used to estimate the total amount of Cr dust found in the homes and on all windowsills (Table 7). The larger living areas in the homes at site 200 provided greater estimates of

Table 6. HCCES – comparison of wipe samples by site: means (SD)

Site	All wipe samples			Window sill samples		
	n	Wipe mass (mg/cm^2)	Wipe Cr (ng/cm^2)	n	Wipe mass (mg/cm^2)	Wipe Cr (ng/cm^2)
100	33	0.56 (0.67)	53.5 (64.4)	19	0.68 (0.78)	65.9 (77.1)
200	15	0.41 (0.48)	73.2 (88.5)	10	0.54 (0.51)	98.9 (93.4)
300	6	0.34 (0.47)	54.5 (66.4)	3	0.63 (0.55)	96.0 (76.0)
400	15	0.12 (0.10)	14.5 (13.8)	11	0.12 (0.10)	12.8 (12.3)

Comparison of dust and Cr levels across sites:

All wipe dust samples:

Wipe mase K-W = 11.58, $p = 0.009$

Wipe Cr K-W = 8.10; $p = 0.044$

Site $400 < 300, 200, 100$

Window sill dust samples:

Wipe mass K-W = 10.64, $p = 0.014$

Wipe Cr K-W = 14.34, $p = 0.002$

Site $400 < 300, 200, 100$

Table 7. HCCES – estimated chromium level in homes based on house area and number of windows: means (SD)

Site	Max. site Cr (mg/km)	Home Cr (mg)	Windowsills Cr (µg)
100	43 700	1.53 (1.11)	184.9 (155.2)
200	14 492	12.94 (9.32)	596.0 (386.9)
300	26 200	3.69 (1.34)	278.2 (219.3)
400	3 900	1.70 (1.07)	107.0 (62.2)

household Cr relative to the other sites than was obtained simply from measured values per unit space. In contrast the smaller sizes of the homes at size 100 reduce the total surface area on which Cr dust can accumulate.

Discussion

Seasonal variations in PM10 and BaP ambient concentrations in THEES can be attributed to community-wide use of heating systems in the winter. While in winter most of indoor concentrations and personal exposure to PM10 and BaP were driven by outdoor ambient concentrations, there were several life-style influences. These included range top cooking, cleaning habits, use of supplementary home heat sources, and ETS. It should be noted that none of the participants in THEES smoked, and that nearly all ETS exposure occurred in the workplace.

The HCCES study was more limited in temporal scope, with only one or two air samples per home over a 7-day period. Use of point estimates of PM10 and Cr concentrations in HCCES limited the detail with which household exposures could be analyzed. However, it provided insights into the

Silverman F, Corey P, Mintz S, Oliver P, Hosien R (1982) A study of effects of ambient urban air pollution using personal samplers. Environ Int 8:311–316

Waldman JM, Buckley TJ, Lioy PJ, Greenberg A, Butler JP, Pietarinen C (1990) Investigations of indoor and outdoor levels of benzo(a)pyrene in a community of older homes. PAC 1:137–149

Wallace LA, Pellizzari ED, Hartwell TD et al. (1985) Personal exposures, indoor-outdoor relationships, and breath levels of toxic air pollutants measured for 355 persons in New Jersey. Atmos Environ 19:1651–1661

Wallace LA, Pellizzari ED, Hartwell TD et al. (1987) The TEAM study: personal exposure of toxic substances in air, water, and breath. Environ Res 43:290–307

Wallace LA (1987) The total exposure assessment methodology (TEAM study), vol 1. US Environmental Protection Agency Report EPA/600/6-87/002a

Disorders in the Olfactory Function and Injury of the Upper Airways of Exposed Workers in Copper-Producing Works

N. GINCHEVA and A. SAVOV

Higher Medical School, Sofia, Dept. of Hygiene, Ecology and Occupational Health, Boul. D. Nestorov 15, 1431 Sofia, Bulgaria

Workers in copper-producing works are exposed occupationally to dust, sulfur dioxide, and aerosols of sulfuric acid, chlorine, hydrogen chloride, nitrogen oxides, lead, selenium, arsenic, etc. (Table 1), which may lead to an injury of the mucous of the upper air ways (UAW) (Alexieva and Kiryakov 1982; Volfkovich 1963; Dimov 1975, 1984; Gamble et al. 1984; WHO 1977, 1979, 1987; Soskone 1984; Tzalev and Zaprianov 1983), including disorders in olfactory function. In determining the threshold limit value (TLV; Table 2) of dust and chemical noxa in the air of the work environment, of special interest is the degree of effect on exposed workers, as well as the rate of disorders in the function of the analyzer and chronic changes involving diseases of the (UAW).

Methods and Materials

Olfactory analyzer function was examined by the method of subjective olfactometry; this is suitable for screening in work conditions (Soldatov et al. 1976) and is used only with workers manifesting no acute symptoms during examination. Both basic functions of the olfactory organ were assessed, determining (a) the threshold of olfactory perception (quantitative) and (b) the threshold of identification (qualitative).. For the former we used the method of Voyachek (Soldatov et al. 1976), using various olfactory stimulants of different degrees (ascending olfactory scale, with 0.5% acetic acid, 95% ethyl alcohol, tincture of valerian, and ammonia). For the latter we used the quantitative method of Kiselevski (Soldatov et al. 1976), using solutions of varying concentrations of the specific stimulants: acetic acid for the trigeminal nerve; concentrated citral, geraniol, and terpineol for the olfactory nerves; and menthol for both nerves. The threshold of perception for acetic acid among healthy persons aged up to 50 years is 0.2% and that for methol is 0.008%.

U. Mohr et al. (Eds.)
Advances in Controlled Clinical
Inhalation Studies
© Springer-Verlag Berlin Heidelberg 1993

Table 1. Chemical pollutants and health conditions at copper-producing works (unpublished data of G. Bobev and V. Dzharova)

Production area	Principal chemical pollutants of the work environment	Hygiene assessment of the chemical factor (overall index of toxicity[a])
Metallurgic (Copper-smelting furnace)	Lead and copper aerosols, arsenic	Dangerous, especially unfavorable, unfavorable, acceptable
	Cadmium and zinc aerosols	Acceptable
	Sulfur dioxide, tellurium	Acceptable
Electrolytic (copper sheet)	Sulfuric acid aerosols	Unfavorable
	Sulfur dioxide	Acceptable
	Copper and lead aerosols	Acceptable, especially dangerous
	Kerosine	Unfavorable
Precious metals	Selenium, lead aerosols, arsenic, tellurium	Unfavorable, especially unfavorable
	Nitrogen oxide, nitrogen, dioxide, chlorine, hydrogen chloride, sulfur dioxide	Dangerous
Sulfuric acid	Sulfuric acid aerosols	Acceptable, unfavorable
	Sulfur dioxide	Especially unfavorable
	Lead aerosol	Unfavorable

[a] Acceptable conditions, below TLV; unfavorable, $1.1–5 \times$ TLV; especially unfavorable, $5.1–10 \times$ TLV; dangerous, $>10 \times$ TLV.

Table 2. Bulgarian TLV for chemical substances in the work environment of copper-producing works

Substance	TLV (mg/m^3)
Copper Vapors	0.5
Copper aerosols	0.1
Zinc	5.0
Cadmium	0.05
Lead	0.01
Arsenic	0.1
Selenium	2.0
Tellurium	0.01
Nitrogen oxide	10.0
Nitrogen dioxide	2.0
Sulfur dioxide	5.0
Sulfuric acid (aerosol)	1.0
Chlorine	1.0
Hydrogen chloride	5.0
Kerosine	300.0

Table 3. Age, duration of employment, and tobacco smoking among workers exposed to pollutants in copper-producing works ($n = 115$)

	n	%
Age		
21–50 years	90	78.3
51–60 years	24	20.9
Duration of employment		
<5 years	25	21.7
5–10 years	24	21.0
10–20 years	37	32.2
>20 years	29	25.2
Tobacco smoking		
Nonsmokers	62	53.9
Smokers	53	46.1
Weak	21	39.6
Moderate	23	43.4
Heavy	9	17.0

Olfactory-taste perception was tested by chloroform, a specific stimulant for the glossopharyngeal nerve. The threshold of identification was determined by the same substances, but at the above threshold concentrations. Clinical study of the UAW was performed using the classic method of otorhinolaryngological examination. In cases requiring clinical methods we used olfactometry with the olfactometer of Dimov and Raykov (1971) and working on the basis described by Elsberg and Levy (1935), roentgeno graphy of the nasal cavities, and allergologic tests.

We examined a total of 115 workers exposed to pollutants. The analysis considered their age, duration of employment at the works, and their tobacco-smoking habits (Table 3). The latter was measured using the index of Belomitzeva (1978); this index is calculated as the product of the number of cigarettes smoked in 24 h and the number of years of smoking, the level of smoking is classified as weak, moderate, or heavy. The control group consisted of 47 employees of the data-processing center, with no dust or chemical exposure. Comparisons between the two groups used either the χ^2 test or Fisher's exact test. Differences in olfactory perception were considered on the basis of the following variables: age, duration of employment, smoking, and previous diseases of the UAW.

Results

More than half of the workers examined (58.3%) had subjective complaints; these included irritation, dryness, burning, itching in the nose and the throat, frequent hemorrhages, frequent colds, crust formation, and occasional olfactory loss. Subjective complaints were most common among non-smokers and heavy smokers. Those employed longer than 5 years showed symptoms that increased in frequency with the duration of employment.

Examination of the olfactory receptor among exposed workers (Table 4) revealed normosmia in 32 (28%), hyposmia in 58 (50%), anosmia partialis in 22 (19%), and anosmia total is in 3 (2.6%). Statistically significant differences were observed between exposed workers and controls ($p < 0.05$) regarding the proportions showing normosmia. These were also significantly larger numbers of exposed workers with anosmia for acetic acid, the test substance for the trigeminal nerve (19% versus 0%; Table 4) and with hyposmia for olfactory irritants (48% versus 12.8%; Table 5). No disorders in olfactory-taste perception were found.

No relationship was seen between changes in olfactory perception and age or duration of employment. A relationship to smoking was observed only in those with partial or total anosmia, these being the moderate and heavy smokers.

Table 4. Olfactory function in exposed workers ($n = 115$) and controls ($n = 47$)

	Exposed		Controls	
	n	%	n	%
Normosmia	32	27.8*	33	70.2
Hyposmia	58	50.4	14	29.8
Anosmia partialis	22	19.1*	0	0
Anosmia totalis	3	2.6	0	0

*$p < 0.05$.

Table 5. Hyposmia in exposed workers ($n = 115$) and controls ($n = 47$)

Substance	Exposed		Controls	
	n	%	n	%
Acetic acid	46	40.0	13	27.7
Menthol	27	23.5	8	17.0
Citral, geraniol, terpineol	55	47.8*	6	12.8

*$p < 0.05$.
Some of the exposed workers, suffering hyposmia, demonstrate hyposmia towards two or three olfactory specific stimulants together.

influences of outdoor air and life-style activities. Smoking exposure and cigarette use were influences on and sources for PM10 concentrations in both HCCES and THEES. Airborne Cr in the home also was influenced by house member smoking habits. While cleaning habits cannot be treated as a source of Cr dust, they clearly influence the amount of Cr to which individuals in the home can be exposed. Analysis of PM10 levels in non-smoker homes found an association between cleaning habits and PM10 similar to that found in THEES. At present, the relationship between dust levels and airborne levels of Cr are not clear, since the size fractions of the dust particles have not been determined.

While the residential levels of Cr found were not found to be as high as in industrial settings, opportunities for exposure did exist from sources within the home or near the home. Differences in air and dust Cr levels existed among the sites which could not be attributed solely to the smoking and cleaning habits of the residents. Generalizations as to the influence of the slag deposits on indoor levels cannot be made until data from control sites have been analyzed. The substantially lower dust levels of Cr in the homes at site 400 may reflect the lower levels of Cr found in the soil at this site (maximum 1600 mg/kg compared to 14 492–43 700 mg/kg found at sites 100, 200, and 300).

Conclusions

Surveys were completed for all households in both THEES and HCCES. These afforded good estimates of time/activity information, availability of exposure sources, and potential routes of exposure. Daily activity logs, because they are "real-time" reportage would give a more accurate measure of time/activity information, exposure sources, and routes of exposure when they were filled out. However, activity logs place regular demands on the participants in the study period and require a level of literacy and motivation which may be lacking in some cases. Use of activity logs in THEES may have been successful because members of the research team were in direct contact with study participants in their homes every day of the study. These participants, most of whom participated in the study for 3 years, were highly motivated, as evidenced by their willingness to provide daily food and urine samples. The use of personal monitors in THEES in combination with personal daily activity logs allowed identification of sources of exposure which would not have been identified if only household monitoring had been carried out. The diaries were able to identify both the sources and locations of exposure.

Use of survey instruments which provide a single estimate of exposure activities should be used only with point estimates of pollution concentration. Such point estimates screen out the variability which may occur within an individual's or household's experiences. The compilation of personal biomonitoring questionnaire information to create a household data file as was used in HCCES should be a more sensitive instrument than the survey instrument and perhaps as sensitive as a daily activity diary when information can be obtained from all members of the household. Since survey instruments rely upon one individual to report on all household members, the reporter makes estimates for all individuals other than herself. Personal reportage from each household member should be more accurate. However, failure to obtain information from significant contributors to household pollution adversely affects the usefulness of this information. The use of repeated measures for each of the study homes in THEES in combination with detailed daily activity information allowed for a more sensitive evaluation of sources and routes of exposure for individuals and for households.

Acknowledgements. The research reported here was supported by the Division of Science and Research of the New Jersey Department of Environmental Protection.

References

Buckley TJ, Waldman JM, Freeman NCG, Marple VA, Turner WA, Lioy PJ (1991) Calibration, intersampler comparison, and field application of a new PM-10 personal air sampling impactor. Aerosol Sci Tech 14:380–387

Chapin L (1984) Human activity patterns. Wiley, New York

Dockery DW, Spengler JD (1981) Personal exposure to respirable particulates and sulfates. JAPCA 31:153–159

Freeman NCG, Waldman JM, Lioy PJ (1991) Design and evaluation of a location and activity log used for assessing personal exposure to air pollutants. J Exposure Anal Environ Epidemiol 1:327–338

Lebowitz MD, Quackenboss JJ, Soczk ML, Colome JD, Lioy PJ (1989) Workshop: development of questionnnaires and survey instruments. Am Soc Test Mater Spec Tech Publ 1002:203–216

Lioy PJ, Wainman T, Turner W, Marple VA (1988a) An intercomparison of the indoor air sampling impactor and the dichotomous sampler for a 10 micron cut size. JAPCA 38:668–670

Lioy PJ, Waldman JM, Greenberg A, Harkov R, Pietarinen C (1988b) The total human environmental exposure study (THEES) to benzo(a)pyrene: comparison of the inhalation and food pathways. Arch Environ Health 43:304–312

Lioy PJ, Waldman JM, Buckley T, Butler J, Pietarinen C (1990) The personal, indoor, and outdoor concentrations of PM-10 measured in an industrial community during the winter. Atmos Environ 24b:57–66

Miguel AH, Friedlander SK (1978) Distribution of BaP with respect to particle size in Pasadena aerosols in the submicron range. Atmos Environ 15:23–30

Quackenboss JL, Kanarek MS, Spengler JD, Letz R (1982) Personal monitoring for nitrogen dioxide exposure: methodological considerations for a community study. Environ Int 8:249–258

Robinson JP (1977) How Americans use their time. Praeger, New York

Sexton K, Spengler JD, Treitman RD (1984) Personal exposure to respirable particles: a case study in Waterbury, Vermont. Atmos Environ 18:1385–1398

Table 6. Diseases of the UAW in exposed workers

	n	%
Diseases of the nose and nasal cavities	66	56.0
Rhinopharyngitis	40	33.9
Rhinitis	6	5.1
Rhinitis sicca anterior, varices septi nasi, deviatio *septi nasi*	20	17.0
Disease of the pharynx and larnyx	59	50.0
Chronic tonsilitis	28	23.7
Chronic pharyngitis	13	11.0
Chronic pharyngolaryngitis	11	9.3
Chronic laryngitis	7	6.0

We also examined whether there was relationship between olfactory disorders and diagnosed diseases of the UAW in exposed workers; the results are presented in Table 6. The very frequent chronic diseases of the nose and nasal cavities, including the diagnosis *deviatio septi nasi*, are one probable cause of the changes in the olfactory perception.

Conclusions

1. High morbidity of the UAW was established in 101/118 exposed workers (86%) at the copper-producing works. The disorders are irritative changes to varying degrees (of different rates) in the mucous of the UAW, affecting the protective function of the nose.
2. Subjective olfactometry revealed a disturbance in the receptor olfactory area of the trigeminal nerve of exposed workers and, to a lesser extent, that of the olfactory nerve. The disorder in olfactory function is of the peripheral type.
3. There was no relationship between olfactory disturbance and age or duration of employment. As regards tobacco smoking, a relationship was found only in exposed workers having most severe disorders in olfactory perception (partial and total anosmia).
4. The high morbidity of the UAW and the disturbances in olfactory function among exposed workers compared to the control group implicate the intensive effect of chemical factors and an unfavorable microclimate.

References

Alexieva C, Kiryakov K (1982) Profesionalna pathologiya (Professional pathology, in Bulgarian). Medicina i Fizkultura, Sofia, pp 33–74

Belomitzeva L (1978) The spread of chronic bronchitis among workers in petro-chemical manufacture (in Russian). Gig Tr Prof Zabol 10:5–9

Dimov D (1975) State of the olfactory function in some chemical intoxications. Hig Zdraveopazvane 1:30–34

Dimov D (1984) Vkus i obonyanie (Taste and smell, in Bulgarian). Bulgarian Medicina i Fizkultura, Sofia, pp 96–99

Dimov D, Raykov Hr (1971) Bulgarian olfactometer (in Bulgarian). Otorinola-ringologiya (Sofia) 3:142

Elsberg S, Levy I (1935) Bull Neurol Inst NY 4/5:20–25

Gamble J, Jones W, Hancock J (1984) Epidemiological environmental study of lead acid battery workers. Environ Res 35:11–29, 30–52

Soldatov I, Danilin V, Mitin Y (1976) Issledovanie obonyatelnovo analizatora (The investigation of olfactory analysis). In: Professionalnaya patologiya VDP v himicheskoy promishlenosti (Professional pathology in the chemical industry, in Russian). Medicina, pp 66–69

Soskone S (1984) Laryngeal cancer and occupational exposure to sulfuric acid. Am J Epidemiol 120:358–365

Tzalev D, Zaprianov Z (1983) Atomic absoption spectrometry in occupational and environmental health practice, vol 1. CRC Press, Boca Raton, pp 87–92, 105–111, 121–127, 137–150, 182–187, 194–196, 209–214

Volfkovich M (1963) Rukovodstvo po oto-rino-laringologii, vol 4 (Manual of oto-rhino-laryngology, in Russian) Medgiz, Moscow

World Health Organisation (1977) Oxides of nitrogen, Environmental health criteria, vol 4. WHO, Geneva

World Health Organisation (1979) Sulfur oxides and suspended particulate matter. Environmental health criteria, vol 8. WHO, Geneva

World Health Organisation (1987) Oxides of nitrogen. Air quality guidelines for Europe. WHO Eur Series 23:297–315

Elevated Bioaerosols in Manufactured/Conventional Homes

C.T. Howlett, Jr., L.R. Newton, T.N. Vire, and J.J. Tice IV

Georgia-Pacific Corporation, 2883 Miller Road, Decatur, GA 30035, USA

Introduction

Georgia-Pacific Corporation has over the years provided users of their building products prompt investigative service of any complaint related to indoor air quality. As a major producer of formaldehyde and wood products containing formaldehyde-based adhesives, Georgia-Pacific initially focused its indoor air quality investigations on formaldehyde. However, as formaldehyde levels within dwellings dramatically decreased with the advent of low formaldehyde-emitting resins, alternate structural wood products, and building materials containing little or no formaldehyde, it became apparent that other causative agents were being overlooked. Specifically, airborne micro-organisms were suspected, but bioaerosol tests of mobile homes and conventional homes were not conducted until January 1989.

Twenty-one investigations of mobile homes and conventional homes were conducted from January 1989 to October 1990 in response to complaints of one or more occupants claiming upper respiratory distress. These dwellings were evaluated for both bioaerosols and formaldehyde. Adequate time was not available to identify an appropriate control unit in the same geographical area as the complaint dwelling.

Our intent here is to share with interested researchers information obtained by Georgia-Pacific from site testing, including the identity of prevalent airborne organisms. Hopefully, this paper will be a starting point for further intensive scientific studies of indoor air quality of homes.

Methods

Formaldehyde Measurement Method and Protocol

Sample locations for formaldehyde measurements were chosen based on two criteria: (a) the amount of time that the occupants spent in each room and (b) the severity of air quality complaints by the occupant in a room. Samples

U. Mohr et al. (Eds.)
Advances in Controlled Clinical
Inhalation Studies
© Springer-Verlag Berlin Heidelberg 1993

were generally obtained in a living room or family room, kitchen, master bedroom, and a second bedroom.

Crystal Diagnostics' AirScan Low Level Formaldehyde-TWA passive monitors were used for formaldehyde measurements in the home. Each location was sampled for a total of 4 h. The passive monitor was hung from the ceiling about 130–150 cm above the floor and in the center of the room. Temperature and relative humidity measurements were obtained at the beginning and end of the sampling period. Due to wide variation of temperature and humidity conditions in our field surveys, formaldehyde concentrations were corrected to 25°C and 50% relative humidity using the Berge equation (Berge et al. 1980). Table 1 summarizes measured formaldehyde concentrations in parts per million (vol/vol) corrected to 25°C and 50% relative humidity.

Bioaerosol Air Sampling Protocol

Area samples of airborne organisms were collected using a Surface Air High Flow Sampler (SAS) manufactured by PBI International (Milan, Italy). The

Table 1. Bioaerosols and formaldehyde investigations

Amplification Bacteria	Fungi	Formaldehyde (ppm at 25C/50% RH)
Conventional houses		
−	−	<0.26
+	−	0.11
−	+	<0.18
+	+	0.06
−	+	0.16
−	−	<0.06
+	−	<0.10
−	−	0.09
−	−	<0.18
+	−	<0.12
−	−	<0.08
Manufactured houses		
+	−	0.10
+	+	<0.26
+	+	<0.18
+	−	<0.16
+	−	<0.26
+	+	<0.18
−	−	0.24
+	+	<0.12
+	+	<0.15
+	−	0.06

air sampling method was based on the bioaerosol protocol recommended by the American Conference of Governmental Industrial Hygienists' (ACGIH) Bioaerosols Committee (1989). The air to be examined was drawn into the SAS sampler at a fixed speed and time through a cover, which had been machinized with multiple small holes of special design. The air flow setting on the SAS sampler for the investigations was 180 l/m for 20, 40, and 60 s. The air flow was directed into the agar surface of the contact plate. After the preset sampling time, the plate was removed and sent to the microbiological lab for incubation.

Generally, three bioaerosol tests were conducted in each complaint mobile home or conventional home: Typically, living room, bedroom, and outside air were sampled. Each location was considered a test site. The SAS sampler was placed in the center and a minimum height of 0.9 m off the floor. The outdoor air sample was obtained at roof level.

Eight plates of three types of agar were used at each test site, including a blank control sample. Before sampling at each site location, the front sieve plate was unscrewed and wiped clean inside and outside with an alcohol sponge. The plate was screwed back on, and the sampler was allowed to run for 20 s to evaporate the alcohol. The specific agar plate was then loaded for sampling. Air was collected at each sample location according to the specifications shown in Table 2.

After the plates were exposed, they were placed into their original plastic bags and packed with the contact plate base containing agar face down. The plates were returned to the microbiological laboratory within 8 h after collection. The bacteria plates were incubated at three temperatures: 20°, 35°, and 56°C. Environmental bacteria grow best at 20°C while human-type bacteria grow best at 35°C. Thermophilic bacteria growth is favored at 56°C.

Fungal amplification was considered to be of concern at concentrations above 100 colony-forming units per cubic meter of air and at least twice (200%) that detected on the outside. In addition, bacterial amplification was

Table 2. Bioaerosol sample collection specifications

Plate	Medium	Sample time (s)	Microbial group
1	MEA	20	Fungi
2	R2A	20	Environmental bacteria
3	TSA	20	Human-associated bacteria
4	MEA	40	Fungi
5	R2A	40	Environmental bacteria
6	TSA	40	Human-associated bacteria
7	TSA	60	Thermophilic bacteria
8	Nonculturable	60	

MEA, Malt extract agar; R2A, R2A agar; TSA, tryptic soy agar.

considered only for environmentally associated bacteria and not those of human origin. Amplification was considered to be of concern when counts were above 200 and exceeded other sites within the building by two times (200%).

Discussion

Table 1 summarizes the 21 sites investigated. A conventional home is built on-site and is constructed using nominal 2-in.-thick framing materials. The amplification column for bacteria and fungi indicates by plus or minus the

Table 3. Frequency of fungi and bacteria

Fungi	Cases	Sites	Bacteria	Cases	Sites
Alternaria	6	11	*Acinetobacter*	1	1
Arthrinium	1	1	*Acinetobacter*-like	2	3
Aspergillus, niger Group	7	6	*Alcaligenes*	1	1
Aspergillus, not *fumigatus*	4	9	*Arthrobacter*-like	14	22
Aureobasidium	2	3	*Bacillus*	20	57
Botryosporium	1	1	*Corynebacteria*	12	30
Candida	1	1	Enterobacteriaceae	5	5
Chaetumium	1	1	*Flavobacterium*	1	1
Cladosporium	21	58	*Micrococcus varians*	10	20
Curvularia	2	2	*Micrococcus kristinae*	2	2
Drechslera	1	1	*Micrococcus luteus*	4	7
Epicoccum	8	12	*Micrococcus lylae*	1	1
Fusarium	7	9	*Micrococcus nishiomiyaensis*	1	1
Monocillium	1	1			
Mycelia Sterilia	1	1	*Micrococcus roseus*	1	1
Nigrospora	1	1	*Micrococcus sendentarius*	4	8
Penicillium	15	37	*Micrococcus,* various spp.	7	16
Pithomyces	1	2	*Pseudomonas,* not *aeruginosa*	6	10
Rhizopus	6	8	*Staphylococcus,* not *aureus*	17	31
Sporotrichum	1	1	*Staphylococcus, aureus*	1	1
Trichoderma	3	5	*Streptomyces*	3	5
Tritirachium	1	3	Thermophilic actinomycetes	1	1
Unidentified	1	1	Unidentified	4	7
Unidentified, nonsporulating	16	36	*Xanthomonas*	2	2
Yeast	3	3			

Seventy air samples referred to as sites in the 21 cases investigated; 21 air samples were the outdoor air control, and 49 tests were conducted indoors.

presence of excess micro-organisms, as detailed above. The last column provides the formaldehyde concentrations in parts per million corrected to 25°C and 50% relative humidity. Table 3 gives the frequency of the various micro-organisms.

The inspections of manufactured homes revealed possible causation factors for the elevated bioaerosols. It is well-known that micro-organisms require adequate culture media and environmental conditions to favor growth. From our observations, there appeared to be inadequate fresh air exchanges within the test homes. One potential source of fungi and/or bacteria is the ground beneath the manufactured home. This space is an ideal environment to culture both fungi and bacteria because of the wetness, darkness, and moderate temperatures. In most cases, we observed actual growth of fungi on both the ground and structural materials beneath the home. In these cases, some wipe samples were obtained to verify the fungal growth observed in the dwelling. Contaminants from this source can potentially enter the home through breaks in the flooring (plumbing, electrical), vents, ducts, and windows/doors. Because these types of structures are so energy efficient, the mere opening and closing of doors can cause sufficient negative pressure to allow entrance of these airborne micro-organisms into the home. In the homes which had a plastic vapor barrier, and/or the ground was dry due to sufficient ventilation ports in the skirting, the level of bioaerosols monitored within the home was not amplified.

The amplified bacteria levels observed in manufactured housing appear to be associated with occupancy density, personal hygiene habits, and housekeeping practices of the occupants. The most prevalent genera observed within the home were of human shed type. Again, this may reflect the inadequacy of fresh make-up air into the dwelling.

The amplified levels of bioaerosols observed in conventional homes appear to coincide with remodeling of a home or room. It is speculated that the removal of old building materials, i.e., carpeting, paneling, flooring, wallpaper, etc. may contribute to the observed elevated levels of airborne micro-organisms. Again, the personal hygiene habits and housekeeping practices of the owners may be a contributing factor to elevated bioaerosols.

Conclusions

Of the 11 conventional and 10 manufactured homes that were investigated for bioaerosols and formaldehyde, none exceeded the United States Department of Housing and Urban Development guideline of 0.4 ppm formaldehyde. The average formaldehyde concentration in the manufactured homes was less than 0.17 ppm, while the average concentration for the conventional homes was less than 0.13 ppm.

Bacterial amplification was observed in 7 of the 21 (33.3%) homes tested for airborne micro-organisms. Fungi amplification was found only in two (9.5%) of the sites surveyed. In some cases, there was selective amplification of airborne fungi within the home. In six (28.6%) of the units monitored, both bacteria and fungi amplification were present.

An examination of Table 3 reveals that the predominant organisms are of common variety and generally do not possess pathogenic properties. This limited data base indicates that there may be a relationship between high levels of common-variety bioaerosols and health complaints of occupants. Any nonpathogenic organism can become an opportunistic organism when it affects an individual susceptible to respiratory irritants. Since none of the occupants underwent a medical examination, there is no objective data on the overall health of the occupants, i.e., preexisting respiratory illness. We suspect that there is a relationship between the occupant's complaint, i.e., upper respiratory distress, and the observed amplification of fungi and/or bacteria in the home. However, we realize that only a true cohort study could confirm these initial observations and measurements.

The owner of a home manufactured to be energy efficient needs to be aware of the potential for microbiological activity. The inspection of crawl spaces for an intact vapor barrier and proper ventilation ports in the skirting or foundation is one way of discouraging microbial activity. Personal hygiene, housekeeping practices, and occupancy density are three other factors of which the homeowner needs to be aware. In addition, the conventional homeowner needs to take precautions during removal of old building materials during remodeling.

Acknowledgements. The microbiological laboratory used by Georgia-Pacific was PathCon, Pathogen Control Associates, Inc., Tucker, Georgia. Dr. George K. Morris (Director of Scientific Activities) and Brian Shelton (Laboratory Manager) performed the identification and counted the colonies of fungi and bacteria.

References

ACGIH: American Conference of Governmental Industrial Hygienists (1989) Guidelines for assessments of bioaerosols in the indoor environment. Publication 3180

Berge A, Mellegard P, Hanetho O, Ormstad E (1980) Formaldehyde from particleboard-evaluation of a mathematical model. Holz als Roh-und Werksoff 38:251–255

Single-Breath Bolus Exposure for Noninvasive Determination of Ozone Dose Distribution

S.C. Hu[1], J.S. Ultman[2], and A. Ben-Jebria[3]

[1] Center for Environmental Medicine and Lung Biology, University of North Carolina, School of Medicine, Campus Box No. 7310, Chapel Hill, NC 27599-7310, USA
[2] Dept. of Chemical Engineering, The Pennsylvania State University, 133 Fenske Laboratory, University Park, PA 16802-4400, USA
[3] Laboratoire de Physiologie, Université de Bordeaux II, 33000 Bordeaux, France

Introduction

Ozone (O_3) resulting from the photochemical reaction of automobile emissions is an urban air pollutant which can have adverse effects on human health, particularly in the lung. Previous laboratory studies in which human subjects were exposed to controlled levels of O_3 have demonstrated that decrements in lung function are possible even during short exposures of 2.5 h at the National Ambient Air Quality Standard of 0.12 ppm O_3 (McDonnell et al. 1983). Morphometric studies of the lungs of animals exposed to low ozone concentrations for 1–6 weeks reveal that there is epithelial cell injury which is far more serious in the bronchoalveolar duct region than in any other lung region (Barry et al. 1985; Mellick et al. 1977). Mathematical model simulations indicate that this nonuniform distribution of cell damage coincides with a nonuniform distribution of O_3 uptake (Miller et al. 1985), leading to the hypothesis that the heterogeneity of cell response is driven by differences in cell dose rather than by differences in cell sensitivity.

As starting point for confirming the hypothesis, this article describes how the longitudinal distribution of O_3 uptake can be measured in intact human lungs by using an ozone bolus-response technique. The specific aims of the research were to: construct a bolus inhalation system for use with human subjects; develop protocols to measure the bolus-response in a safe and effective manner; and measure the distribution of O_3 absorption on four previously unexposed subjects during quiet breathing.

U. Mohr et al. (Eds.)
Advances in Controlled Clinical
Inhalation Studies
© Springer-Verlag Berlin Heidelberg 1993

Mathematical Model

To estimate the risk of bolus inhalation relative to the risk of a conventional continuous inhalation experiment, we employed a computer simulation based on fundamental diffusion theory (Hu et al. 1992). By viewing the lung as a symmetrically branching structure in which the longitudinal distributions of ozone concentration and absorption are the same along all possible paths from the airway opening to the alveolar sacs, the transport of O_3 was described by a single mass conservation equation written for the gas phase:

$$\frac{\partial F_{O_3}}{\partial t} + \frac{\dot{V}}{A}\frac{\partial F_{O_3}}{\partial y} = \frac{1}{A}\frac{\partial}{\partial y}\left(D_{eff}A\frac{\partial F_{O_3}}{\partial y}\right) - KaF_{O_3} \qquad (1)$$

were F_{O_3} is the mole fraction of O_3 which is a function of time, t, and longitudinal distance from the airway opening, y; $\dot{V}$ is respiratory flow, A is the cross-section available for flow, D_{eff} is the longitudinal dispersion coefficient, K is the mass transfer coefficient for lateral absorption, and a is the ratio of local absorption surface to gas volume.

In order to specify the geometric functions, $A(y)$ and $a(y)$, the lower airways were represented by Weibel's anatomic model (Weibel 1963) scaled to a total volume of 2.65 l, and the upper airways were represented by an equivalent cylinder whose length, mean cross-section, and mean hydraulic diameter were matched to the actual oropharyngeal path (Fredberg et al. 1980). Previous estimates of mucus thickness and O_3 reactivity in mucus were used to compute a distribution of K values (Miller et al. 1985), D_{eff} was equated to the molecular diffusion coefficient of O_3 in air, and a constant respiratory flow of 250 ml/s at a breathing frequency of 15 min^{-1} was employed.

Equation 1 was constrained by an initial condition and two boundary conditions. At the start of the simulation, we assumed that no O_3 was present; at the lips, a specific O_3 concentration pattern was prescribed during inspiration, and the gradient of O_3 concentration was assumed to be zero during expiration; and at the distal end of the lung, the diffusional flux of O_3 was equated to the KaF_{O_3} product. Digital computer simulations were implemented by using orthogonal collocation on finite elements, a numerical technique that was selected because of its inherent numerical efficiency and stability. One set of simulations using a bolus input curve similar to those employed in human subject experiments was carried out at alternative penetrations from 50 to 400 ml. A simulation of the continuous inhalation of an O_3-air mixture was also performed.

Methods

The four healthy male nonsmokers used in this pilot study had the following characteristics: age 31.5 ± 5.2 years, height 173 ± 6 cm, and weight = 67 ± 9 kg.

The bolus inhalation apparatus originated with a short stainless steel mouthpiece assembly containing a proximal injection port connected to a bolus generator (Ben-Jebria et al. 1991) and two distal sampling ports connected to a chemiluminescent O_3 analyzer (Ben-Jebria et al. 1990) and to a carbon dioxide (CO_2) analyzer (McGaw RMS-6 Respiratory Mass Spectrometer). The rapid response of the O_3 analyzer (i.e., 10%–90% step response in 110 ms) was critical to the success of the bolus-response measurements. A rubber mouthpiece through which the subject breathed was mounted on the distal end of the stainless steel assembly, and a pneumotachograph (Fleisch, no. 1) was mounted on the proximal end of the assembly. The differential pressure from the pneumotachograph was converted to a flow signal by a transducer (Validyne, MP45) and demodulator (Validyne, CD19), and the flow signal was processed by an analog integrator (Validyne, FV156) to obtain a respired volume signal. The flow and both gas analyzer signals were recorded by a computerized data acquisition system (Keithley 570 driven by a Zenith 386 workstation), and the respired volume signal was displayed on an x-y monitor (Tektronix, 603 storage monitor). Drawn on the viewing surface of this monitor was a triangular volume pattern equivalent to a 500 ml inspiration in 2 s followed by a 500-ml expiration in 2 s.

Seated comfortably on a stool and wearing noseclips, the subject grasped the rubber mouthpiece and initiated a test breath by depressing a switch which simultaneously activated the time sweep of the x-y monitor, reset the flow integrator, and initiated data collection by the data acquisition system. Beginning at FRC, the subject attempted to match his respired volume to the pattern drawn on the surface of the x-y monitor. The data acquisition system automatically triggered bolus injection at a preset inhaled volume, and by reversing his respired flow at the correct end-inspiration point, the subject ensured that the bolus would penetrate to a desired volume. A peak O_3 bolus concentration of 3–4 ppm was used to maximize the signal-to-noise ratio of the ozone analyzer output. During a complete experimental session, bolus injection occurred at 19 penetration volumes from 20 to 200 ml in increments of 10 ml with each measurement replicated approximately five times.

The raw digitized data consisted of respired flow, O_3 fraction (F_{O_3}) and CO_2 fraction (F_{CO_2}) versus time. The first steps in processing the data were to numerically integrate the flow data to obtain respired volume (V) and to shift the time axes of both sets of gas fraction data to account for the time delays of the instruments. Next, each O_3 data point was corrected for CO_2 interference by dividing F_{O_3} by the factor of $1 + 3.8F_{CO_2}$, and the corrected O_3 data were smoothed by a 20-Hz low-pass filter and cross-plotted against respired volume (Fig. 1).

The F_{O_3} data obtained during the inspiratory (subscript I) and expiratory (subscript E) phases of a test breath were separately integrated to determine the amount of O_3 (M) in the inhaled bolus and in the exhaled response:

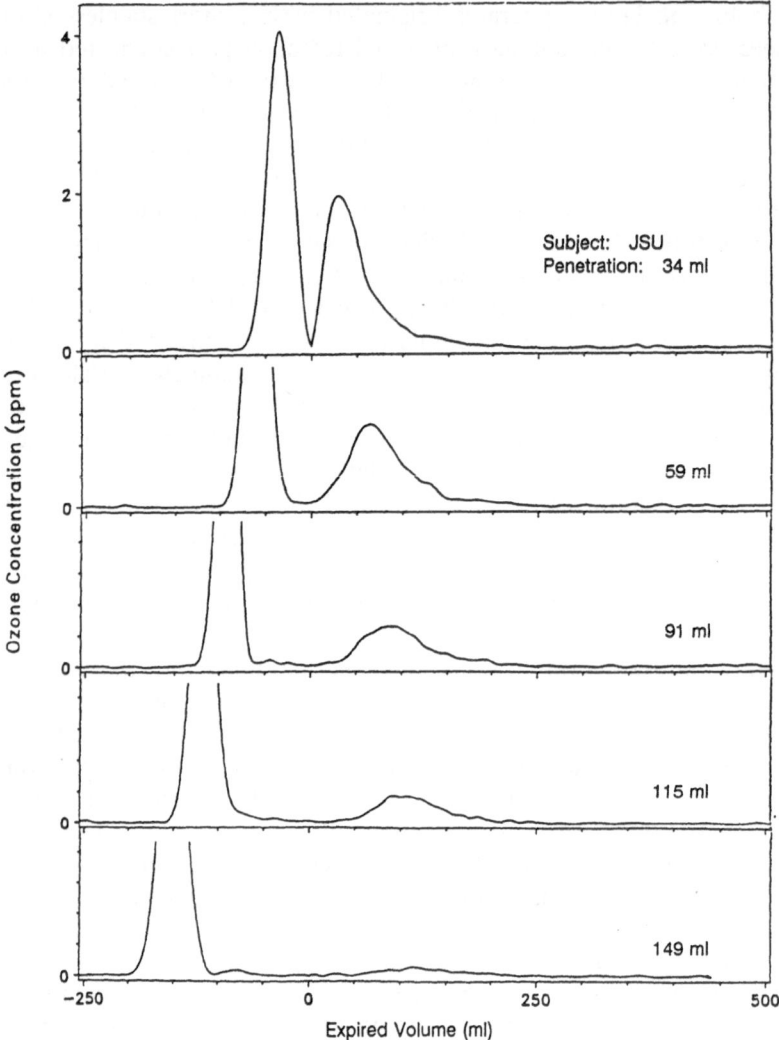

Fig. 1. Representative bolus-response data from subject JSU at progressively increasing bolus penetration volumes. Negative values of expired volume correspond to inspiration, and the origin corresponds to the beginning of expiration

$$M_I = \int (F_{O_3})_I dV \qquad (2)$$

and

$$M_E = \int (F_{O_3})_E dV \qquad (3)$$

The fraction of inhaled O_3 absorbed within the test breath was then computed from the equation:

$$\Lambda = 1 - M_E/M_I \qquad (4)$$

and the corresponding bolus penetration was represented by the mean volume of the inhaled F_{O_3} data:

$$V_p = (1/M_I) \int (F_{O_3})_I V dV \qquad (5)$$

The Λ values obtained for each subject were subdivided into 10-ml increments of V_p, and the mean and standard error in each increment were determined for the pooled data from all subjects (Fig. 2).

Results and Discussion

In Table 1, simulations for the continuous inhalation of 0.4 ppm O_3, often used in controlled chamber studies (e.g., Colucci 1983), are compared to simulations of the bolus-response protocol when the peak inhaled concentration is 4 ppm. For ease in presentation, the lung has been subdivided into five sequential tissue regions: region 1 contains the mouth, trachea, primary and secondary bronchi; region 2 contains bronchial generations 3–9; region 3 contains bronchial generations 10–16; region 4 contains the transition airways where the alveolarization begins; and region 5 contains fully alveolated ducts and sacs. Each entry in this table is a local tissue dose expressed as the amount of O_3 absorbed per breach per unit area of airway surface.

The predicted O_3 dose to each tissue region is greater for a 0.4-ppm continuous inhalation than it is for a 4-ppm bolus inhalation at all of the penetrations that were simulated. This may be explained by the fact that during continuous inhalation, tissue is constantly exposed to fresh O_3, and diffusion through the mucus blanket to the tissue surface is relatively complete. During bolus inhalation, however, O_3 passes through each lung region in such a short time that diffusion is relatively incomplete. These simulations

Table 1. Computer simulations of ozone dose to tissue during continuous and during bolus inhalation

	Region 1	Region 2	Region 3	Region 4	Region 5
Generations	0–2	3–9	10–16	17–19	20–23
Volume (ml)	95	14	56	158	2360
Continuous inhalation at a 0.4-ppm O_3 concentration and a 500 ml tidal volume					
	0.27	4.11	17.13	8.05	0.31
Bolus inhalation at a 4.0-ppm O_3 peak concentration and penetrations of 50–400 ml					
50 ml	0.11	0.02	0.01	0.01	0.01
100 ml	0.21	2.00	1.16	0.05	0.01
200 ml	0.14	2.53	12.08	5.27	0.19
300 ml	0.13	2.35	11.36	5.99	0.24
400 ml	0.13	2.35	11.35	6.00	0.24

Units of dose are given as micrograms of ozone absorbed per $100 \, m^2$ tissue surface.

suggest that our bolus inhalation protocol is comparatively safe. In point of fact, none of the four subjects we tested reported any O_3-related symptoms.

, The principal variable observed in this study was the fraction of O_3 absorbed when an inhaled bolus transverses an airway region extending from the lips to a particular penetration volume. Figure 2 indicates that no absorption occurred for the first 20 ml of penetration, corresponding to the volume of the mouthpiece assembly between the lips and the O_3 sampling port. On the other hand, 54% of inhaled O_3 was absorbed at a penetration of 70 ml, which roughly corresponds to the upper airways. This is within the range of absorbed fractions previously measured in the upper airways by using direct pharyngeal sampling during continuous inhalation of O_3 (Gerrity et al. 1988). Figure 2 also demonstrates that absorption was essentially complete at a penetration of 160 ml, which is within the broncho-alveolar transition region at about the 18th generation of airway branching.

The variation of absorbed fraction data within each 10-ml increment of bolus penetration was characterized in two ways. The standard deviation about the mean of each subject's data was averaged among the four subjects to characterize intrasubject variation, SD_{intra}. Then, the standard deviation of the four means was computed as a measure of intersubject variation,

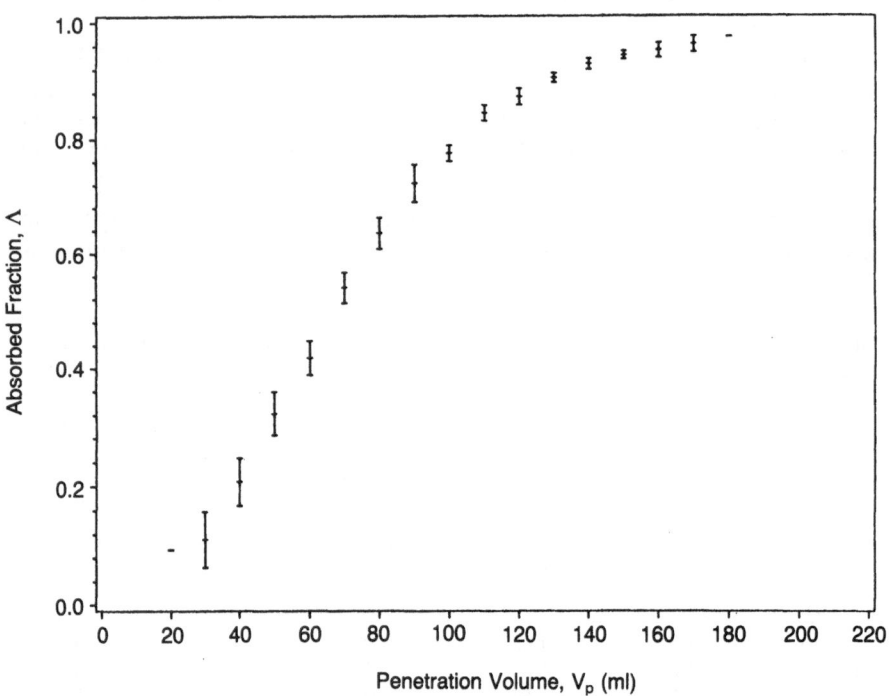

Fig. 2. Absorbed fraction distribution pooled for four subjects. The Λ values collected for all subjects were sorted into 10-ml penetration volume increments. The mean $\pm$ 2 standard errors within each increment is represented by the data points and their associated error bars

SD_{inter}. The intersubject variation was somewhat larger than the intra-subject variation (e.g., $SD_{intra} = \pm 0.044$ and $SD_{inter} = \pm 0.076$ for the 75- to 85-ml increment). This suggests that the precision of the data would be more improved by adding subjects than by increasing the number of test breaths taken by each subject.

In conclusion, it is becoming increasingly apparent that the extrapolation of exposure-response data from animals to people, from high concentrations to low concentrations, and from non-susceptible to susceptible populations requires a better understanding and improved quantification of the relationship between inhaled dose and the dose to target tissue. The results of this pilot study indicate that the bolus-response method is a promising technique with which to noninvasively map out the longitudinal distribution of O_3 absorption in intact human lungs. Under quiet breathing conditions, the sensitivity and dynamic response of the inhalation system we developed is adequate to obtain reliable values of absorbed fraction over the first 200 ml of lung volume.

Acknowledgement. Research described in this article was conducted under contract to the Health Effects Institute (HEI), an organization jointly funded by the United States Environmental Protection Agency (EPA) (Assistance Agreement X-812059) and automobile manufacturers. The contents of this article do not necessarily reflect the views of the HEI, nor do they necessarily reflect the policies of EPA or automobile manufacturers.

References

Barry BB, Miller FJ, Crapo JD (1985) Effects of inhalation of 0.12 and 0.25 parts per million ozone on the proximal alveolar region of juvenile and adult rats. Lab Invest 53:692–704

Ben-Jebria A, Hu S-H, Ultman JS (1990) Improvements in a chemiluminescent analyzer for respiratory applications. Rev Sci Instrum 61:3435–3439

Ben-Jebria A, Hu S-H, Kitzmiller EL, Ultman JS (1991) Ozone absorption into excised sheep trachea by a bolus-response method. Environ Res 56:144–157

Colucci AV (1983) Pulmonary dose/effect relationships in ozone exposure. In: Lee SD, Mustafa MG, Mehlman MS (eds) Advances in modern environmental toxicology, vol V. Princeton Scientific, Princeton

Fredberg JJ, Wohl ME, Glass GM, Dorkin HL (1980) Airway area by acoustic reflections measured at the mouth. J Appl Physiol 48:749–758

Gerrity TR, Weaver RA, Berntsen J, House DE, O'Neil JJ (1988) Extrathoracic and intrathoracic removal of ozone in tidal breathing humans. J Appl Physiol 65:393–400

Hu S-C, Ben-Jebria A, Ultman JS (1992) Simulation of ozone uptake distribution in the human airways by orthogonal collocation on finite elements. Comp Biomed Res 25:264–278

McDonnell WF, Horstman DH, Hazucha MJ, Seal E, Haak ED, Salaam SA, House DE (1983) Pulmonary effects of ozone exposure during exercise: dose-response characteristics. J Appl Physiol 54:1345–1352

Mellick PW, Dungworth DL, Schwartz LW, Tyler S (1977) Short term morphologic effects of high ambient levels of ozone on lungs of Rhesus monkeys. Lab Invest 36:82–90
Miller FJ, Overton JH, Jaskot RH, Menzel DB (1985) A model of the regional uptake of gaseous pollutants in the lung. Toxicol Appl Pharmacol 79:11–27
Weibel E (1963) Morphometry of the human lung. Academic, New York

Problems of Regulating Outdoor Ozone Levels

A.D. Kappos[1], G. Koss[1], I. Tesseraux[1], and P. Bruckmann[2]

[1] Behörde für Arbeit, Gesundheit und Soziales, Amt für Gesundheit,
Tesdorpfstraße 8, 2000 Hamburg 13, FRG
[2] Minsterium für Umwelt, Raumordnung und Landwirtschaft NRW,
Schwannstraße 3, 4000 Düsseldorf 30, FRG

Introduction

Tropospheric ozone (O_3) levels have been rising with increasing industrialization during this century. The yearly rate of increase is estimated to be 1%–2%. During summer in Germany the outdoor O_3 levels at multiple measuring sites repeatedly exceed the values of the air quality guidelines set forth by the WHO. Recent studies have shown that the range between natural O_3 concentrations and first health effects is very narrow. This paper discusses the problems of regulating outdoor O_3 levels and presents the efforts of FRG health and pollution control authorities concerned with this subject.

Formation of Ozone and Outdoor Ozone Levels

It is now well understood that the O_3 formation in the sun-lit troposphere proceeds via photochemical reactions involving volatile organic compounds and nitrogen oxides (NO_x) as precursors (Finlayson and Pitts 1976; Bruckmann 1983; Güsten 1986). The mechanism shown in Fig. 1 explains the typical cycle of O_3 and other photochemical oxidants and also the fact that O_3 concentrations typically are lower in the vicinity of strong NO sources, such as downtown areas or crowded highways, and are often higher in otherwise nonpolluted rural areas.

Health Effects in Different Population Groups

The established pathophysiological responses to the inhaled irritant gas O_3 are reviewed elsewhere (Kappos and Koss 1991). An overview of the lowest O_3 concentrations producing significant pathophysiological alterations after acute exposure is given in Fig. 2. Significant effects are observed at low O_3

U. Mohr et al. (Eds.)
Advances in Controlled Clinical
Inhalation Studies
© Springer-Verlag Berlin Heidelberg 1993

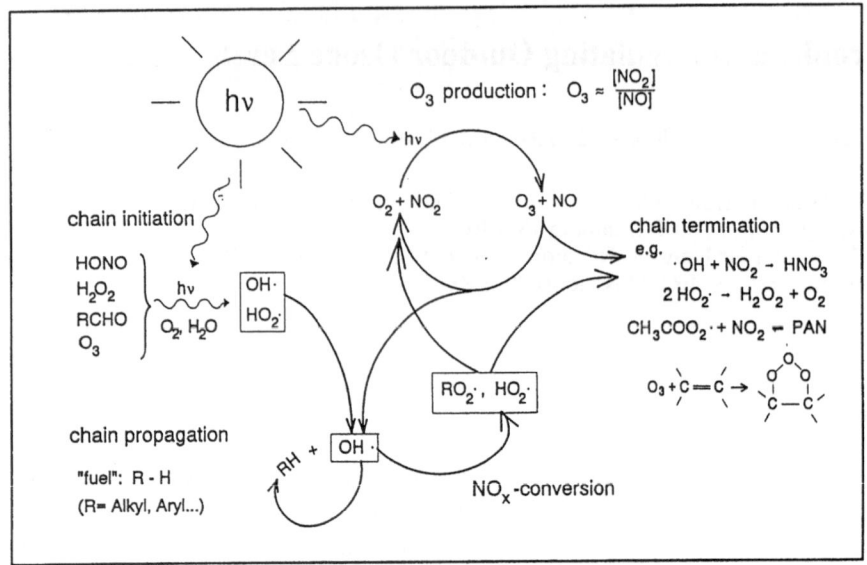

Fig. 1. Formation of O_3 in the troposphere

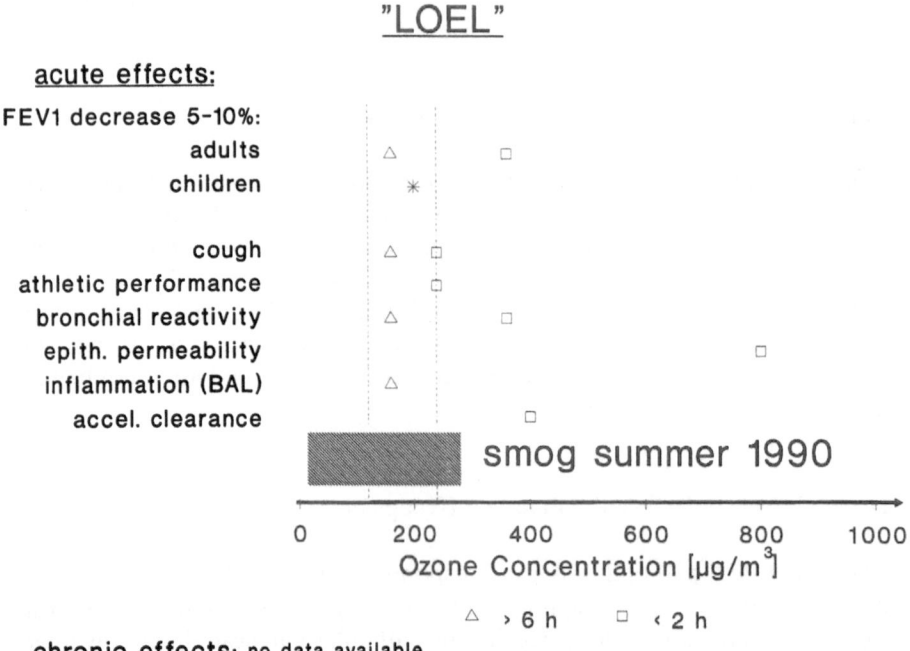

Fig. 2. Lowest O_3 concentration at which effects on humans are observed. (Modified from Lippmann 1989)

concentrations, occasionally down to $120\,\mu g/m^3$ if the exposure time exceeds 6 h (Folinsbee et al. 1988), during heavy exercise (Hazucha 1987), and in studies under natural exposure conditions (Spektor et al. 1988a,b; Gong et al. 1986). For the latter it is supposed that other photooxidants than O_3 may contribute significantly to the effects observed.

Lung function losses of 10% are accompanied by lower respiratory symptoms (cough, sputum production, dyspnea, substernal irritation, and chest tightness; Ostro and Lippsett 1989), except in studies with children (McDonnell et al. 1985a). In spite of a great variance in the sensititivity of healthy young adults (McDonnell et al. 1985b) or healthy children (Kinney et al. 1989) to ozone, there are apparently no special risk groups. Asthmatics or patients with chronic obstructive bronchitis are not more sensitive to O_3 than healthy subjects. Populations of major concern relevant to regulatory measures are healthy adults and children exercising outdoors.

Regulation of Ozone

The existing standards or guideline values relevant to FRG or Europe are listed in Table 1. In Germany pollution control and health authorities have developed a concept of information and "warning values" for the general public. Most states in the FRG provide a daily information service on the current O_3 concentration. The necessity of "public warning" is a matter of ongoing discussion. The proposed threshold concentrations for such warning are given in Table 2. A preliminary air quality guideline of the European Community proposes a value of $110\,\mu g/m^3$ as 8-h mean and a threshold value for warning of $174\,\mu g/m^3$ as 30-min mean. To achieve a significant reduction in the O_3 levels several short-term regulation measures have been adopted in the United States and Japan (automobile traffic restrictions to reduce NO_x and limitation of petrochemical emissions). It has been estimated that the reduction in hydrocarbon emissions is more effective than the local reduction in NO_x in decreasing the O_3 maxima (US Environmental Protection Agency 1987). Measures such as summer smog regulations for

Table 1. Ozone standards in Europe

Standard	Ozone concentration ($\mu g/m^3$)	Exposure conditions
FRG occupational exposure limit	200	8 h/day
FRG ambient air guideline	120	30-min mean
WHO air quality guidline	150–200	1 h
	100–120	8 h
EC air quality guideline (proposed)	110	8 h
Swiss air pollution prevention guideline	100	30-min mean
	120	1-h mean

320   A.D. Kappos et al.

Table 2. Proposed public warning thresholds in the FRG

Ozone mean concentration ($\mu g/m^3$)	Recommendation	Issuing agency
180 30-min	Avoid unnecessary heavy outdoor exercise	GMK
180 2-h	Avoid outdoor exercise	UMK
240	Subjects sensitive to ozone should not exercise outdoors	BGA
360	General recommendation not to exercise outdoors	BGA

GMK, Conference of Ministers of Health; UMK, Conference of Ministers of the Environment; BGA, Federal Health Authority.

cities have been shown to have little or no effect in reducing the O_3 level of the city itself, mainly because they start when the air is already polluted (Lindsay et al. 1989). Long-term regulations are considered to be much more effective to achieve lower ambient O_3 levels in the future. These should consist of (a) technical measures, such as those for the entire European Community regarding catalysts for new and old cars, lowering the limit values for diesel exhaust, and reducing vapor emissions during refueling; and (b) traffic concepts, such as improvement of public transport systems. All these regulations require interregional and international cooperation.

References

Bruckmann P (1983) Bildung von Säuren und Oxidantien durch Gasphasenreaktionen. VDI Ber 500:21–33
Finlayson BJ, Pitts N Jr (1976) Photochemistry of the polluted troposphere. Science 192:111–119
Folinsbee LJ, McDonnell WF, Horstman DH (1988) Pulmonary function and symptom responses after 6.6 hours exposure to 0.12 ppm ozone with moderate exercise. JAPCA 38:28
Gong H, Bradley PW, Simmons MS, Tashkin DP (1986) Impaired exercise performance and pulmonary function in elite cyclists during low-level ozone exposure in a hot environment. Am Rev Respir Dis 134:726–733
Güsten H (1986) Formation, transport and control of photochemical smog. In: Hutzinger O (ed) Air pollution. Springer, Berlin Heidelberg New York, pp 53–105 (Handbook of environmental chemistry, vol 4A)
Hazucha MJ (1987) Relationship between ozone exposure and pulmonary function changes. J Appl Physiol 62:1671–1680
Kappos AD, Koss G (1991) Gesundheitliche Wirkungen des Ozons als Bestandteil des Sommersmogs. Off Gesundheitswes 53:16–22
Kinney PL, Ware JH, Spengler JD, Dockery DW, Speizer FE, Ferris Jr BG (1989) Short-term pulmonary function change in association with ozone levels. Am Rev Respir Dis 139:56–61

Lindsay RW, Richardson JL, Chameides WL (1989) Ozone trends in Atlanta, Georgia: have emission controls been effective? JAPCA 39:40–43

Lippmann M (1989) Health effects of ozone. A critical review. JAPCA 39:672–695

McDonnell WF, Chapman RS, Leigh MW, Strope GL, Cullier AM (1985a) Respiratory responses of vigorously exercising children to 0.12 ppm ozone exposure. Am Rev Respir Dis 132:875–879

McDonnell WF, Horstmann DH, Abdul-Salam S, House DE (1985b) Reproducibility of individual responses to ozone exposure. Am Rev Respir Dis 131: 36–40

Ostro BD, Lipsett MJ (1989) Predicting respiratory morbidity from pulmonary function tests: a reanalysis of ozone chamber studies. JAPCA 39:1313–1318

Spektor DM, Lippmann M, Lioy PJ, Thurston GD, Citak K, James DJ, Bock N, Speizer FE, Hayes C (1988a) Effects of ambient ozone on respiratory function in active, normal children. Am Rev Respir Dis 137:313–320

Spektor DM, Lippmann M, Thurston GD, Liouy PJ, Steko J, O'Connor G, Garshik E, Speizer FE, Hayes C (1988b) Effect of ambient ozone on respiratory function in healthy adultsexercising outdoors. Am Rev Respir Dis 138:821–828

US Environmental Protection Agency (1987) US EPA national air quality and emission trends report. EPA-450/4-87-001

Inhalation Studies with Airborne Particulates in Rodents: Cytotoxic and Genotoxic Effects on Alveolar Macrophages and Bone Marrow Cells

A. Kiell, W. Hadnagy, N.H. Seemayer, H. Behrendt, and R. Tomingas

Medizinisches Institut f. Umwelthygiene an der Heinrich-Heine-Universität, Gurlittstraße 53, 4000 Düsseldorf 1, FRG

Introduction

Industrialization, traffic, and urbanization are the most important factors causing contamination of the atmosphere with particulate and gaseous pollutants. These represent a very complex chemical mixture composed of several hundreds of mostly organic compounds (Helmes et al. 1982; Schlipköter 1983). In previous studies it has been repeatedly reported that organic extracts are cytotoxic, mutagenic, and carcinogenic in a number of short-term bioassays using rodent and human tissue culture cells (Hadnagy et al. 1986, 1989; Motykiewiecz et al. 1991; Seemayer et al. 1984, 1988, 1989). Airborne particulates with a diameter of less than 5 µm are of special importance as they can reach the bronchoalveolar space in human lung by respiration. Macrophages in alveoli come into direct contact with noxious particles and gases as well as with diverse pathogenic microorganisms.

Cytotoxic effects of airborne particulates to macrophages have been repeatedly reported. A dose-dependent loss of cell viability of mouse macrophages (line IC-21) by extract and various fractions of airborne particulates was observed (Seemayer and Manojlovic 1980). Loss of cell viability and an increased release of lactate dehydrogenase of rat alveolar macrophages exposed to airborne particulates have been described by Liu et al. (1987). Alterations in macrophage functions by various environmental chemicals were presented by Loose et al. (1981) and Gardner (1984). Gulyas et al. (1990) reported noxious effects of airborne particulates and fly ashes on rabbit alveolar macrophages which were correlated with arsenic, lead, and antimony contents. Profound alterations in morphology of human macrophages by extracts of particulates has been shown by Behrendt et al. (1986, 1990).

In addition, inhaled noxious substances may also be absorbed and distributed to remote tissues and organs. Inhalation studies with mice exposed

U. Mohr et al. (Eds.)
Advances in Controlled Clinical
Inhalation Studies
© Springer-Verlag Berlin Heidelberg 1993

to aerosols of several genotoxic chemicals demonstrated cytotoxic and genotoxic effects on bone marrow cells (Odagiri et al. 1986).

This paper reports the results of inhalation experiments on rats with aerosols containing substances from extracted particulates of a highly industrialized region. Data showing cytotoxic and genotoxic effects on bronchoalveolar cells and bone marrow cells are presented.

Material and Methods

Airborne Particulate Sampling and Extraction. Airborne particulates were collected in the city of Duisburg (FRG) in 1983–1984 with a high-volume sampler (Draeger Box Micron Filter MB 1700) on ten membrane filter lamellae of $1.5\,m^2$. The collection was conducted at an air flow rate of $1500\,m^3/h$ for a period of 215 h corresponding to a total air volume of $322\,000\,m^3$. Particulates were extracted with methanol. For inhalation experiments extract was quantitatively transferred to Lutrol E 400 (polyethylene glycol, mol. wt. 400, Roth, Karlsruhe). This represents the global extract (GEX).

Animals. Female rats 6–8 weeks old (Wistar or brown Norway) were used for inhalation experiments. Food and water were given ad libitum.

Inhalation Conditions. Inhalation equipment for "nose-only exposure" was obtained from TSE (Kronberg, FRG) and consists of an inhalation chamber and an aerosol-generating system (compressor, pump with calibrated syringe, nozzle). For aerosol generation test extract in Lutrol E 400 (2 ml/h) was mixed with the air stream (600 l/h) utilizing a nozzle. The stock solution consisted of extracted substances from particulates corresponding to $648\,m^3$ air. Vehicle control was performed with Lutrol E 400 only. The inhalation conditions were controlled by a Multi-Function Unit (TSE), registering temperature (°C), humidity (%), pressure (mB), O_2 (%), CO_2 (%), and flow rate (l/h) throughout inhalation. The aerosol concentration in the inhalation chamber was monitored by aerosol deposition on membrane filters at an air flow rate of 30 l/h and gravimetric measurement. Animals were kept in plastic tubes inserted into the inhalation chamber in such a way that the nose was in contact with the GEX aerosol or the vehicle aerosol only. In general, exposure time per day was 5 h. Wistar rats were exposed to aerosols produced from the stock solution for 1, 2, 3, and 4 days. Exposure of brown Norway rats was performed with diluted stock solution (1:4) for 6 or 11 days. Each control and exposure group consisted of four animals.

Bronchoalveolar Lavage Cells. Immediately after inhalation animals were sacrificed by sodium pentobarbital anesthesia. Alveolar macrophages were obtained by bronchoalveolar lavage (BAL) with sterile physiological saline

(1 × 2 ml, 2 × 3 ml) utilizing a plastic tubing (canula Braun, Melsungen Article, no. 420 757/2, 2-G14 Luer) introduced into the trachea. Aspirated cells were suspended in siliconized centrifuge tubes containing RPMI-1640 medium supplemented with 10% fetal calf serum and antibiotics (penicillin/streptomycin). Cell number was determined by hemocytometry and with a Coulter counter (Coulter Electronics, Model ZB). Cell viability was performed by the dye exclusion test with trypan blue. Cytological analysis of BAL cells was carried out from cytocentrifuge preparations by determination of the proportion of macrophages, granulocytes, and lymphocytes. For studies on phagocytic properties of macrophages, BAL cells were seeded into fibronectin-coated Lab-Tek tissue culture chambers (no. 4808) at a density of 4×10^5 cells/cm^2. After a cultivation period of 2 or 24 h Polychromatic Fluoresbrite Microspheres (Latex) with a diameter of 5.72 μm were added to the cultures at a ratio of five particles per seeded cell. Following an incubation period of 2 h cultures were carefully rinsed three times with phosphate-buffered solution, fixed with Bouin's solution, and stained with Mayer's hematoxylin and eosin. Phagocytosis of particles was evaluated microscopically by determination of the phagocytic activity (percentage of phagocytizing cells) and the phagocytic capacity (number of phagocytized particles per cell) from 400 cells (100 cells per replicative culture). For analysis by transmission electron microscopy BAL cells were centrifuged at 150 g, fixed with buffered glutaraldehyde for 30 min, washed, and post-fixed with osmium tetraoxide. After dehydration in graded series of ethanol, cells were embedded in Araldite. Ultrathin sections were stained with uranyl acetate and lead citrate and analyzed in a Phillips TEM 400 electron microscope (Behrendt et al. 1986, 1987b).

Bone Marrow Cells. The femur of each animal was removed. The bone marrow cells were flushed out with 1 ml fetal calf serum, suspended, and centrifuged at 100 g for 10 min. After resuspending the pellet, smears were prepared on slides, air dried, and fixed with methanol. Giemsa-stained bone marrow cell preparations (5% Giemsa in Sörensen's buffer, pH 6.8, 10 min) were analyzed for the percentage of polychromatic erythrocytes (PCEs) from 1000 total erythrocytes per slide and two replicatives per animal. For the micronucleus assay smears were stained with Mayer's hematoxylin and eosin according to Pascoe and Gatehouse (1986) to discriminate between DNA-containing micronuclei and mast cell granules. One thousand PCEs per slide were scored microscopically for the presence of micronucleated polychromatic erythrocytes (MPCEs) from two replicatives per animal at a magnification of ×1250.

Results

Monitoring of the concentration in the inhalation chamber was based on gravimetric measurements of membrane filters. Taking into consideration the inhalation conditions, filter weights, and respiratory volume of rats of about 5 l/h, Wistar rats were exposed to aerosols containing extractable substances of airborne particulates equivalent to $1\,m^3$ air per hour. Brown Norway rats received a four times lower concentration.

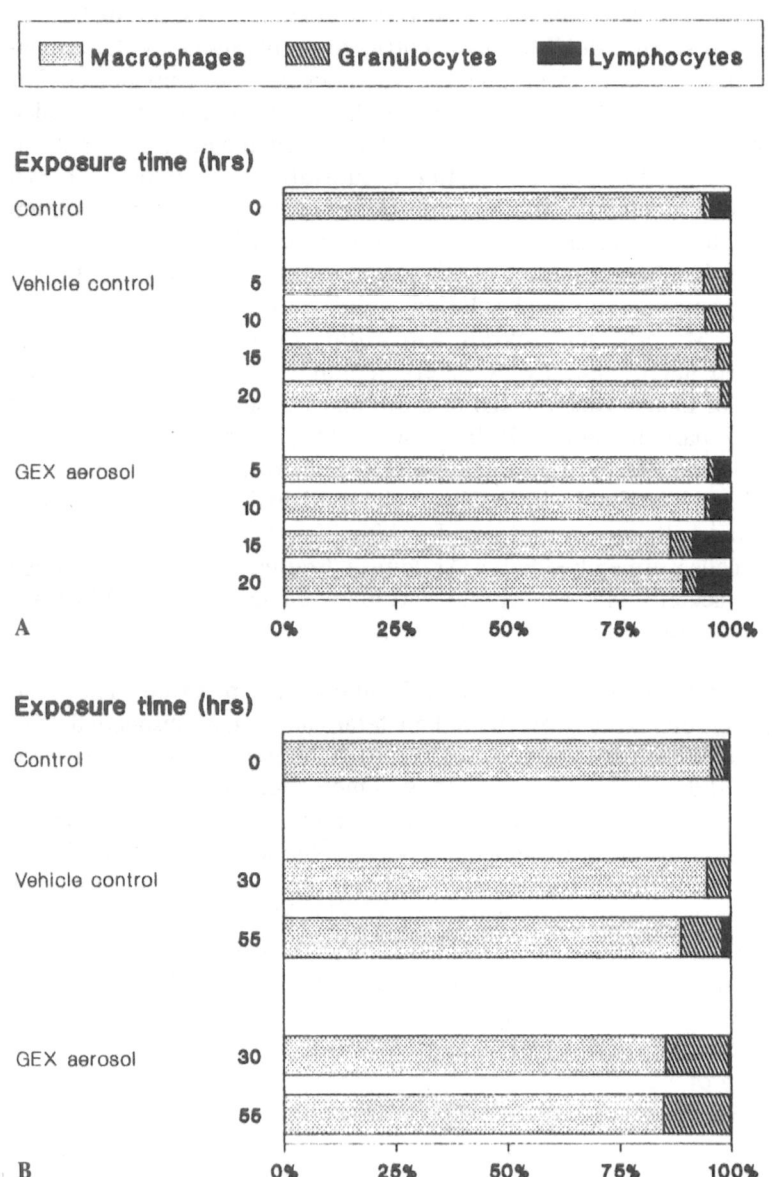

Fig. 1A,B. Cytology of BAL cells of control, vehicle control, and GEX aerosol rats. **A** Wistar rats; **B** brown Norway rats

After exposure BAL was performed, and obtained cells were analyzed for cytotoxic effects. Generally, BAL yielded a cell number of $5-10 \times 10^6$ cells. This range was for Wistar and brown Norway rats regardless of control and exposed animals and within the animal groups. Figure 1 presents the results of the cytological analysis of BAL cells. For Wistar rats a moderate increase in granulocytes and lymphocytes after 15 and 20 h of exposure to GEX aerosols was obtained as compared to the control. The percentage of granulocytes of exposed brown Norway rats was increased by a factor of about 4, indicating an inflammatory reaction. Utilizing the trypan blue dye exclusion test, cell viability of macrophages remained unchanged for control and exposed groups (Wistar, brown Norway), revealing a survival rate of about 90%.

Fig. 2 presents the data of the phagocytosis assay after addition of Fluoresbrite microspheres to macrophage cultures. Wistar rats' phagocytotic activity remained unchanged for the vehicle controls up to 20 h of exposure. In contrast, macrophage cultures obtained from GEX aerosol exposed animals revealed a concentration- and time-dependent reduction in phagocytic activity. This effect was especially pronounced for macrophages after a culture period of 2 h. After an inhalation period of 20 h phagocytic activity was reduced to values of nearly 10% as compared to the controls. For macrophage cultures cultivated 24 h activity of macrophages recovered up to values of 70%–80%. These values still differed from the vehicle control values, showing an activity of 97%–98%. Based on the results of phagocytic capacity macrophage cultures of GEX aerosol exposed Wistar rats revealed a strong concentration- and time-dependent reduction after a cultivation period of 2 or 24 hours (Fig. 3). Phagocytic capacity of macrophages from vehicle controls was also reduced as compared to nonexposed animals but did not differ in dependency on the exposure time. A recovery effect as shown for phagocytic activity was not observed for the 24-h macrophage cultures. Similar results with the phagocytosis assay were obtained after exposure of brown Norway rats (Figs. 4, 5). The 2-h macrophage cultures obtained from animals exposed for 30 and 55 h showed a remarkable reduction in phagocytic activity and capacity. In comparison to Wistar rats, which were exposed to a four times higher concentration but shorter exposure time, macrophages of brown Norway rats revealed a better recovery rate in the 24-h cultures.

Bone marrow preparations from the femura of control, vehicle control and GEX aerosol exposed Wistar and brown Norway rats were evaluated for cytotoxic and genotoxic effects. Fig. 6 shows the frequency of PCEs expressed as a percentage of total erythrocytes. No considerable influence on the percentage of PCEs were obtained for the vehicle control of Wistar or brown Norway rats as compared to the control. After exposure to GEX aerosols a concentration- and time-dependent reduction in the frequency of PCEs was observed for both rat strains, indicating an inhibition of erythropoiesis. This cytotoxic effect was more clearly expressed in brown

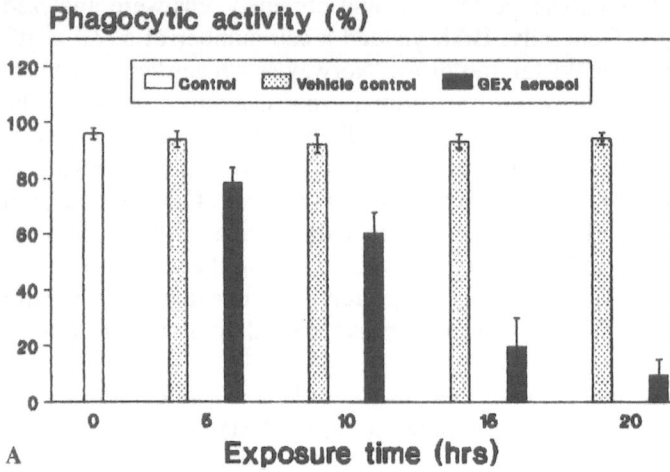

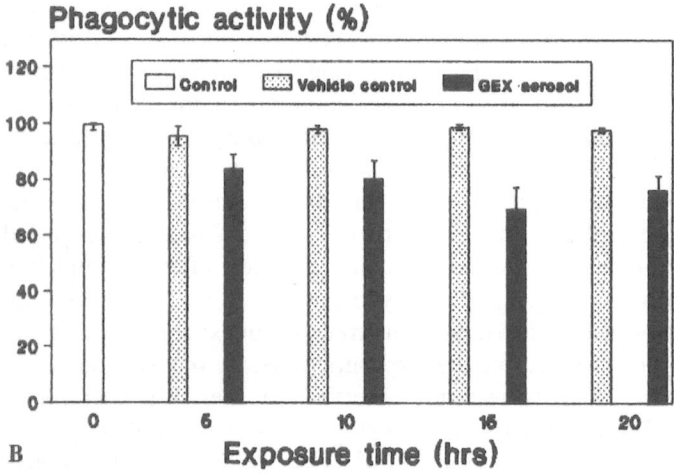

Fig. 2A,B. Phagocytic activity (percentage) of alveolar macrophages of control, vehicle control, and GEX aerosol exposed Wistar rats. **A** Cultivation of 2h; **B** cultivation of 24h

Norway rats. Preliminary results also indicate an increase in MPCEs after exposure to GEX aerosols (Fig. 7), suggesting a genotoxic and/or epigenetic effect of inhaled aerosols on bone marrow cells.

Morphological alterations in alveolar macrophages of Wistar rats exposed to GEX aerosols for 5–20h were analyzed by transmission electron microscopy. A concentration- and time-dependent increase in electron-dense granules was found, indicating a lysosomal activation. Furthermore, vacuoles in the cytoplasm may reflect an injury of the intracytoplasmatic membrane

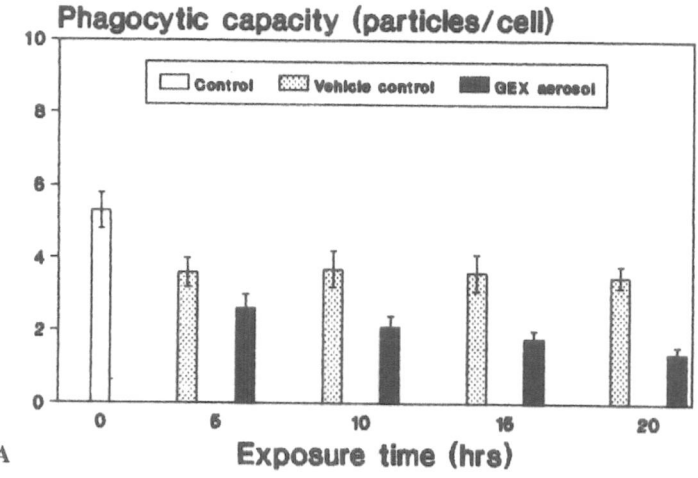

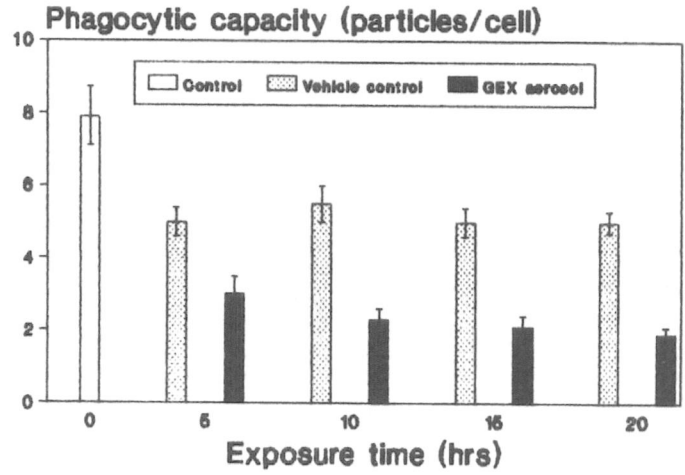

Fig. 3A,B. Phagocytic capacity (particles/cell) of alveolar macrophages of control, vehicle control, and GEX aerosol exposed Wistar rats. **A** Cultivation of 2 h; **B** cultivation of 24 h

system, as earlier described for mouse macrophages exposed in vitro to extract of airborne particulates (Behrendt et al. 1986).

Discussion

Airborne particulates with a diameter of less than 5 µm have a great potential for tracheobronchial and alveolar deposition (Lippmann et al.

Phagocytic activity (%)

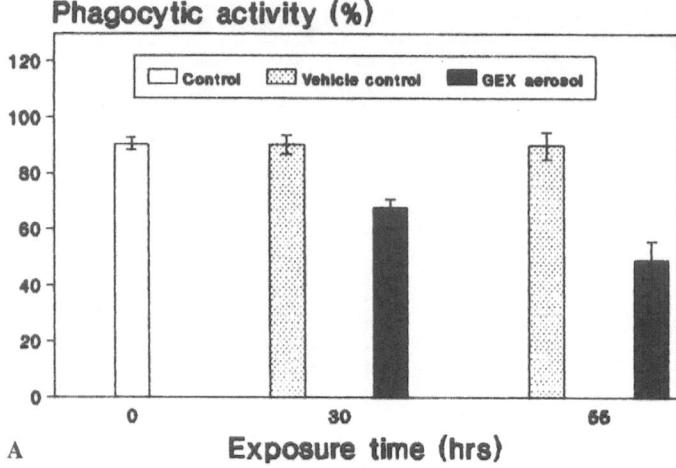

A

Phagocytic activity (%)

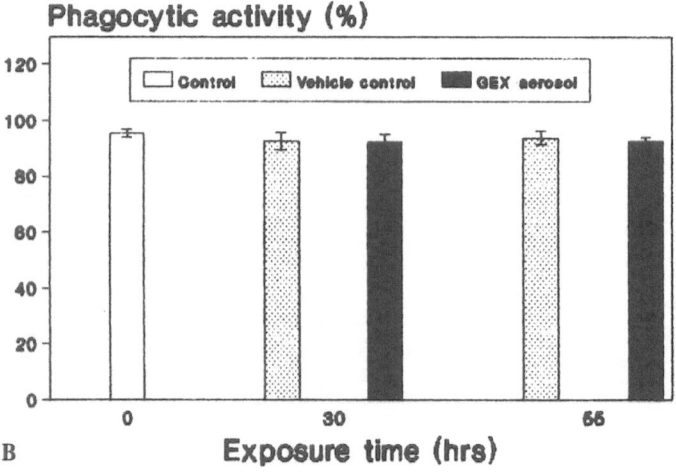

B

Fig. 4A,B. Phagocytic activity (percentage) of alveolar macrophages of control, vehicle control, and GEX aerosol exposed brown Norway rats. **A** Cultivation of 2 h; **B** cultivation of 24 h

1979). Alveolar macrophages play a pivotal role in the pulmonary defense mechanism eliminating particulates, bacteria, viruses, etc. from the alveolar unit by phagocytosis (Brain 1986; Dannenberg 1977; Green et al. 1977). Our combined in vivo/in vitro experiments demonstrate that aerosols containing extractable substances from airborne particulates collected in a highly industrialized region can profoundly affect functions of alveolar macrophages of exposed animals. Results obtained indicate that phagocytic activity and capacity of alveolar macrophages is reduced in a concentration- and time-dependent manner after inhalation showing no considerable strain dif-

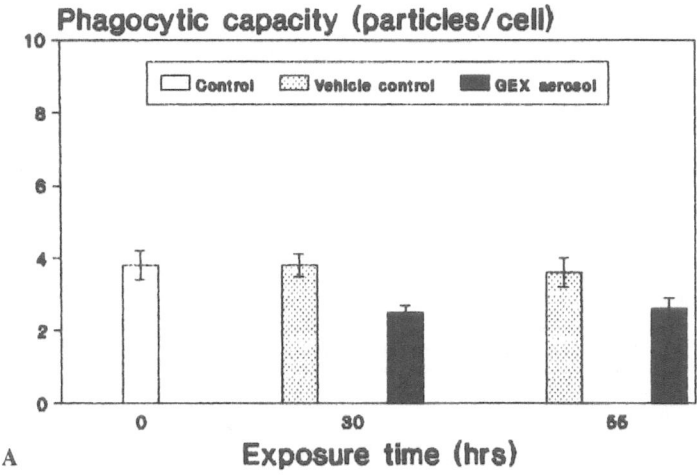

A

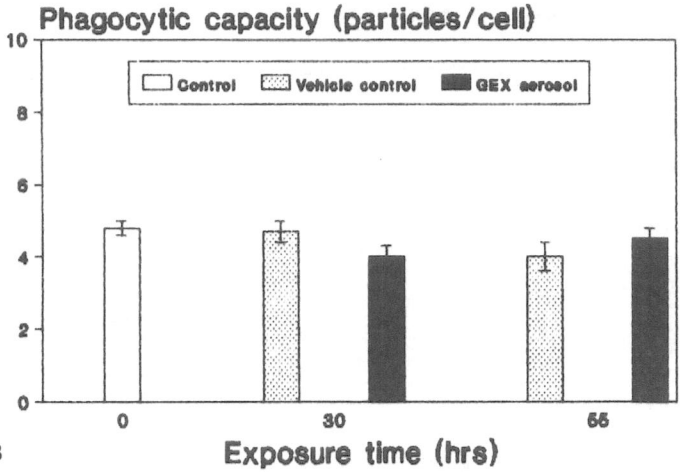

B

Fig. 5A,B. Phagocytic capacity (particles/cell) of alveolar macrophages of control, vehicle control, and GEX aerosol exposed brown Norway rats. **A** Cultivation of 2 h; **B** cultivation of 24 h

ferences between Wistar and brown Norway rats. On the other hand, it is remarkable that the cell viability of macrophages was not affected. These results confirm our in vitro studies with cultures of rat and human macrophages utilizing the same sample of extract of particulate matter (Seemayer et al. 1990). In this study substances from particulates of 0.8–1.6 m^3 air impaired phagocytosis, while cell viability of macrophages was not considerably influenced. Inhibition of phagocytosis was also reported in other studies. Extracts of outdoor airborne particulates inhibited phagocytosis of rat macrophages in a dose-dependent manner at concentrations of 6–

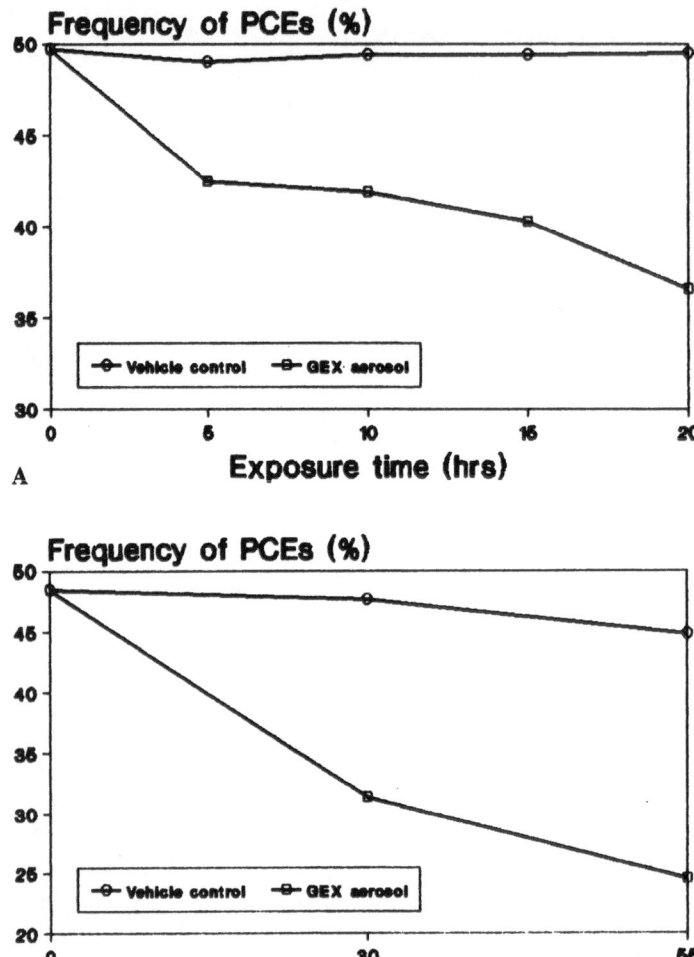

Fig. 6A,B. Frequency of polychromatic erythrocytes (*PCEs*) in rats following inhalation exposure to vehicle and GEX aerosol. **A** Wistar rats; **B** brown Norway rats

$60\,m^3$ air, while indoor air polluted by wood smoke or cigarette smoke were highly toxic at concentrations below $2\,m^3$ air (van Houdt and Rietjens 1988). Beck et al. (1988) reported a 65% inhibition of phagocytized gold particles to hamster alveolar macrophages after instillation of particulate emissions of space heaters burning automotive waste oil. Hatch et al. (1985) reported an impairment of pulmonary host defense caused by airborne particulates from various locations in the United States and Germany (St. Louis, Washington, Düsseldorf, Bochum). Mice pretreated with airborne particulates showed a high excess mortality after infection with aerosolized streptococci. Castranova

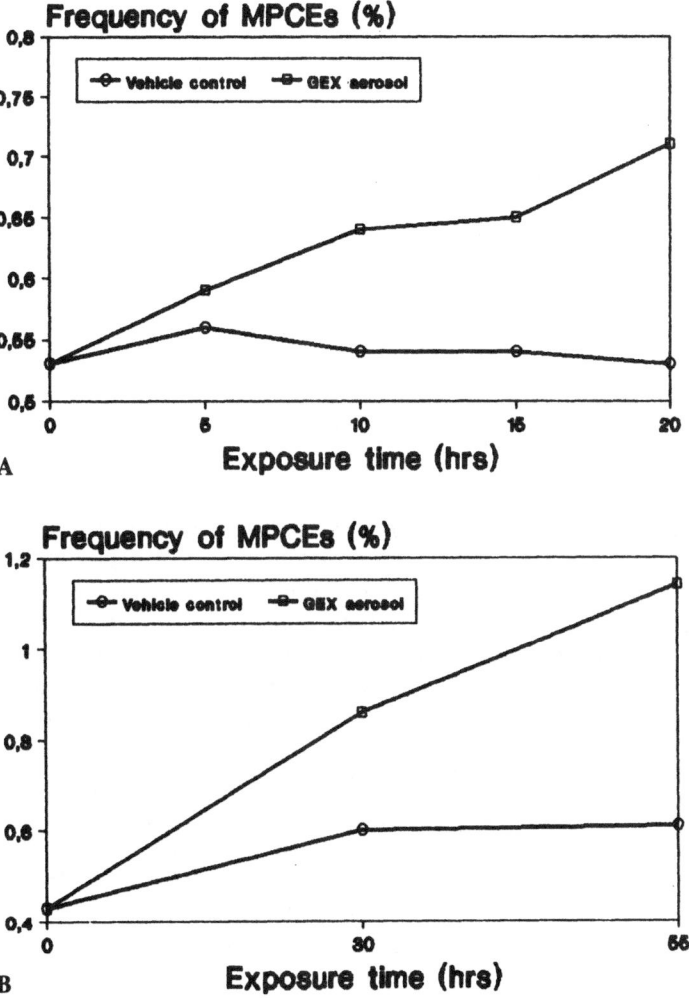

Fig. 7A,B. Frequency of micronucleated polychromatic erythrocytes (*MPCEs*) in rats following inhalation exposure to vehicle and GEX aerosol. **A** Wistar rats; **B** brown Norway rats

et al. (1985) studied the response of rat alveolar macrophages to chronic inhalation of diesel exhaust. While chronic inhalation of diesel exhaust did not affect viability of alveolar macrophages, the phagocytic activity and chemiluminescence of these cells were depressed. Ruiz et al. (1988) found that peripheral blood macrophages of school children from a highly polluted city (Santiago, Chile) showed a lower phagocytic index than those from a rural village.

In addition to effects of airborne particulates on the primary target cells of the respiratory tract, distant organs may also be affected. This is shown in the present study by a concentration- and time-dependent depression of bone marrow maturation. The reduced frequency of PCEs suggests sytemic effects of inhaled aerosols. This assumption is also supported by the occurrence of micronucleated PCEs, indicating damage to genetic material and/or the spindle apparatus essential for identical distribution of chromosomes to progeny cells. The effects on bone marrow cells may be due to the absorption of dissoluted substances from aerosols into the systemic circulation. Blood passing from the lung to the heart and then into the peripheral circulation can carry substances directly to other tissues and organs without passing through the detoxification process of the liver (WHO 1978).

The calculation of inhaled doses on the basis of the test substance concentration in the aerosol and the respiratory volume can only be regarded as a rough approximation. This does not take into account uptake, deposition, and clearance of inhaled aerosol. Nevertheless, under the given inhalation conditions animals were exposed to extractable substances from airborne particulates equivalent to $1\,m^3$ air per hour (Wistar rats) or $0.25\,m^3$ air per hour (brown Norway rats). In comparison human beings have a respiratory volume of $12-14\,m^3$ air per day in rest, corresponding to a respiratory volume of $0.5-0.6\,m^3$ air per hour. Accordingly, the obtained effects on alveolar macrophages and bone marrow cells in animal inhalation experiments suggest that human exposure to airborne particulates is associated with potential health hazards. Apart from this, airborne particulates may also induce a number of other effects. Sugiri et al. (1985) observed an increase of multinucleated cells after exposition of mouse macrophages (line IC-21) to an extract of airborne particulates. This effect was dose dependent, reaching maximum values of 31% while control values were between 7.5% and 9%. Furthermore, extract of airborne particulates can also affect formation and release of surfactant from human type II pneumocytes of cell line A549 in vitro (Behrendt et al. 1987a). Additionally, preexisting diseases could be a major risk factor when high levels of air pollution occur, such as in smog episodes (Lave and Seskin 1970; Sweeny et al. 1988). The burden of exogeneous chemical substances with which individuals must cope may be far higher than normal and may exceed their ability to detoxify (Repace 1982). This could be a critical factor in triggering or maintaining environmentally related diseases, especially human cancer (Carnow 1978; Doll 1978; Tomatis 1990).

Acknowledgements. This work was supported in part by Bundesministerium für Forschung und Technologie, contract no. 07 ALL 04 9.

References

Beck B, Brain JD, Wolfthal SF (1988) Assessment of lung injury produced by particulate emissions of space heaters burning automotive waste oil. Ann Occup Hyg 32:257-265

Behrendt H, Seemayer NH, Tomingas R (1986) Evidence for specific ultrastructural alterations of macrophages induced by airborne particulates. AEROSOL: Formation and reactivity. 2nd international aerosol conference, Berlin. Pergamon, New York, pp 212–214

Behrendt H, Seemayer NH, Holle A, Dehnen W (1987a) Effect of extract of airborne particulates and of Ca^{++}-ionophore A 23187 on formation and release of surfactant from human type II pneumocytes. J Aerosol Sci 18:705–708

Behrendt H, Seemayer NH, Braumann A, Nissen M (1987b) Electron microscopy investigations on the effect of quartz dust DQ 12 on human monocyte/ macrophages in vitro. Silicosis report North-Rhine Westfalia, vol 16. Steinkohlebergbauverein, Essen, pp 171–183

Behrendt H, Seemayer NH, Happel A, Tomingas R (1990) Dust induced alterations of human macrophages. In: Seemayer NH, Hadnagy W (eds) Environmental hygiene II. Springer, Berlin Heidelberg New York, pp 195–198

Brain JD (1986) Toxicological aspects of alterations of pulmonary macrophage function. Annu Rev Pharmacol Toxicol 26:547–565

Carnow BW (1978) The "urban factor" and lung cancer: cigarette smoking or air pollution. Environ Health Perspect 22:17–21

Castranova V, Bowman L, Reasor MJ et al. (1985) The response of rat alveolar macrophages to chronic inhalation of coal dust and/or diesel exhaust. Environ Res 36:405–419

Dannenberg AM (1977) Influence of environmental factors on the respiratory tract. J Reticuloendothel Soc 22:273–289

Doll R (1978) Atmospheric pollution and lung cancer. Environ Health Perspect 22:23–31

Gardner DE (1984) Alterations in macrophage functions by environmental chemicals. Environ Health Persp 55:343–358

Green GM, Jakab GJ, Low RB, Davis GS (1977) Defense mechanisms of the respiratory membrane. Am Rev Respir Dis 115:479–514

Gulyas H, Labedzka M, Geertz R, Gercken G (1990) Alveolar macrophage damage by dusts in vitro is correlated with arsenic, lead and antimony contents. In: Seemayer NH, Hadnagy W (eds) Environmental hygiene II. Springer, Berlin Heidelberg New York, pp 191–194

Hadnagy W, Seemayer NH, Tomingas R (1986) Cytogenetic effects of airborne particulate matter in human lymphocytes in vitro. Mutat Res 175:97–101

Hadnagy W, Seemayer NH, Tomingas R, Ivanfy K (1989) Comparative study of sister-chromatid exchanges and chromosomal aberrations induced by airborne particulates from an urban and a highly industrialized location in human lymphocyte cultures. Mutat Res 225:27–32

Hatch GE, Boykin E, Graham JA, Lewtas J, Pott F, Loud K, Mumforce, JL (1985) Inhalable particles and pulmonary host defense: in vivo and in vitro effects of ambient air and combustion particles. Environ Res 36:67–80

Helmes CT, Atkinson DL, Jaffer J, Sigman CC, Thompson KL, Kelsey MI, Kraybill HF, Munn JI (1982) Evaluation and classification of the potential carcinogenicity of organic air pollution. J Environ Sci Health A17:321–389

Lave LB, Seskin EP (1970) Air pollution and human health. Science 169:723–733

Lippmann M, Albert R, Yeates D (1979) Effects of inhaled particles on human and animals: deposition, retention and clearance. In: Air particles. National Research Council. University Park Press, Baltimore, pp 107–145

Liu WK, Tam NFY, Wong MH, Cheung YH (1987) Cytotoxicity of airborne particles from roadside urban gardens. Sci Total Environ 59:267–276

Loose LD, Silkworth JB, Charbonneau T, Blumenstock F (1981) Environmental chemical-induced macrophage dysfunction. Environ Health Perspect 39:79–82

Motykiewicz G, Hadnagy W, Seemayer NH, Szeliga J, Tkocz A, Chorazy M (1991) Influence of airborne suspended matter on mitotic cell division. Mutat Res 260:195–202

Pascoe S, Gatehouse D (1986) The use of a simple haematoxylin and eosin staining procedure to demonstrate micronuclei within rodent bone marrow. Mutat Res 164:237–243

Odagiri Y, Adachi S, Katayama H, Takemoto K (1986) Detection of the cytogenetic effect of inhaled aerosols by the micronucleus test. Mutat Res 170:79–83

Repace JL (1982) Indoor air pollution. Environ Int 8:21–36

Ruiz F, Videla LA, Parra MA, Trier A, Silvia C (1988) Air pollution impact on phagocytic capacity of peripheral blood macrophages and antioxidant activity of plasma among school children. Arch Environ Health 43:286–291

Schlipköter H-W (1983) Lufthygienische Probleme der Großstadt. Arcus 5:244–250

Seemayer NH, Manojlovic N (1980) Cytotoxic effects of air pollutants on mammalian cells in vitro. Toxicology 17:177–182

Seemayer NH, Manojlovic N, Schürer C-C, Tomingas R (1984) Cell cultures as a tool for detection of cytotoxic, mutagenic and carcinogenic activity of airborne particulate matter. J Aerosol Sci 15:426–430

Seemayer NH, Manojlovic N, König H, Tomingas R (1988) Comparative investigation of carcinogenic and mutagenic activity of airborne particulate matter from polluted areas using human and rodent tissue culture cells. Ann Occup Hyg 32:247–256

Seemayer NH, Hadnagy W, Tomingas R (1989) Assessment of health risks by air pollutants from in vitro cytotoxicity and genotoxicity testing on mammalian cells: a longitudinal study from 1975 until now. In: Brasser LJ, Mulder WC (eds) Man and his ecosystem, vol 2. Proceedings of the 8th world clean air congress 1989, The Hague, The Netherlands, 11–15 September 1989. Elsevier, Amsterdam, pp 137–142

Seemayer NH, Happel A, Behrendt H, Hadnagy W, Tomingas R (1990) Comparison of cytotoxicity of airborne particulates to rat and human macrophages. J Aerosol Sci 21:387–391

Sugiri D, Behrendt H, Seemayer NH (1985) Biological effects of city smog extract: IX. Quantitative cytological investigation on the cytotoxic effect of city smog extracts on macrophages in vitro. Zentralbl Bakteriol Parasitenkd Infektionskr Hyg Abt I Orig Reihe B 181:226–239

Sweeny TD, Brain JD, Godlewski JJ (1988) Preexisting disease. In: Brain JD et al. (eds) Variation in susceptibility to inhaled pollutants. John Hopkins Press, Baltimore, pp 142–158

Tomatis L (ed) (1990) Air pollution and human cancer. Springer, Berlin Heidelberg New York

Van Houdt JJ, Rietjens IMCM (1988) Toxicity of airborne particulate matter to rat alveolar macrophages: a comparative study of five extracts collected indoors and outdoors. Toxical In Vitro 2:121–123

World Health Organization (1978) Environmental health criteria: 6. Principles and methods for evaluating toxicity of chemicals, part 1. WHO, Geneva

Assessment of Pollutant-Induced Impairment of the Pulmonary Surfactant System by High-Performance Liquid Chromatography

R. Klingebiel, H.D. Winkeler, F. Drenk, and U. Heinrich

Fraunhofer-Institut für Toxikologie und Aerosolforschung, Nikolai-Fuchs-Straße 1, 3000 Hannover 61, FRG

Introduction

The pulmonary surfactant system, consisting mainly of phospholipids and associated glycoproteins, is of importance in inhalation toxicology for several reasons. This system is a characteristic metabolic product of the type II pneumocyte and thus yields information about the metabolic status of the type II cells. It covers the alveolar surface and protects the epithelium mechanically from direct contact with penetrating agents (Morgenroth and Newhouse 1988). Its surface activity assures alveolar stability (Clements and Chambers 1957; Pattle 1955; von Neergard 1929), and the well-known volume changes of the alveoli during inspiration and expiration push surface fluids and particles up to the bronchioli, from where they may be cleared by virtue of the mucociliary escalator (Morgenroth and Newhouse 1988). Surfactant has been shown to act as an opsonin by coating inhaled foreign bodies. Phagocytosis and clearance of inhaled material by alveolar macrophages is enhanced (Juers et al. 1976; LaForce et al. 1973; O'Neill et al. 1984). After the uptake of the particle into the macrophage, cytotoxic effects are prevented as long as the particle stays coated by surfactant (Wallace et al. 1988). It serves as a boundary between the mucus and the sol phase, thus keeping the ciliae from being immobilized by sticking to the mucus phase (Morgenroth and Newhouse 1988). Furthermore, it has been argued that surfactant also constitutes a layer above the mucus phase, extending to the upper airways and thus facilitating penetration of particles into the mucus layer and further down to the bronchoalveolar epithelium (Schürch et al. 1990).

Briefly summarizing, one could say that surfactant may serve as a marker for alveolar injury, is an important factor for the fate of foreign particles penetrating the lung, and is a target of inhaled toxic substances which may impair mechanical stability and nonspecific defense mechanisms of the alveoli by altering the surfactant system.

U. Mohr et al. (Eds.)
Advances in Controlled Clinical
Inhalation Studies
© Springer-Verlag Berlin Heidelberg 1993

Based upon what is described in the literature, an improved high-performance liquid chromatography (HPLC) method has been recently developed in our laboratory that permits separation and quantification of all surfactant phospholipids. The main features of the HPLC method are presented here as well as its application for determining exposure-related changes in the rat lung exposed to a monomeric methylene diphenyl diisocyanate (MDI) aerosol.

Assessment of Surfactant Phospholipids by HPLC

Two-dimensional thin-layer chromatography is still the analytical method of choice for phospholipid separation and quantification in many surfactant laboratories. This method does not require expensive analytical equipment but is time consuming, and it is difficult to achieve satisfactory recovery, especially of the smaller phospholipid fractions (phosphatidylinositol, PI; phosphatidylserine, PS; phosphatidylethanolamine, PE; sphingomyelin, SPH). In the meantime several publications on phospholipid analysis in biological matrices by HPLC have appeared (Becart et al. 1990; Breton et al. 1989; Heinze et al. 1988; Kuhnz et al. 1985; Pison et al. 1986).

The HPLC procedure described here combines the advantages of more accurate quantification by means of mass detection with the well-known separation performances of the convenient HPLC solvents for UV detection. A complete phospholipid profile of the lung lavage fluid (LLF) of small laboratory animals (rat, guinea pig) can be achieved accurately and reproducibly. To obtain these performances we modified the analytical procedure described in the literature with regard to the solvents, column configuration, flow rate, and solvent gradient and by introducing methylamine as the pH determining agent of solvent A (publication in preparation).

Equipment, Reagents, and Standards

The HPLC separations were carried out on HPLC equipment from Waters/ Millipore (Eschborn, FRG) consisting of two HPLC pumps (model 510), an autosampler (model 712 WISP), and the Waters system interface module. Data acquisition and processing was performed using the Waters/Millipore chromatography software Maxima 820 installed on a 386/20 personal computer. Detection was achieved by the evaporative light-scattering detector Sedex 45 from Sedere (Vitry, France). Separation was performed on a Serva silica 60, 5-μm column followed by a Merck Diol 250/4, 5-μm column. The column temperature was kept permanently at 45°C by a column oven, model K-1, from Techlab (Erkerode, FRG). Degassing of the eluents was achieved by using the online degasser A1010 from Knauer (Bad Homburg, FRG). The following phospholipids were purchased from Sigma (Munich, FRG):

PI, PS, PE, SPH, phospatidylcholine (PC), and lysophosphatidylcholine (LPC). HPLC-grade water of the HPLC solvent, methylamine (40%), acetonitrile, and chloroform and methanol used for the phospholipid extraction were obtained from Riedel-de-Haen (Seelze, FRG).

Material and Lipid Extraction

The material was collected from small laboratory rodents (rats and guinea pigs) by lung lavage (Creutzenberg et al. 1989). The method was also applied to samples collected from ventilated newborn infants by tracheal aspiration and from adult patients by bronchoalveolar lavage. The results of these surveys will be presented elsewhere in full detail. The results from investigations with rat LLF are reported here as this material is of most interest in inhalation toxicology.

Following anesthesia by an intraperitoneal injection of sodium pentobarbital, the animal was killed by exsanguination via the abdominal aorta. The lung was excised from the thorax, and the trachea was cut just below the larynx. A cannula was introduced into the trachea, and the lung was lavaged twice with 7 ml sodium chloride (0.9%), yielding about 12 ml altogether. The two lavage fluid aliquots were pooled, centrifugated at 50 g (4°C, 10 min) to sediment cells, and then submitted to the phospholipid extraction or stored at −70°C until being analyzed.

Lipid extraction was achieved using a modification of the method of Folch et al. (1957). Methanol 10 ml and chloroform 20 ml were added to the supernatent. In between, the sample was stirred vigorously. A second centrifugation step was then performed at 900 g (4°C, 10 min). The chloroform layer was removed and dried by nitrogen in a water bath heated to 50°C. Subsequently, resuspension in 100 μl chloroform methanol solution (2:1) was performed.

Chromatographic Analysis

The chromatograhic mobile phase was composed of solvent A – acetonitrile, water, methylamine (78.5% : 20% : 1.5%) – and solvent B – acetonitrile. The gradient applied was nonlinear, following Table 1. The flow rate was kept constant at 1.6 ml/min and the column oven temperature at 45°C. The stationary phase consisted of a silica 60, 5-μm column followed by a Diol 250/4, 5-μm column. Detection was achieved by means of an evaporating light-scattering detector (mass detector). The nitrogen pressure determining the nebulizer gas flow rate was 2 bars and the evaporation temperature was 50°C. The calibration curve corresponded to a quadratic regression and the coeffecient of correlation was ≥99% for concentrations in the range from

Table 1. HPLC gradient

Time	Flow	Eluent %A	Eluent %B
0.0	1.6	10.0	90.0
2.0	1.6	30.0	70.0
3.0	1.6	30.0	70.0
15.0	1.6	80.0	20.0
18.0	1.6	80.0	20.0
20.0	1.6	10.0	90.0
28.0	1.6	10.0	90.0

0.5–20 µg (PC: 200 µg). Detection limits, assessed by diluting the standard mixture until a signal/noise ratio of 3 was reached, ranged from 0.1 µg (PE, PC) to 0.2 µg (PI), 0.5 µg (PG, SPH), and 1.5 µg (PS). The in-between run coefficient of variation (day to day) was in the range of 5%–20% depending on the respective phospholipid. Due to the uneven distribution of phospholipids in the LLF and the detector response limitation two analytical runs with different injection volumes (10 and 40 µl) were performed. The run time for a single sample was 30 min. Figure 1 shows a chromatogram of a mixture of phospholipid standards.

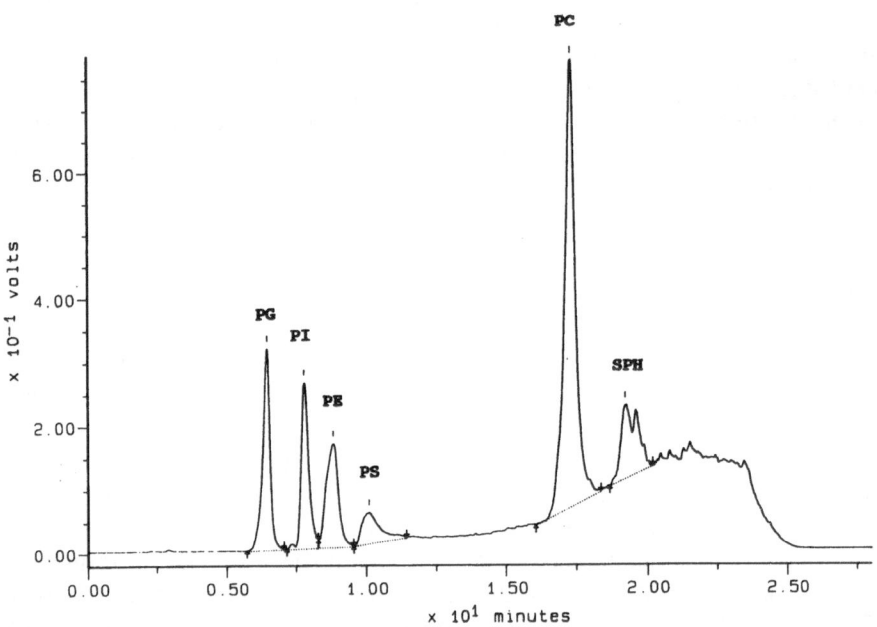

Fig. 1. Chromatogram of a mixture of phospholipid standards

Application of the Method

One group of inhalative pollutants whose detrimental health effects in exposed workers has raised concern in recent decades is that of the isocyanates (Karol 1986; Musk et al. 1988). Isocyanates comprise various highly reactive chemicals characterized structurally by the so-called isocyanate group R – N=C=O. This isocyanate group tends to react with hydroxyl-, sulfhydryl- and amino- groups of proteins and is important for isocyanate toxicity in the respiratory tract. Monoisocyanates are used for the synthesis of herbicides and insecticides whereas the diisocyanates are of great importance for the manufacturing process of polyurethane (Karol 1986). Affection of the respiratory tract subsequent to diisocyanate exposure extends from "chest tightness", to soreness of the throat, cough, and rhinitis through obstructive alterations in mechanical lung function to allergic asthma with immediate and late-onset reactions and to hypersensitivity pneumonitis (Karol 1986; Musk et al. 1988).

To evaluate isocyanate surfactant interactions adult male Wistar rats were exposed to $1.0\,mg/m^3$ monomeric MDI for 18 hours/day, 5 days/week for 12 weeks (mass median aerodynamic diameter, MMAD, of the MDI aerosol: $1.1\,\mu m$). At end exposure LLF was collected, cell count performed, and surfactant phospholipid content determined by HPLC. In a satellite group mechanical lung function parameters were measured in a whole-body plethysmograph (Heinrich and Wilhelm 1985). Total phospholipid content of LLF was significantly reduced ($p < 0.05$, Wilcoxon test) whereas the relative PI content was increasd ($p < 0.05$) in the MDI group compared to the clean air group. The relative PC content was reduced, but the change was not statistically significant ($p = 0.053$). Figure 2 shows the chromatogram of LLF phospholipids of a rat exposed subchronically exposed to MDI.

The LLF cell content was elevated in the exposure group ($p < 0.05$) as well as lung weight ($p < 0.01$). The percentage of alveolar macrophages in the LLF cell count was diminished in exposed animals ($p < 0.01$) whereas the relative lymphocyte concentration was augmented ($p < 0.01$). No statistically significant alterations in lung resistance or compliance were observed in the exposure group.

These results are in good agreement with a former investigation from our laboratory using thin-layer chromatography for LLF phospholipid analysis in rats subsequent to 4 weeks of exposure to MDI. Total phospholipid content as well as the relative PC content in rat lung lavagate were significantly reduced after 4 weeks of exposure to $3.0\,mg/m^3$ monomeric MDI. The percentage of all other surfactant phospholipids was significantly increased, with the PS/PI fraction showing the highest level of significance ($p \leqslant 0.01$).

Obviously the degree of biochemical changes in surfactant phospholipids subsequent to MDI exposure varies according to the concentration applied, which seems to be a more decisive factor for the extent of phospholipid

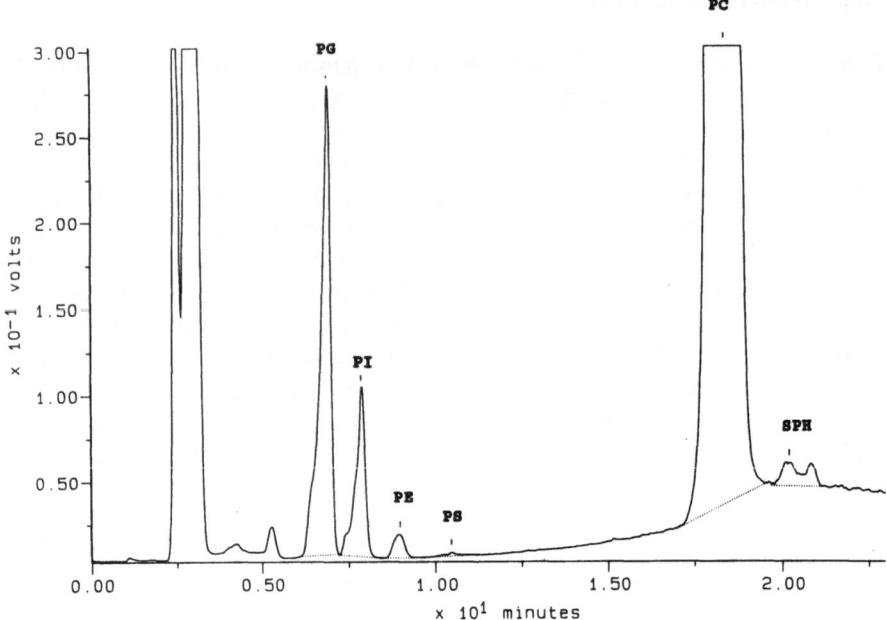

Fig. 2. Chromatogram of LLF phospholipids of a rat exposed subchronically to MDI

concentration changes in LLF with regard to MDI than the duration of exposure.

Discussion

Considering the variety of aspects and data that surfactant analysis may yield for the assessment of toxicological processes in the lung periphery, the question arises why this parameter is rarely addressed by biochemical investigations of LLF in inhalation toxicity studies. One reason may that high-performance analytical equipment has not been available to scientists until recently. Surfactant phospholipid separation and quantification by HPLC has been described in several publications in recent years, but satisfactory results on all major phosphoplipids were often lacking or were restricted due to the use of UV detection. UV detection results vary according to the degree of fatty acid saturation in the phospholipid molecule. Faced with these difficulties, we decided to introduce modifications in the conventional analytical set up.

The HPLC method described in here permits separation and quantification of all surfactant phospholipids. By the use of an autosampler up to 48 samples may be analyzed without the need for the operator to work on the equipment after calibration has been accomplished and the analytical program started. Thus a great number of samples can be analyzed, demanding only low manpower at the start of analysis. This method was applied to the occupational and indoor pollutant MDI, which may cause slight or severe pulmonary affections in exposed persons. The results obtained are in good agreement with the outcome of a preceding investigation in which thin-layer chromatography was used for phospholipid determination. Differences between the phospholipid concentrations found in these two studies may be explained by differences in the concentrations of the pollutant used.

References

Becart J, Chevalier C, Biesse JP (1990) Quantitative analysis of phospholipids by HPLC with a light scattering evaporating detector – application to raw materials for cosmetic use. J High Resolut Chromatogr 13:126–129

Breton L, Serkiz B, Volland J-P (1989) A new rapid method for phospholipid separation by high performance liquid chromatography with light-scattering detection. J Chromatogr 497:243–249

Clements JA, Chambers WH (1957) Surface tension of lung extracts. Proc Soc Exp Biol Med 95:170–172

Creutzenberg O, Muhle H, Bellmann B (1989) Reversibility of biochemical and cytological alterations in broncho-alveolar lavagate upon cessation of dust exposure. Exp Pathol 37:243–247

Folch J, Lees M, Sloane-tanley GH (1957) Simple method for the isolation and purification of total lipids from animal tissues. J Biol Chem 226:497–509

Heinrich U, Wilhelm A (1985) Lung function tests on hamsters and rats using the whole body plethsmograph. In: Bass R, Grosdanoff P, Hackenberg U (eds) Problems in inhalation toxicity studies. BGA-Schriften 5/84. MVV, Munich, pp 255–266

Heinze T, Kynast G, Dudenhausen JW, Schmitz C, Saling E (1988) Quantitative determination of phospholipids in amniotic fluid by high-performance liquid chromatography. Chromatographia 256:497–503

Juers JA, Rogers RM, McCurdy JB, Cook WW (1976) Enhancement of bacterial capacity of alveolar macrophages by human alveolar lining material. J Clin Invest 58:271–275

Karol MH (1986) Respiratory effects of inhaled isocyanates. Crit Rev Toxicol 16/4:349–379

Kuhnz W, Zimmermann B, Nau H (1985) Improved separation of phospholipids by high–perfomance liquid chromatography. J Chromatogr 344:309–312

LaForce FM, Kelly WJ, Huber GL (1973) Inactivation of staphylococci by alveolar macrophages with preliminary observations on the importance of alveolar lining material. Am Rev Respir Dis 108:784–790

Morgenroth K, Newhouse M (1988) The surfactant system of the lungs. de Gruyter, Berlin

Musk AW, Peters JM, Wegman DH (1988) Isocyanates and respiratory disease: current status. Am J Ind Med 13:331–349

O'Neill S, Lesperance E, Klass DJ (1984) Rat lung lavage surfactant enhances bacterial phagocytosis and intracellular killing by alveolar macrophages. Am Rev Respir Dis 130:225–230

Pattle RE (1955) Properties, function and origin of the alveolar lining layer. Nature 175/4469:1125–1126

Pison U, Gono E, Joka T, Obertake U, Obladen M (1986) High-performance liquid chromatography of adult human bronchoalveolar lavage: assay for phospholipid lung profile. J Chromatogr 377:79–89

Schürch S, Gehr P, Im Hof V, Geiser M, Green F (1990) Surfactant displaces particles toward the epithelium in airways and alveoli. Respir Physiol 80:17–32

von Neergard K (1929) Neue Auffassungen über einen Begriff der Atemmechanik. Die Retraktionskraft der Lunge, abhängig von der Oberflächenspannung in den Alveolen. Z Gesamte Exp Med 66:373–381

Wallace WE, Keane MJ, Vallythan V (1988) Suppression of inhaled particle cyto-toxicity by pulmonary surfactant and re-toxification by phospholipase: distinguishing properties of quartz and kaolin. Ann Occup Hyg 32:291–298

Assessment of 2,4-Dichlorophenoxyacetic Acid Exposure in the Chemical Industry by Biological Monitoring

D. Knopp[1], G. Richter[2], M. Skerswetat[3], H. Hermenau[3], and E. Stottmeister[3]

[1] Institut für Wasserchemie und Chemische Balneologie der TU München, Marchioninistraße 17, 8000 München 70, FRG
[2] Chemie AG Bitterfeld, 4400 Bitterfeld, FRG
[3] Institut für Wasser-, Boden- und Lufthygiene des Bundesgesundheitsamtes, Forschungsstelle Bad Elster, 9933 Bad Elster, FRG

Somewhat conflicting results about a possible association between specific types of cancer and occupational exposure to phenoxy herbicides, especially 2,4-dichlorophenoxyacetic acid (2,4-D) have been reported in a number of case reports and epidemiological studies (Anonymous 1986; Lilienfeld and Gallo 1989). A main drawback of almost all of these studies is the lack of individual pesticide exposure data. Such data have been published in some reports for applicators in agriculture and forestry in recent years (Frank et al. 1985; Grover et al. 1986a,b; Knopp and Glass 1991; Kolmodin-Hedman and Erne 1980; Lavy et al. 1982; Libich et al. 1984; Taskar et al. 1982), however data on occupational exposure to 2,4-D in herbicide production plants are very limited (Anonymous 1986; Vural and Burgaz 1984). Related studies have generally only measured herbicide concentrations in the air at the workplace. A proper assessment of the potential hazard to workers during herbicide production requires reliable estimates, however, of the amount of herbicide absorbed under these conditions.

Immunochemical assays for small molecules (haptens), such as pesticides, are gaining increasing acceptance among analytical chemists (Hammock et al. 1987; Knopp et al. 1989). These methods are rapid, sensitive, and cost effective. Therefore, a radioimmunoassay (RIA) for 2,4-D was developed at our laboratory (Knopp et al. 1985). This was used in a 5-year biological monitoring study of 27 male and 18 female, occupationally exposed employees engaged in the manufacture, formulation, or packaging of 2,4-D and related salts.

Urinary 2,4-D concentrations in spot samples delivered during the last 3 h of a working shift varied substantially, from only a few micrograms to several milligrams per liter. Further, the herbicide urinary concentration profile at weekly intervals showed an increase in 2,4-D exposure over the week, cumulating on Friday, with a decrease on the work-free week-end but

U. Mohr et al. (Eds.)
Advances in Controlled Clinical
Inhalation Studies
© Springer-Verlag Berlin Heidelberg 1993

not reaching the zero level in any case. A strong correlation was found between the 2,4-D urinary concentration and the eliminated herbicide amount, adjusted for endogenous creatinine. After an interruption of production for 3 weeks, 2,4-D was no longer detected in urine.

From 2,4-D air concentration levels at the workplace it was concluded that the respiratory route of absorption could not be the sole route of 2,4-D entry into the body. Dermal exposure also seemed to play an important role. Workers, on average, absorbed below 0.1 mg 2,4-D/kg body weight per day. This level was sometimes markedly exceeded, presumably owing to inappropriate working conditions and neglectful hygienic behavior.

References

Anonymous (1986) Occupational exposures to chlorophenoxy herbicides. IARC Monogr 41:357–406

Frank R, Campbell RA, Sirons GJ (1985) Forestry workers involved in aerial application of 2,4-dichlorophenoxyacetic acid (2,4-D): exposure and urinary excretion. Arch Environ Contam Toxicol 14:427–435

Grover R, Cessna AJ, Muir NI, Riedel D, Franklin CA, Yoshida K (1986a) Factors affecting the exposure of ground-rig applicators to 2,4-D dimethylamine salt. Arch Environ Contam Toxicol 15:677–686

Grover R, Franklin CA, Muir NI, Cessna AJ, Riedel D (1986b) Dermal exposure and urinary metabolite excretion in farmers repeatedly exposed to 2,4-D amine. Toxicol Lett 33:73–83

Hammock BD, Gee SJ, Cheung PYK, Miyamoto T, Goodrow MH, van Emon J, Seiber JN (1987) Utility of immunoassays in pesticide trace analysis. In: Greenhalgh R, Roberts TR (eds) Pesticide science and biotechnology. Blackwell, London, pp 309–316

Knopp D, Glass S (1991) Biological monitoring of 2,4-dichlorophenoxyacetic acid exposed workers in agriculture and forestry. Int Arch Occup Environ Health 63:329–333

Knopp D, Nuhn P, Dobberkau H-J (1985) Radioimmunoassay for 2,4-dichlorophenoxyacetic acid. Arch Toxicol 58:27–32

Knopp D, Degenkolb H, Dobberkau H-J (1989) Immunoassays. Leistungsfähige Analysenmethoden für die unwelttoxikologische Forschung und Praxis. Z Gesamte Hyg 35:122–125

Kolmodin-Hedman B, Erne K (1980) Estimation of occupational exposure to phenoxy acids (2,4-D and 2,4,5-T). Arch Toxicol Suppl 4:318–321

Lavy TL, Walstad JD, Flynn RR, Mattice JD (1982) (2,4-Dichlorophenoxy)acetic acid exposure received by aerial application crews during forest spray operations. J Agric Food Chem 30:375–381

Libich S, To JC, Frank R, Sirons GJ (1984) Occupational exposure of herbicide applicators to herbicides used along electric power transmission line right-of-way. Am Ind Hyg Assoc J 45:56–62

Lilienfeld DE, Gallo MA (1989) 2,4-D, 2,4,5-T, and 2,3,7,8-TCDD: an overview. Epidemiol Rev 11:28–58

Taskar PK, Das YT, Trout JR, Chattopadhyay SK, Brown HD (1982) Measurement of 2,4-dichlorophenoxyacetic acid (2,4-D) after occupational exposure. Bull Environ Contam Toxicol 29:586–591

Vural N, Burgaz S (1984) A gas chromatographic method for determination of 2,4-D residues in urine after occupational exposure. Bull Environ Contam Toxicol 33:518–524

Assessment by Aerosol Recovery Technique of Site of Airway Constriction During Intravenous Histamine Challenge

M. Meyer[1] and A. Rahmel[2]

[1] MPI für Experimentelle Medizin, Abteilung Physiologie, Hermann-Rein-Straße 3, 3400 Göttingen, FRG
[2] MPI für Experimentelle Medizin Abteilung Physiologie, Hermann-Rein-Straße 3, 3400 Göttingen, FRG
Jetzt: Universitätskliniken, Innere Medizin C, Albert-Schweitzer-Straße 33, 4400 Münster/Westf, FRG

Introduction

Assessment of airway dimensions based on the analysis of deposition and recovery of monodisperse aerosols in the respiratory tract during breath holding, originally introduced by Palmes et al. (1967), has recently been refined (single-breath aerosol recovery technique) and applied in spontaneously breathing normal human subjects (Heyder 1989) and in anesthetized, mechanically ventilated dogs with normal airway geometry (Rahmel et al., this volume). The technique has been demonstrated to facilitate the determination of effective airway diameters in vivo which were in close agreement with morphometric data of human and canine lungs.

In the present study, the feasibility of the aerosol recovery technique for detection of magnitude and site of acute experimentally induced airway constriction was analyzed by determination of aerosol-derived airway diameters in dogs with airways maintained in sustained constriction by intravenous infusion of histamine. Simultaneously, the effects of histamine on airway diameters and lung mechanics were studied.

Methods

The measurements were performed in nine anesthetized, paralyzed supine beagle dogs (mean body wt. 15.2 kg, range 12.5–19 kg). After premedication with 0.5 mg atropine, 75 mg pitritramide and 5 mg droperidol, the dogs were anesthetized with pentobarbital sodium (initial dose 120 mg intravenously, supplemented as needed) and paralyzed by continuous infusion of alcuronium (0.8 mg/h). The dogs were intubated with a cuffed endotracheal

U. Mohr et al. (Eds.)
Advances in Controlled Clinical
Inhalation Studies
© Springer-Verlag Berlin Heidelberg 1993

tube and connected to a computerized ventilatory servo system designed for lung function testing in experimental animals (see Meyer and Slama 1983). To produce a state of sustained constriction of pulmonary airways histamine was infused intravenously. The histamine infusion rate was adjusted to prevent mean arterial blood pressure from decreasing below 60 mmHg. The average histamine dose for all dogs was 1.7 mg/kg per hour.

Functional residual capacity (FRC) was determined by the helium dilution technique. The volume after static inflation of the lung at an airway opening pressure of +20 mmHg was defined as total lung capacity (TLC). Similarly, deflation of the lung to −10 mmHg airway opening pressure yielded the expiratory reserve volume (ERV). The total compliance (C) of the respiratory system (comprising lungs and chest wall) was determined for static and dynamic (breathing frequency 15/min) conditions before and during histamine infusion from the change of lung volume (ΔV_L) per unit alveolar (P_A) to ambient (P_B) pressure difference [$\Delta(P_A - P_B)$]. Expiratory airway resistance (R_{aw}) was determined by an interrupter technique from simultaneous measurements of alveolar pressure (P_A) and expiratory airflow ($\dot{V}_E$) at the point of flow interruption (see Bates et al. 1988).

Effective aerosol-derived airway diameters were determined by the single-breath aerosol recovery technique described in more detail elsewhere in this volume (Rahmel et al.). Only a brief account of the principle and procedures are presented here for convenience (Fig. 1). Monodisperse, nonhygroscopic, di-(2-ethyl-hexyl) sebacate particles (density $0.912 \, g/cm^3$; mean aerodynamic diameter ±SD, $1.17 \pm 0.13 \, \mu m$) were inhaled in a single breath with inspired volume normalized to 50% FRC and exhaled after varying periods of breath holding (0–10 s, 2-s steps). The instantaneous aerosol concentration was continuously monitored with a miniature in-line light-scattering aerosol photometer incorporated into the respiratory gas stream. Airway diameters were calculated for local (volumetric) penetration depths of test particles normalized to the individual's actual TLC (5%–43% TLC, 2% steps). The local aerosol recovery ($R_{(V,t)}$) underlying the determination of airway radius was calculated from the local ratio of instantaneous expiratory ($CE_{(V,t)}$) and (constant) inspiratory aerosol concentration ($CI_{(V,t)}$).

$$R_{(V,t)} = \frac{CE_{(V,t)}}{CI_{(V,t)}} \qquad (1)$$

The recovery of particles from the lung decreases exponentially with time of breath holding. The effective airway radius (r) or airway diameter is calculated from the slope of the corresponding recovery function ($R_{(V,t)}$) for any volumetric depth (V) according to the following equation,

$$r = \frac{2v}{\pi d[\ln(R_{(V,t)})]/dt} \qquad (2)$$

where v is the settling velocity of the particles determined independently in a convection-free sedimentation cell. The magnitude and intrapulmonary

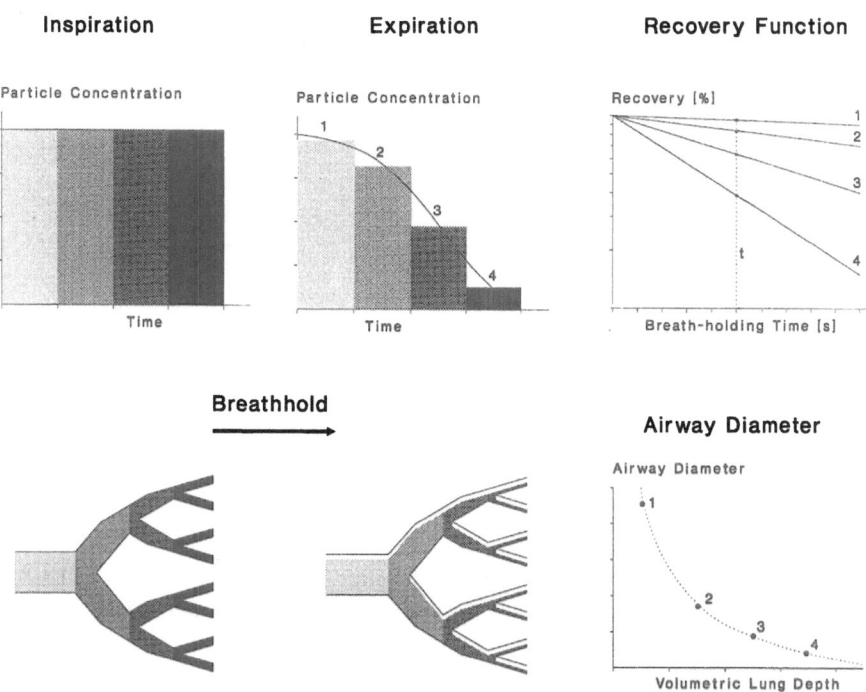

Fig. 1. Single-breath aerosol recovery technique – principle. During inspiration (*upper left*) volume fractions (*shaded areas*) with *constant* concentration of particles are inspired. At the end of inspiration (*lower left*) particles are homogeneously distributed throughout the airways, penetrating to a volumetric depth that corresponds to the inspired volume. During breath holding (*lower middle*) the intrapulmonary particle concentration decreases as a result of gravitational settlement. Particle concentration during expiration (*upper middle*) exhibits a characteristic pattern because particle loss from intrapulmonary locations (*1–4*) is inversely related to airway size. The rate of decrease in particle recovery as a function of breath holding (*upper right*) is faster for small airways (*location 4*) as compared to larger airways (*locations 3–1*). The recovery function is used to determine the effective airway diameter as a function of volumetric depth (*lower right*). See text for details

location of airway constriction elicited by histamine was calculated from the change in airway diameters for the same normalized volumetric lung depth (% TLC) before and during histamine infusion.

Results

The effects of histamine infusion on lung mechanics are summarized in Fig. 2. Whereas the residual volume (RV = FRC − ERV) remained practically unchanged as a result of histamine challenge, FRC (−11%) and TLC (−25%) were markedly reduced. The series (Fowler) dead space (V_D)

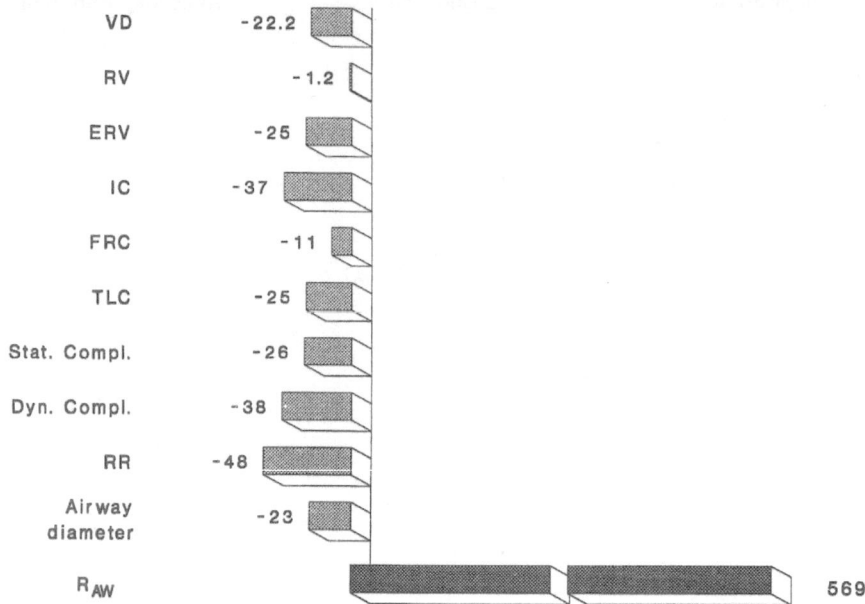

Fig. 2. Lung mechanics, blood pressure, and aerosol-derived airway dimensions during histamine infusion. *VD*, series dead space; *RV*, residual volume; *ERV*, expiratory reserve volume; *IC*, inspiratory capacity; *FRC*, functional residual capacity; *TLC*, total lung capacity; *RR*, mean arterial blood pressure; R_{aw}, airway resistance

calculated from single-breath helium washout was reduced by 22%. Airway resistance (R_{aw}) was increased during histamine infusion by a factor of 5.7 on the average, but the response of individual animals was highly variable (range 2.5–9). The static and dynamic compliances of the respiratory system were markedly decreased upon histamine infusion and remained constant during the infusion period. The difference between static and dynamic compliances was increased significantly during histamine infusion ($p < 0.01$).

The effective airway diameters as a function of normalized volumetric lung depth during control and histamine-induced airway constriction are shown in Fig. 3. In control conditions the diameter of the proximal airways decreased rapidly from about 4000 μm at 5% TLC to 200–250 μm at 25% TLC and remained constant in deeper lung regions. During histamine challenge proximal airway diameters were markedly reduced compared to control conditions, but no bronchoconstrictory effects were detectable in more distal airways (>25% TLC). The magnitude and site of airway constriction by histamine can be analyzed in more detail by the relative (to control) change of airway diameters for different volumetric lung depths (Fig. 3, insert). In the most proximal airways (corresponding to 5%–9% TLC) airway diameters were reduced by half, but constriction was con-

Airway Diameter [µm]

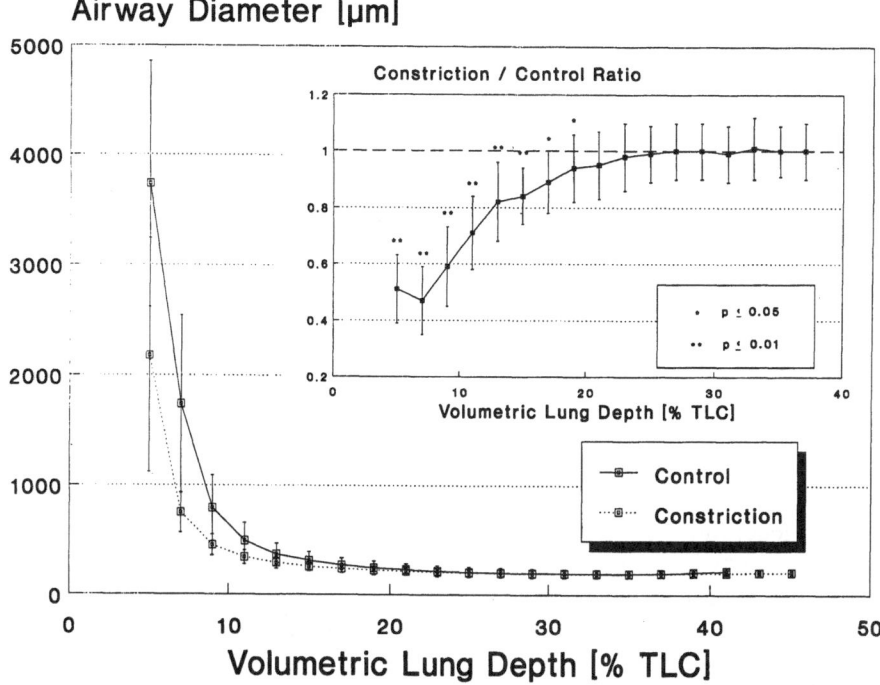

Fig. 3. Airway diameters of dog lungs during control and histamine-induced airway constriction. *Insert*, airway diameters displayed as ratio relative to control values

tinually fading toward more peripheral airways, and beyond a volumetric depth of 19% TLC no significant differences from control values were discernible.

Discussion

In the present study, the sensitivity of the single-breath aerosol recovery technique (Rahmel et al., this volume) to histamine-induced airway constriction was analyzed and compared with conventional indirect indices for changes in airway geometry. Since inhalation of aerosolized histamine would not produce steady constriction of airways for prolonged periods, intravenous infusion of histamine was used, allowing for adverse side effects of histamine and hemodynamic compromise.

The measurements of aerosol-derived airway diameters revealed a characteristic pattern for the distribution of histamine-induced airway constriction in dog lungs. Airway constriction was most pronounced in the proximal airways, with a maximum decrease of airway diameters of 50% at a volumetric depth of about 7% TLC. Airway narrowing rapidly diminished toward peripheral lung regions, and beyond 19% TLC no significant difference was detectable.

The comparison of airway dimensions in normal and constricted lungs is complicated by the fact that airway volume is decreased during constriction. Hence, for the same inspired volume, inhaled particles penetrate into deeper lung regions and eventually deposit in smaller airways, which would exaggerate the extent of airway constriction detected by the aerosol recovery technique. To correct for this effect, airway diameters quantified in terms of volumetric lung depth were related to the individual's current TLC (normalized volumetric lung depth) before and during histamine-induced airway constriction. Normalization implies that airway constriction by histamine was homogeneously distributed throughout the lung, and that the ensuing (volumetric) lung contraction was isomorphic (see below).

The marked increase in airway resistance during histamine infusion is attributable mainly to constriction of proximal airways because more than 80% of the total resistance to airflow is located in the first five to seven airway generations (Jaffrin and Kesic 1974). The more distal airways would not be expected to contribute materially to overall airway resistance. The series dead space, which reflects mainly the volume of the conducting airways, was markedly reduced by histamine. This finding suggests that the proximal airways were indeed constricted as a result of histamine infusion.

The results from the present study suggest that infused histamine had little if any effect on distal airways, or, alternatively, changes of peripheral airway dimensions were not detectable by the aerosol recovery technique. The lack of evidence for peripheral effects of histamine appears to be intriguing with respect to histological findings that pulmonary airways way down to alveolar ducts are surrounded by smooth muscle networks. Smooth muscle fibers distributed throughout the interstitial lung tissue have been demonstrated to contract upon histamine exposure, but narrowing of alveolar ducts and alveoli was inhomogeneously distributed (Colebatch and Engel 1974; Fredberg et al. 1985). Whereas some alveoli and alveolar ducts were closed almost completely, histologically giving rise to the formation of local microatelectasis, other regions had normal dimensions or showed compensatory enlargement (von Hayek 1970).

The action of histamine in proximal airways is mediated by two interacting mechanisms: (a) binding of histamine to H_1 receptors of airway smooth muscle results in muscle contraction and airway constriction; (b) histamine is known to activate irritant receptors in the airways, leading to vagally mediated bronchoconstriction (Sellick and Widdicombe 1971). Moreover, the vagal action on airway smooth muscle is enhanced by histamine due to augmented release of acetylcholine from histamine receptors located on cholinergic nerves (Antonissen et al. 1980). Vagal innervation is restricted to the conducting airways, and bronchoconstriction induced by vagal stimulation rapidly decreases toward the lung periphery (Yanta et al. 1981; Barnes et al. 1983). Both direct and vagally mediated effects of histamine lead to narrowing of the conducting airways, which is most pronounced in airways that are short of firm cartilaginous support. Hence, the major decrease in airway diameters is expected to be distal of the segmental bronchi, i.e., in airways with an average normal diameter of about 2 mm (Shioya et al. 1987). Accordingly, the expected pattern of histamine-induced airway constriction has been observed by tantalum bronchography (Kessler et al. 1973), and the results of the present series derived from aerosol recovery techniques have yielded a similar pattern.

An increasing difference between static and dynamic lung compliances has been suggested as a sensitive index for the presence of inhomogeneous peripheral airway constriction (Fredberg et al. 1985), attributable to time-constant inhomogeneity of different lung compartments due mainly to inhomogeneous distribution of flow resistances within the lung (Otis et al. 1956; Mead 1969). In the present experiments the total compliance of the

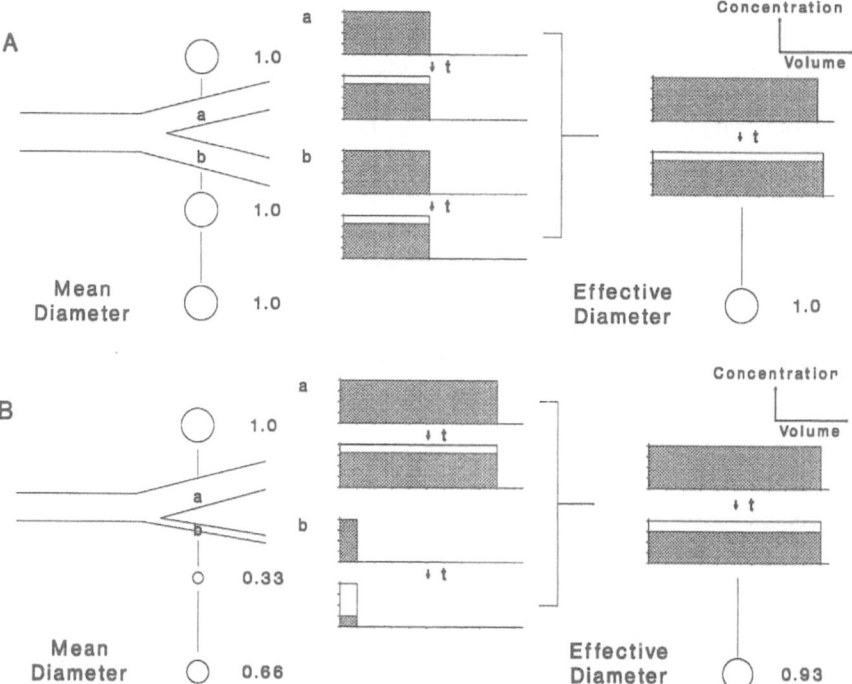

Fig. 4. Mean and effective airway diameters distal to an airway branchpoint for equal (**A**) and unequal (**B**) distribution of airway diameters. Geometric airway diameters and their arithmetic means (*left panels*). The aerosol volume of the two parallel pathways and the aerosol concentration at the end of inspiration and after breath holding (*t*) is displayed schematically (*middle panels*). The volume-weighted means of aerosol concentration from parallel daughter branches after breath holding with reference to the initial aerosol concentration is shown along with the effective airway diameter (*right panels*). **A** Equal diameter of branches *a* and *b*. **B** Airway diameter of *b* is one third that of *a*; volume of *b* is one ninth that of *a*

respiratory system was determined comprising both lung and chest wall compliances. The changes in total compliance due to histamine can be interpreted to reflect mainly changes in lung compliance because chest wall compliance would be unaffected by histamine. Therefore, the increase in the difference between static and dynamic compliances during histamine infusion strongly suggests that airway constriction in the lung periphery was present and was inhomogeneously distributed. Finally, the marked decrease of TLC (-25%) would not be accounted for by proximal airway constriction alone and, in contrast to lack of evidence by the aerosol recovery technique, would further support the presumption that peripheral airway constriction had been present during histamine infusion.

The explanation for this apparent discrepancy could reside in the fact that the model underlying the calculation of effective airway diameters strictly applies to an idealized symmetrical lung with identical diameters of parallel airways (Heyder 1975). If this assumption were applicable to real lungs, effective aerosol-derived airway diameters would correspond to the average anatomical diameter. On the other hand, in the presence of parallel airways with widely different diameters the effective airway diameter determined by the aerosol method would differ from the mean anatomical diameter of these airways. This is because larger airways, according to their relative contribution to the total volume of all airways located in a given volumetric depth, have a more pronounced effect on the effective airway diameter than smaller airways. The effect of unequal distribution of airway size in a given volumetric depth on the effective airway diameter recovered by the aerosol single-breath method is illustrated in Fig. 4 by simple modeling. The experimental findings, in line with theoretical model predictions, appear to suggest that the aerosol single-breath recovery technique is insensitive to marked peripheral airway constriction elicited by histamine infusion.

References

Antonissen LA, Mitchell RW, Kroger EA, Kepron W, Stephens NL, Bergen J (1980) Histamine pharmacology in airway smooth muscle from a canine model of asthma. J Pharmacol Exp Ther 213:150–155

Barnes PJ, Basbaum CB, Nadel JA (1983) Autoradiographic localization of autonomic receptors in airway smooth muscle. Am Rev Respir Dis 127:758–762

Bates JHT, Baconnier P, Milic-Emili J (1988) A theoretical analysis of interrupter technique for measuring respiratory mechanics. J Appl Physiol 64:2204–2214

Colebatch HJM, Engel LA (1974) Constriction of the lung by histamine before and after adrenalectomy in cats. J Appl Physiol 37:798–805

Fredberg JJ, Ingram RH, Castile RG, Glass GM, Drazen JM (1985) Nonhomogeneity of lung response to inhaled histamine assessed with alveolar capsules. J Appl Physiol 58:1914–1922

Heyder J (1975) Gravitational deposition of aerosol particles within a system of randomly oriented tubes. Aerosol Sci 6:133–137

Heyder J (1989) Assessment of airway geometry with inert aerosols. J Aerosol Sci 2:89–97

Jaffrin MY, Kesic P (1974) Airway resistance: a fluid mechanical approach. J Appl Physiol 36:354–361

Kessler G-F, Austin JHM, Graf PD, Gamsu G, Gold WM (1973) Airway constriction in experimental asthma in dogs: tantalum bronchographic studies. J Appl Physiol 35:703–708

Mead J (1969) Contribution of compliance of airways to frequency-dependent behavior of lungs. J Appl Physiol 26:670–673

Meyer M, Slama H (1983) A versatile hydraulically operated respiratory servo system for ventilation and lung function testing. J Appl Physiol 55:1023–1030

Otis AB, McKerrow CB, Bartlett RA, Mead J, McIlroy MB, Selverstone NJ, Radford EP (1956) Mechanical factors in distribution of pulmonary ventilation. J Appl Physiol 8:427–443

Palmes ED, Altshuler B, Nelson N (1967) Deposition of aerosols in the human respiratory tract during breath holding. In: Davies CN (ed) Inhaled particles and vapours II. Pergamon, London, pp 339–347

Sellick H, Widdicombe JG (1971) Stimulation of lung irritant receptors by cigarette smoke, carbon dust, and histamine aerosol. J Appl Physiol 31:15–19

Shioya T, Solway J, Munoz NM, Mack M, Leff AR (1987) Distribution of airway contractile responses within the major diameter bronchi during exogenous bronchoconstriction. Am Rev Respir Dis 135:1105–1111

von Hayek H (1970) Die menschliche Lunge. Springer, Berlin Heidelberg New York

Yanta MA, Loring SH, Ingram RH, Drazen JM (1981) Direct and reflex bronchoconstriction by histamine aerosol inhalation in dog. J Appl Physiol 50:869–873

Attempted Selective Deposition of Aerosols Using Differently Sized Particles in Man

S.P. Mohammed[1], R.W. Barber[2], and T.W. Higenbottam[1]

[1] Regional Pulmonary Physiology Laboratory, Papworth Hospital, Papworth Everad, Cambridge CB3 8RE, UK
[2] Department of Nuclear Medicine, Addenbrooke's Hospital, Hills Road, Cambridge CB2 2QQ, UK

Introduction

Therapeutic aerosols are widely used to treat respiratory disorders. To obtain good therapeutic responses it is essential to deposit an adequate amount of the aerosol in the lungs. By altering the factors that influence aerosol deposition, such as particle size and the inhalation mode, it is possible to modify the deposition of therapeutic and also pharmacological aerosols deliberately. The selective deposition pattern may then be related to changes in large and small airway function and inferences made about the distribution of receptor sites within the lung (Ruffin et al. 1978, 1981).

Conventionally, two-dimensional gamma scintigraphy has been used to visualise the deposition of radioaerosols in the human respiratory tract. However, Phipps and colleagues (1989) recently showed the three-dimensional method of single photon emission computed tomography (SPECT) to be more sensitive for discriminating between aerosol deposition in large and small airways than two-dimensional gamma scintigraphy. In this study the authors examined the penetration index of two differently sized aerosol droplets in normal subjects. Although the authors modified particle size and carefully controlled variations in inhalation mode, the two nebuliser generating systems were unmatched in terms of the flow rate of compressed gas through the device. This could lead to differences in aerosol output and differences in aerosol deposition.

In the present study we have examined the deposition of two aerosols, which have been matched for volume output but differ in terms of particle size, in normal subjects using the technique of SPECT.

Method

Aerosol Generation and Inhalation. A large-particle aerosol was produced using a DeVilbiss ultrasonic nebuliser (USN; DeVilbiss Healthcare,

U. Mohr et al. (Eds.)
Advances in Controlled Clinical
Inhalation Studies
© Springer-Verlag Berlin Heidelberg 1993

Feltham, UK) with a power setting of 5 and vent fully open. The aerosol passed through corrugated tubing 1 m long, into a 1-l cone-shaped dead space to ensure continuous supply of "similarly" aged aerosol. Each subject breathed from the cone through a two-way low-resistance valve (Godden et al. 1986). The small-particle aerosol was generated using four acorn jet nebulisers (JET; Medic Aid, Pagham, UK) connected in parallel with two Y pieces and short lengths of plastic tubing. The output from all four nebulisers passed through the same system as described above for the USN. The JET system was run from a pressurised gas cylinder. The airflow was controlled by two needle valves and measured by two floating ball flowmeters. The airflow through each needle valve was kept at $15 \, l \, min^{-1}$.

Aerosol Output. A corrugated anaesthetic filter (Pall Biomedical, Portsmouth, UK) was placed on the inspiratory end of the two-way valve. The USN and JET nebulisers were loaded with 50 ml and 4×5 ml of the radiopharmaceutical technetium-99m diethylene triamine penta acetic acid (^{99m}Tc DTPA) in 0.9% saline, respectively. The activity in 1 ml solution, removed from the nebuliser reservoir, was measured prior to nebuliser operation. The quantity of radioactivity trapped on the filter was measured having run the nebuliser for 1 min. The volume output from the nebuliser was calculated in millilitres of liquid produced as aerosol particles per minute of operation of the nebuliser system.

Particle Size. A May cascade impactor (Biral, Bristol, UK) was used to determine the particle size characteristics of the aerosols produced by the two nebuliser systems. The aerosols were sampled from the dead space cone via the inspiratory end of the two-way cone. As above, the nebuliser reservoir contained approximately 50 MBq ^{99m}Tc DTPA in 0.9% saline. A calibrated scintillation counter was used to measure the quantity of radioactivity deposited on each plate of the cascade impactor. It was assumed that each particle contained radioactivity proportional to its mass, and the activity distribution was treated as if it were a mass distribution. The mass distribution was fitted to a log normal distribution, from which the mass median aerodynamic diameter (MMAD) and the geometric standard deviation (GSD) of the two aerosols were calculated.

Distribution Study Using Radioaerosol. Four healthy, nonsmoking male volunteers participated in this study (Table 1). District Ethical Committee approval was obtained for the study. Each subject gave informed consent. The USN nebuliser was loaded with approximately 7000 MBq ^{99m}Tc DTPA in 50 ml saline and the JET with approximately 5000 MBq ^{99m}Tc DTPA in 20 ml saline. Each subject inhaled the radioerosol from both nebuliser systems, the order of inhalation from the nebulisers being randomised, with an interval of at least 1 week between the two visits. On each occasion, subjects breathed normally for 1 min from the nebuliser. Subjects received

Table 1. Subject details

Subject	Age (years)	Height (cm)	FEV$_1$ (l)	FVC (l)	FEV$_1$ (% of Pred)	FVC (% of Pred)
1	40	175	4.3	5.7	117	123
2	31	178	4.4	5.8	106	114
3	27	178	4.8	5.9	105	113
4	22	168	3.9	4.8	104	107

FEV$_1$, Forced expiratory volume in 1 s; FVC, forced vital capacity; Pred, predicted.

approximately 20 MBq ^{99m}Tc DTPA for each study, giving a total radiation dose for the two studies combined of 0.2 mSv effective whole-body dose equivalent. Immediately following aerosol inhalation the subject rinsed the mouth to remove excess aerosol and was placed supine on a tomographic imaging couch. Subjects were imaged using a large field-of-view gamma camera with a low-energy general purpose collimator (IGE400AT, International General Electric Medical Systems, Slough, UK). The gamma camera was connected to an on-line computer (Nodecrest, Byfleet, UK). For the 20 s, 64 × 64 word images were acquired at each of 64 angles around the subject. Since ^{99m}Tc DTPA deposited in the lungs and airways is lost by a number of absorptive and non-absorptive processes (Bennet and Ilowite 1989; Lippman et al. 1980), by looking at the number of counts in the first and last frames a correction factor was determined, and this applied to each frame of the study assuming exponential removal. Transaxial slices were reconstructed using standard Nodecrest filtered back-projection software; attenuation correction was applied using a mean attenuation coefficient obtained from transmission studies. Transverse and coronal mid-lung images were formed from the reconstructed transaxial dataset as described by Phipps et al. (1989) (See Fig. 1). Right and left lungs were both assessed. The boundary of each lung was defined as the contour drawn at 20% of the maximum count in that lung. A separate region was created to incorporate extrapulmonary and extrathoracic airways (excluding mouth). A central region was defined which included intrapulmonary airways down to segmental bronchi, as well as extrapulmonary and extrathoracic airways (excluding mouth). A peripheral region was defined which included intrapulmonary airways from the segmental bronchi to the alveoli. In each subject the region defined for the JET was used for the USN images. From the anterior lung view, the quantity of radioactivity deposited in the lungs and airways was calculated using a gamma camera counter efficiency factor. The volume of liquid output deposited in the lungs and airways was calculated using the following equation:

$$\frac{\text{MBq of radioactivity in the lungs and airways}}{\text{MBq of radioactivity aerosolised as liquid volume output}}$$

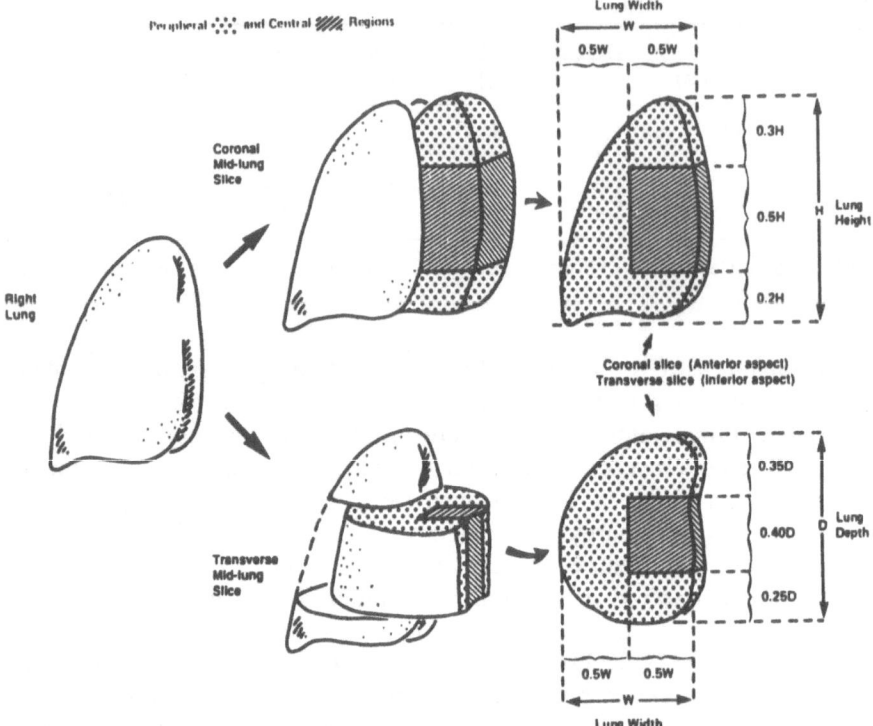

Fig. 1. Diagram of peripheral and central regions and mid-lung slicing

Data Analysis. Paired data were analysed using paired Student *t* test. All results are expressed as actual values or percentages ± standard error of the mean.

Results

The USN and JET nebuliser systems were matched for liquid volume output in 1 min: USN = 0.85 ± 0.01 ml (*n* = 18) and JET = 0.86 ± 0.01 ml (*n* = 16). Although both systems produced heterodispersal aerosols (USN GSD = 2.12; JET GSD = 2.91), the nebuliser systems produced quite different droplet-sized aerosols. The USN produced an aerosol with a MMAD of 7.9 ± 0.7 μm (*n* = 8), compared with 3.83 ± 0.53 μm (*n* = 7) with the JET.

There was no significant difference between peripheral and central deposition with the USN for coronal or transverse lung sections (coronal peripheral 45.5% ± 7.1%, central 54.4% ± 7.1%; transverse peripheral 54.5% ± 5.5%, central, 45.5% ± 5.5%). However, with the JET peripheral

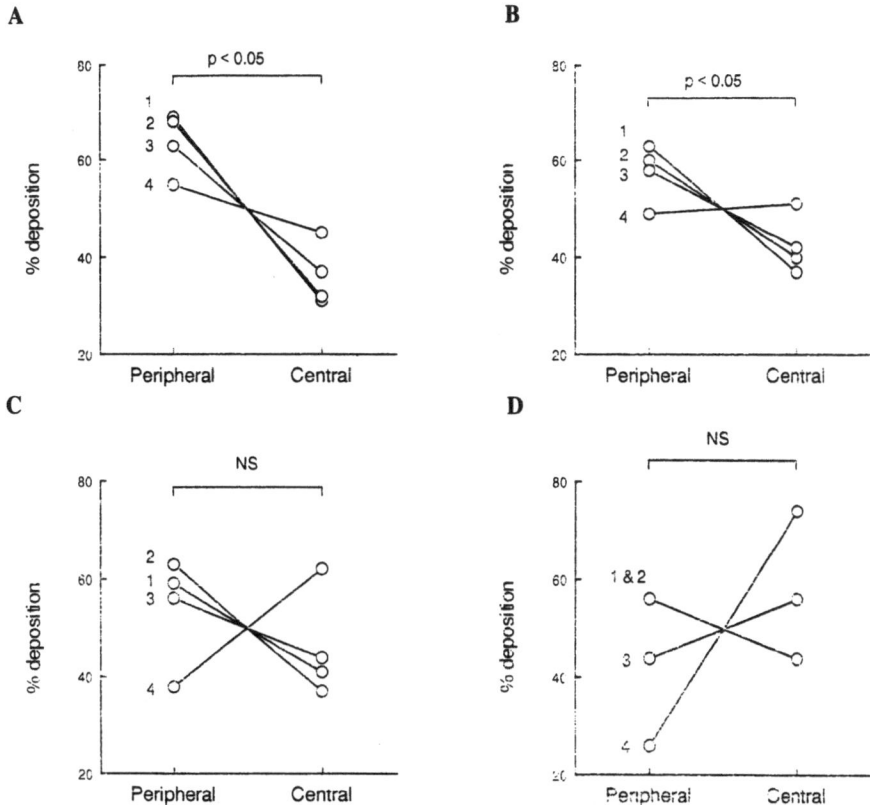

Fig. 2A–D. Percentage of peripheral and central deposition for individual subjects using USN and JET nebulisers. **A,B** Transverse and coronal lung sections for the JET. **C,D** Transverse and coronal lung sections for the USN

and central deposition differed significantly ($p < 0.05$) for coronal and transverse lung slices (coronal peripheral 57.5% ± 3.0%, central 42.5% ± 3.0%; transverse peripheral 63.8% ± 3.2%, central 36.2% ± 3.2%). Individual values for each subject are shown in Fig. 2.

The volume of liquid output deposited in the entire lungs and airways was significantly ($p < 0.05$) higher with the USN than with the JET nebuliser system. For the USN and JET systems the mean liquid volume output deposited in the lungs and airways was 0.14 ± 0.01 and 0.09 ± 0.01 ml, respectively. Individual values for each subject are shown in Fig. 3.

Conclusion

The present study demonstrates that regional deposition of aerosols in the lungs and airways can be changed by altering aerosol particle size. With the

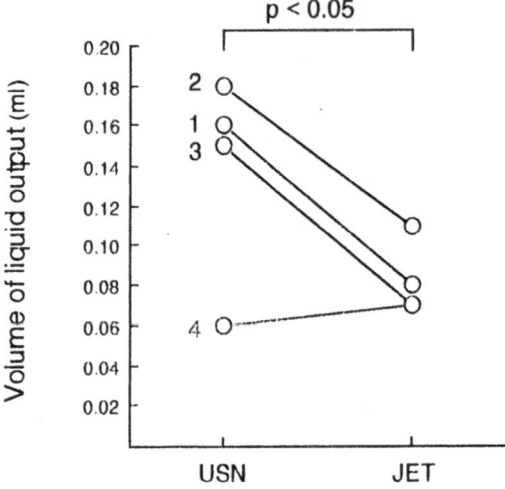

Fig. 3. Individual values for the volume of liquid output deposited in the lungs and airways using the USN and JET nebulisers

USN there was no significant difference between central and peripheral deposition in coronal and transverse lung slices. However, with the JET there was a significant difference in central and peripheral deposition in coronal and transverse mid-lung slices, which favoured peripheral deposition. Since the JET produces a "small" droplet-sized aerosol, a large percentage of these particles are able to penetrate into the periphery of the lung, which would account for the regional difference obtained with the JET. Although the USN produces a "large" droplet-sized aerosol, approximately half of the aerosol is deposited peripherally. However, since the USN generates a heterodispersal aerosol, deposition of the smaller particles in the periphery of the lung could account for this finding. In addition, it has been shown that particles with a diameter of 5 µm can penetrate down to alveolar level (Agnew et al. 1985). Alternatively, the high peripheral deposition could be a consequence of the definition of peripheral the central airways in this study. In most studies of aerosol deposition the lung is divided into three main regions: (a) a central region which incorporates mainly large conducting airways, (b) a peripheral region which includes small airways and alveoli, and (c) an intermediate region which bridges central and peripheral airways (Sanchis et al. 1972). However, these lung divisions have two drawbacks. Firstly, the criteria for defining these regions are based partly on the lung generations described in the Weibel model of the respiratory tract. Although this model is extremely useful in mathematical deposition studies (Morrow and Yu 1985), it must be remembered that the lung is a three-dimensional structure. Secondly, aerosol deposition in the intermediate region is usually overlooked. In the current study we have defined only two regions within the lungs and airways, peripheral and central regions. This definition allows us to simplify regional aerosol deposition since there is no intermediate region to complicate matters. Although our definition of central and peripheral airways differs from that of other investigators, such inconsistency in the literature will remain until a definition for central and peripheral airways is standardised for use by scientists and clinicians.

There are a considerable number of nebuliser systems available which produce a smaller particle-sized aerosol than the JET system used in the current sutyd. However, such nebulisers would have been unable to match the USN system for liquid volume output. Since one of the main aims of the study was to match the nebulisers for this variable, the full extent to which differences in the size of aerosol particles generated using the USN and JET could be exploited was compromised.

Although, the USN and JET were matched for liquid volume output, there was a significantly ($p < 0.05$) higher volume of aerosol deposited in the lungs and airways with the USN compared with the JET. Large aerosol droplets deposit in the lungs by inertial impaction whereas smaller particles deposit primarily by the mechanisms of sedimentation and diffusion. Deposition by impaction occurs simultaneously whereas particle deposition by sedimentation is a time-dependent process [9]. With the latter method the collection efficiency in an airway increases with particle residence time in the airway. In the current study, there was no change in the mode of inhalation of the aerosols between visits. Consequently means of enhancing deposition by sedimentation were not employed. The above differences in aerosol retention can be explained by a greater number of particles being exhaled with the JET compared with the USN.

Planar measurements of aerosol deposition suffer from the problem of the inclusion of overlying peripheral airways in the central airway region (Logus et al. 1984). The major advantage of SPECT is the ability to distinguish between peripheral and central airways (Phipps et al. 1989; Dolovich et al. 1985). In this study the use of SPECT also allows us to overcome this problem. Since a longer period of time is required for acquisition of tomographic images (up to 20 min) compared with conventional planar scintigraphy (3-4 min), dynamic changes to the inhaled aerosol (absorption and muociliary clearance: Bennet and Ilowite 1989; Lippman et al. 1980) would have some effect on aerosol redistribution. Consequently, a correction factor was applied to each frame of the tomographic study, assuming exponential removal of the inhaled radioaerosol.

From this study we conclude that by altering aerosol particle size we can select aerosol deposition patterns within the lung. This is essential in the treatment of respiratory diseases. Secondly, in studies using aerosols with different droplet sizes to investigate the site of action of therapeutic and pharmacological aerosols, investigators should take into account possible differences in the volume of aerosol deposited in the lungs before inferences about receptor distributions are made.

References

Agnew JE, Pavia D, Clarke SW (1985) Factors affecting the "alveolar deposition" of 5 µm inhaled particles in healthy subjects. Clin Phys Physiol Meas 6/1:27–36

Bennet WD, Ilowite JS (1989) Dual pathway clearance of ^{99m}Tc-DTPA from the bronchial mucosa. Am Rev Respir Dis 139:1132–1138

Dolovich MB, Coates G, Hargreave F, Newhouse MT (1985) Aerosols in diagnosis: ventilation, airway penetrance, airway reactivity, epithelial permeability and mucociliary transport. In: Moren F, Newhouse MT, Dolovich MB (eds) Aerosols in medicine. Principles, diagnosis and therapy. Elsevier, Amsterdam, pp 225–59

Godden DJ, Borland C, Lowry RH, Higenbottam TW (1986) Chemical specificity of coughing in man. Clin Sci 70:301–306

Lippman M, Yeates DB, Albert RE (1980) Deposition, retention and clearance of inhaled particles. Br J Med 37:337–62

Logus JW, Trajan M, Hooper HR, Lentle BC, Mann SFP (1984) Single photon emission tomography of the lungs imaged with Tc-labeled aerosol. J Can Assoc Radiol 35:133–138

Morrow PE, Yu CP (1985) Aerosols in diagnosis: models of aerosol behaviour in airways. In: Moren F, Newhouse MT, Dolovich MB (eds) Aerosols in medicine. Principles, diagnosis and therapy. Elsevier, Amsterdam, pp 149–191

Phipps PR, Gonda I, Bailey DL, Borham P, Bautovich G, Anderson SD (1989) Comparison of planar and tomographic gamma scinitigraphy to measure the penetration index of inhaled aerosols. Am Rev Respir Dis 139:1516–1523

Ruffin RE, Dolovich MB, Wolff RK, Newhouse MT (1978) The effects of preferential deposition of histamine in the human airway. Am Rev Respir Dis 117:485–492

Ruffin RE, Dolovich MB, Oldenburg FA, Newhouse MT (1981) The preferential deposition of inhaled isoproterenol and propranolol in asthmatic patients. Chest 80 [Suppl]:904–906

Sanchis J, Dolovich M, Chalmers R, Newhouse MT (1972) Quantitation of regional aerosol clearance in the normal human lung. J Appl Physiol 33/6:757–762

Acute Effects of Ambient Ozone in Physically Active Adults

H.-G. Mücke, U. Ranft, and M.S. Islam

Medizinisches Institut für Umwelthygiene an der Heinrich-Heine-Universität, Gurlittstraße 53, W-4000 Düsseldorf 1, FRG

Introduction and Aim

Ozone occurs as a natural component of the atmosphere. There is a distinction in its occurrence between upper atmosphere (stratosphere; 20–50 km above sea level) and lower atmosphere (troposphere; up to 10 km above sea level) as well as biological consequences. Stratospheric ozone is known to protect life from harmful cosmic radiation. In contrast, tropospheric ozone is a toxic environmental oxidant and plays a role as the key substance in photochemical smog. Important primary components of the photochemical reactions include nitrogen oxides, carbon monoxide, and volatile organic compounds which are typical traffic-induced air pollutants (Becker 1977; Ehhalt 1987; Lippmann 1989b; Moussiopoulos et al. 1989). In addition to sufficiently high concentrations of these chemicals, formation of ambient ozone depends on specific meteorological situations such as stable high pressure conditions with intense isolation, high temperatures, low wind speed, and low relative humidity (Guichert 1989). During the summer in Germany we register on bright, sunny days increasing ambient ozone, with maximum concentrations in the afternoon between 3 and 6 p.m. The geographic distribution of mean ozone concentrations typically shows higher levels in rural areas and alpine/subalpine mountains, while peak concentrations are higher in urban areas (Fricke 1983; Georgii et al. 1977). In summer months, ozone concentrations reach to 200 ppb (30-min mean value). The annual average levels are around 15–20 ppb.

The toxicity of ozone has been widely studied to examine its potential effects on materials, plants, animals, and human health (Bruch and Schlipköter 1977; Lippmann 1989b; Tingey and Taylor 1982). The toxic effects on the lung are well known. Several laboratory and epidemiological studies investigate the transient responses of respiratory function to acute ozone exposure (Kinney et al. 1988, 1989), and it has been claimed that ozone exposure affects the function and structure of the respiratory tract in various ways (Lippmann 1989a,b). It is well established that the inhalation of ozone causes concentration-dependent decrements in lung volumes and

U. Mohr et al. (Eds.)
Advances in Controlled Clinical
Inhalation Studies
© Springer-Verlag Berlin Heidelberg 1993

flow rates during forced expiratory maneuver (Danuser 1988; Lippmann 1989a). These effects have been shown in human experimental studies to an exposure of 100 ppb (Horstman et al. 1989). It is also well established that volunteers engaged in a daily program of outdoor exercise inhale more ozone and deeper because of a higher ratio of respiratory minute ventilation (Danuser 1988; Lippmann 1989b).

Furthermore, it has been reported that the biological effects of ozone are attributed to its ability to cause biochemical oxidation and peroxidation of membrane proteins and lipids directly and/or by free radical chain reactions (Danuser 1988; Mustafa 1990). In this case laboratory research observed a significant fall in arterial blood oxygen pressure (von Nieding et al. 1977; Solic et al. 1982).

In Germany a threshold value for the maximum concentration of ozone (MIK; Guidelines VDI, Part 15) of 60 ppb (30-min mean value) has been proposed (Verein Deutscher Ingenieure 1987). The World Health Organization Task Group recommends a 1-h exposure limit of 50–100 ppb ozone for the protection of public health (World Health Organization 1977). However, it is still an open question at what ozone concentration level under actual photochemical smog conditions, especially in urban areas, measurable acute health effects are to be expected.

The aim of this epidemiological field study was to investigate short-term (acute) health effects of ambient ozone exposure during physically active outdoor work in an urban area. For this we examined pulmonary function and partial pressure of arterial blood gases once in the morning (between 7 and 9 a.m.) at the time with lowest ozone concentrations and again in the afternoon (between 1 and 3 p.m.) when the concentration reaches 80%–90% of the daily maximum after 6–7 h of physically active outdoor work with moderately higher ratio of respiratory minute ventilation. The study area was the city of Düsseldorf (FRG), and the measurements were made in 1989.

Materials and Methods

We examined 50 healthy adult males (horticulturists and cemetery gardeners) without known disease under actual working conditions. They were aged between 18 and 60 years and had an average weight of 82 kg and height of 1.77 m. This field study was conducted in phases at different ozone concentrations, i.e., we investigated on bright, sunny days in summer with distinctly increased ozone concentrations and on cloudy days in autumn with low concentrations.

The pulmonary function test measured the parameters: airway resistance (R_{aw}), intrathoracic gas volume, inspiratory vital capacity, and total lung capacity. Measurements were performed with the help of a volume-constant bodyplethysmograph BYS II with lung function computer (Jaeger,

Germany) installed in a mobile pulmonary function laboratory. The partial pressure of the arterial blood gases (arterial blood oxygen, P_aO_2; arterial blood carbon dioxide, P_aCO_2) was measured with an Analyser ABL 2 Acid-Base Laboratory (Radiometer, Denmark).

The volunteers were interviewed by a questionnaire to obtain information regarding general health condition and smoking habits. In addition, they were requested to give a subjective evaluation of symptoms such as eye irritation, cough, etc. after having had the environmental ozone exposure.

The evaluation of acute health effects on pulmonary function and partial pressure of arterial blood gases was based on the relative daily deviation of the afternoon value (a) after exposure from the morning value (b): ($a - b/b$) × 100. We tested paired comparisions at various ambient ozone concentrations (2-h mean value 1–3 p.m.) by Wilcoxon test (Figs. 2, 3). Figure 4 shows the difference between morning and afternoon values tested by the sign test.

Results

Figure 1 shows the maximum ozone concentrations exceeding the short-term MIK value of 60 ppb ozone as a 30-min mean value in July and August.

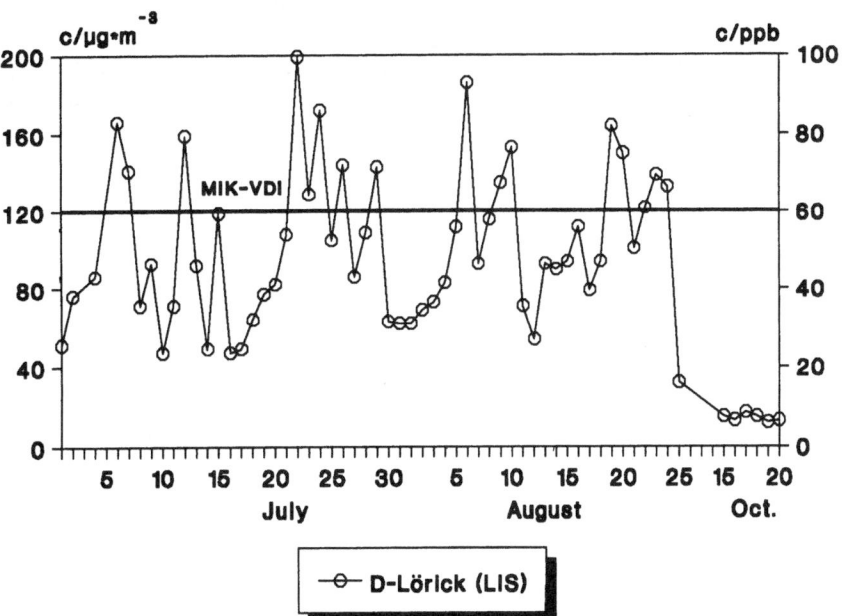

Fig. 1. Maximum ozone concentrations in Düsseldorf (1989). The recommended maximum ozone concentration (*MIK-VDI*) (Verein Deutscher Ingenieure 1987) and the days of investigation are indicated

Table 1. Ozone concentrations (ppb) between 1 and 3 p.m. in Düsseldorf and numbers of volunteers on days of investigation

Date	2-h average	30-min maximum	n
18 July	23	32	11
19 July	31	38	8
20 July	37	41	12
7 Aug.	39	47	11
16 Aug.	32	56	12
20 Aug.	56	61	9
16 Oct.	12	13	11
17 Oct.	15	17	7
19 Oct.	9	12	10

Peak concentrations reached 100 ppb. Table 1 shows the ozone concentrations on days of investigation.

We found an average 10% increase in R_{aw} (Fig. 2) and an average 5% reduction in P_aO_2 (Fig. 3a) on days with higher ambient ozone compared to no average increase or no average reduction, respectively, on days with lower concentrations. On days with ambient ozone above 25 ppb a statistically significantly greater proportion of volunteers ($p < 0.01$) reacted with a decrease in P_aO_2 (Fig. 4). Figure 3a shows the lack of P_aO_2 effect on the relative daily deviation on days with ozone concentrations below 15 ppb (2-h mean value between 1 and 3 p.m.), whereas days with greater than 30 ppb ozone were associated with a significant ($p < 0.05$) decrease in the

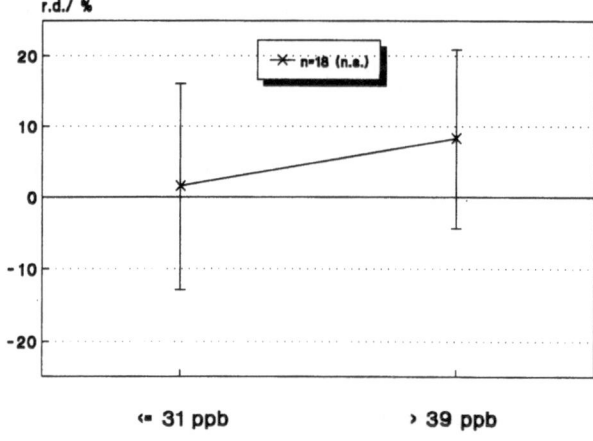

Fig. 2. Comparision of R_{aw} relative deviation ($r.d.$) of afternoon value after 6–7 h exposure from morning value on days at various ambient ozone; 95% confidence interval and paired comparisons tested by the Wilcoxon test

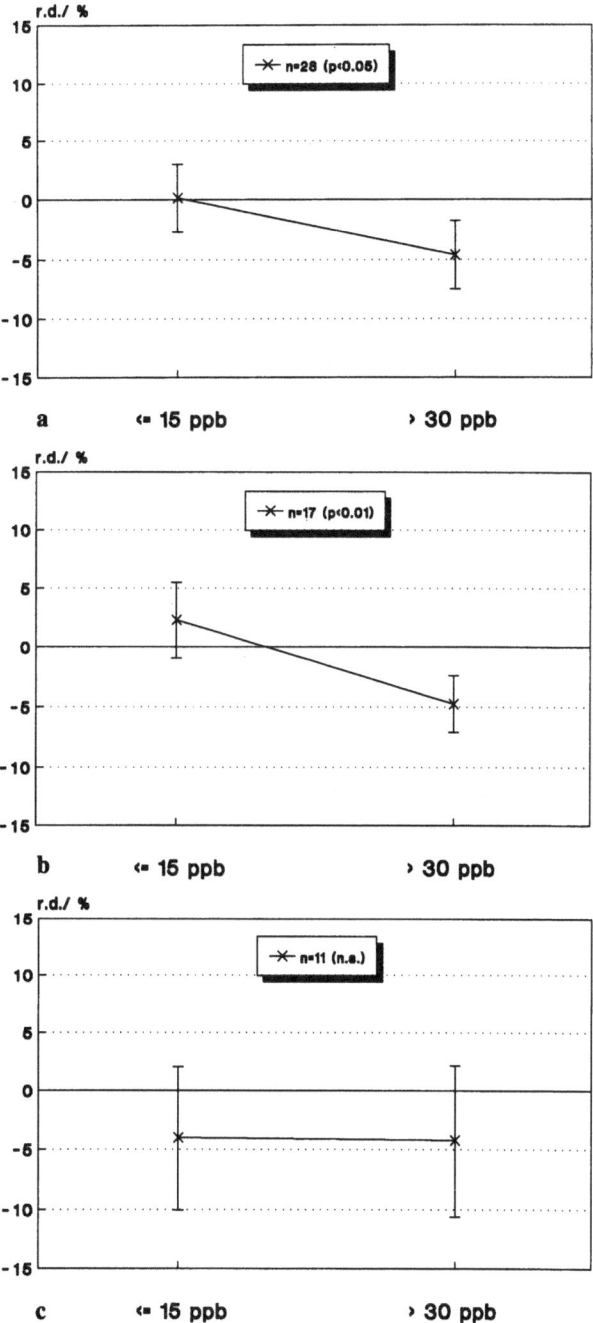

Fig. 3a-c. Comparision of P_aO_2 relative deviation ($r.d.$) of afternoon value after 6–7h exposure from morning value on days at various ambient ozone; 95% confidence interval and paired comparisons tested by the Wilcoxon test. **a** All subjects ($n = 28$); **b** nonsmokers ($n = 17$); **c** smokers ($n = 11$)

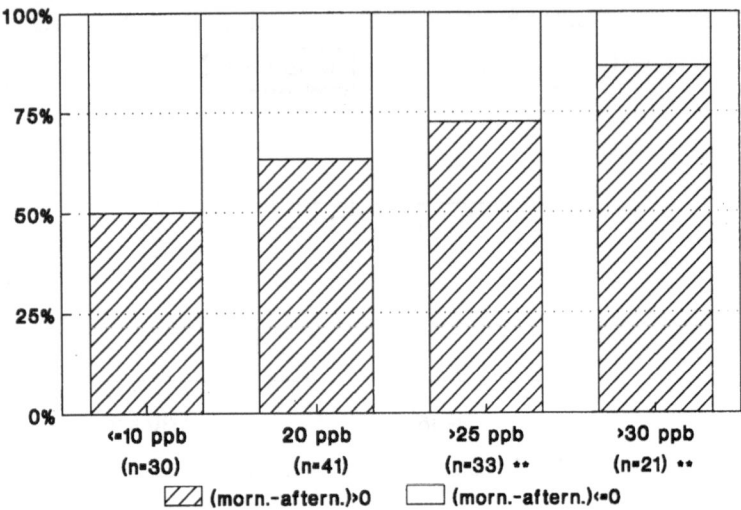

Fig. 4. Distribution of decreased (morning minus afternoon value greater zero) and increase (morning minus afternoon value less zero) P_aO_2 values after 6–7 h exposure on days at various ambient ozone; tested by the sign test

relative daily deviation of P_aO_2. This effect can be attributed mainly to the more sensitive nonsmoking volunteers ($p < 0.01$) as opposed to smokers (not significant; Fig. 3b,c).

The other parameters of pulmonary function and partial pressure of the arterial blood gases demonstrated no specific acute effects of ambient ozone. Thus, no subjective irritations were registered by the questionnaire.

Discussion and Conclusions

It can be concluded from our results that increased ambient ozone concentrations during a sunny summer day adversely affect R_{aw} and P_aO_2 in physically active adults with increased respiratory minute ventilation after 6–7 h outdoor work. Furthermore, it can be concluded that nonsmoking volunteers are more sensitive than smokers.

During the summer the ambient ozone concentrations on our days of investigation ranged between 30 and 60 ppb and only once exceeded the short-term MIK value of 60 ppb (30-min mean value). In laboratory studies the acute effects of peak concentrations have been widely studied (Horstman et al. 1989; Kinney et al. 1989; von Nieding et al. 1977). For example, a 2-h exposure to 100 ppb ozone caused a significant fall in partial pressure of arterial blood in healthy volunteers (von Nieding et al. 1977). Compared to these laboratory findings, it can be concluded from our results that an increase in ambient ozone above 30 ppb on a summer day (between

7 a.m. and 2 p.m.) is enough to induce these biochemical reactions in healthy volunteers after 6–7 h outdoor activities. The acute effects that we have described are most likely reversible. Sustained effects following the exposure to increased ambient ozone during 1 day are not within the scope of this study and are also not well explored at this moment.

Therefore the results of human field studies, especially of physically active persons such as children, outdoor laborers, and athletes who are exposed to ozone in complex ambient mixtures for more than 6 h and laboratory studies in animals indicate that such effects need to be considered in establishing a margin of safety for any future ozone air quality guideline.

References

Becker KH (1977) Ozon und Begleitsubstanzen in photochemischen Smog. VDI Ber 270:7–12

Bruch J, Schlipköter HW (1977) Tierexperimente über die chronische Wirkung von Ozon – morphologische und funktionelle Veränderungen. VDI Ber 270:111–117

Danuser B (1988) Die Wirkung von Ozon auf den Respirationstrakt. Zbl Arbeitsmed 38:62–73

Ehhalt DH (1987) Grundlagen der stratosphärischen Ozonchemie. Promet 1/2:41–44

Fricke W (1983) Großräumige Verteilung und Transport von Ozon und Vorläufern. VDI Ber 500:55–62

Guicherit R (1989) Concentrations and patterns of ozone in western Europe. Environmental Protection Agency US-Dutch 3rd international symposium. In: Schneider T et al. (eds) Atmospheric ozone research and its policy implications, vols 9–13. Elsevier, Amsterdam, pp 167–176

Georgii, H-W, Fricke W, Rudolf W, Deimel M, Becker KH, Schurath U (1977) Bildung und Transport von Photooxidantien im Raum Bonn-Köln und Frankfurt/M. VDI Ber 270:19–24

Horstman DH, McDonnell W, Kehrl H, Delvin R, Abdul-Salaam S, Ives P, Koren H (1989) Current US EPA research concerning more prolonged exposure (>6-hr) of humans to near ambient ozone concentrations (<0.12 ppm). In: Brasser, Mulder (eds) Man and his ecosystem. Proceedings of the 8th world clean air congress 1989, Den Haag. Elsevier, Amsterdam

Kinney PL, Ware JH, Spengler JD (1988) A critical evaluation of acute ozone epidemiology results. Arch Environ Health 43/2:168–173

Kinney PL, Ware JH, Spengler JD, Dockery DW, Speizer FE, Ferris BG (1989) Short-term pulmonary function change in association with ozone levels. Am Rev Respir Dis 139/1:56–61

Lippmann M (1989a) Health effects of ozone. A critical review. JAPCA 39/5:672–695

Lippmann M (1989b) Effects of ozone on respiratory function and structure. Annu Rev Public Health 10:49–67

Moussiopoulos N, Oehler W, Zellner K (1989) Kraftfahrzeugemissionen und Ozonbildung. Springer, Berlin Heidelberg New York

Mustafa MG (1990) Biochemical basis of ozone toxicity. Free Radic Biol Med 9:245–265

Solic JJ, Hazucha MJ, Bromberg PA (1982) The acute effects of 0.2 ppm ozone in patients with chronic obstructive pulmonary disease. Am Rev Respir Dis 125/64:664–669

Tingey DT, Taylor GE (1982) Variation in plant response to ozone; a conceptual model of physiological events. In: Unsworth MH, Ormrod DP (eds) Effects of gaseous air pollution in agriculture and horticulture. Butterworth, London, pp 113–138

Verein Deutscher Ingenieure (1987) Reinhaltung der Luft 2310: Maximale Immissions-Werte zum Schutze des Menschen; maximale Immissionskonzentrationen für Ozon (und photochemische Oxidantien). Blatt 15. Verein Deutscher Ingenieure, Düsseldorf

von Nieding G, Wagner M, Löllgen H, Krekeler H (1977) Zur akuten Wirkung von Ozon auf die Lungenfunktion des Menschen. VDI Ber 270:123–129

World Health Organization (eds) (1977) Air quality guidelines for Europe. Ozone and other photochemical oxidants. WHO Reg Publ Eur Ser 23:315–393

Respiratory Injuries in Workers from the Coke Chemical Industry

E. Petrova[1] and V. Hristeva[2]

[1] Higher Medical School, Sofia, Dept. of Hygiene, Ecology and Occupational Health, Boul. D. Nestorov 15, 1431 Sofia, Bulgaria
[2] National Center of Hygiene and Medical Ecology, Boul. D. Nestorov 15, 1431 Sofia, Bulgaria

The combination of pneumotropic aerosols in the coke chemical industry, including mineral dusts, coal dust, sulfuric oxides, hydrogen sulfide, carbon monoxide, benzene derivatives, and naphthalines, entail clear irritative and sometimes fibrosogenic effects on the respiratory system of workers employed in this industry. We have studied the harmful effects of these factors in the air of the work environment of those involved in ore preparation, blast furnaces, and alloy and steel production. A number of publications (e.g., Bourilkov et al. 1983) deal with the occupational pathology regarding the lungs of these workers. The synergic effect of coal dust and quartz leads to the develoment of benign pneumoconioses. This was also the finding, for example, Irmscher (1961).

The purpose of this study was to determine the injuries to the respiratory system of employees from different work places in the coke chemical production of the metallurgic industry of Bulgaria. We present recommendations for the timely detection, tracing, and prevention of these harmful effects.

Material and Methods

The study included 315 employees from the coke chemical production of the metallurgic enterprise Kremikovtsi. We distinguished the following nine groups on the basis of the area of employment in the plant: coal preparation ($n = 36$), coke batteries ($n = 95$), catching and processing of chemical products (CPCP; $n = 44$) benzene shop ($n = 18$), tar distillation and naphthaline division ($n = 22$), deep sulfur purification ($n = 24$), plant and electrical repair and control-measuring equipment for coke chemical products ($n = 32$) vapor production ($n = 11$), and administration ($n = 33$). All subjects were given clinical (anamnestic, physical) and functional examinations and fluorographic surveys of the respiratory system. Tobacco

U. Mohr et al. (Eds).
Advances in Controlled Clinical
Inhalation Studies
© Springer-Verlag Berlin Heidelberg 1993

smokers accounted for 95% of those examined. The following indices of respiratory function were studied: vital capacity, index of Tiffeno, index of aerial velocity, maximal expiratory capacity of forced vital capacity, and peak expiratory capacity. There were three types of respiratory defects: restrictive, obstructive, and mixed type; in addition, we considered obstruction of the small airways with a diameter of less than 2 mm. Toxicological measurement of the air, blood and urinewas carried out in the Department of Chemcial Factors and Industrial Toxicology of the Institute of Hygiene and Occupational Healh, Bulgarian Medical Academy, Sofia.

Results and Discussion

Table 1 presents the clinical pulmonary disorders (subjective complains plus positive symptoms) in the different age groups of workers. This shows a gradual increase in the lung disorders with increasing age. Among those aged over 50 years there was a particular occurrence of essential pulmonary emphysema, previous lung diseases, and some accompanying chronic pulmonary processes.

There was no tendency for direct influence of the duration of exposure on the appearance of lung clinical defects; however, one should not underestimate the subjective lung complains of workers with a longer length of employment. There was a comparatively hign proportion of workers showing clinical changes and more pronounced clinical symptoms among those employed in the coke batteries, CPCP, benzene shop, and deep sulfur purification. Table 2 presents the distribution of funetional respiratory disorders in terms of the duration of exposure. These increased with the

Table 1. Lung disorders by age group

	n	%
≤30 years ($n = 35$)	21	6.67
31–40 years ($n = 78$)	24	7.61
41–50 years ($n = 131$)	26	8.25
≥51 years ($n = 71$)	35	11.11

Table 2. Lung disorders by duration of employment

	n	%
≤2 years ($n = 45$)	23	7.30
3–5 years ($n = 46$)	26	8.26
6–10 years ($n = 78$)	38	12.06
≥11 years ($n = 146$)	78	24.76

length of employment. These were most common among workers in the coke batteries (14.60%), coal preparation (8.57%), CPCP (7.93%), tar distillation and naphthaline division (5.72%), deep sulfur purification (4.45%), and administration (4.45%).

The type of respiratory defect most characteristic of the various divisions in the plant differed. That most common in coal preparation workers was obstruction of the small airways with a diameter of less than 2 mm (33.33%) and, to a lesser extent, the obstructive type of respiratory insufficiency. Similar functional changes were seen in employees in the coke batteries, CPCP, and deep sulfur purification. In the remaining areas, early obstruction of the small airways was most common.

The fluorographic tests of the chest cells revealed: in six persons from the coke chemical production a reinforced pulmonary drawing; in five persons organic pneumofibrosis; in ten persons metatuberculous calcificates in the hilus lymphatic ganglions and the pulmonary parenchyma; in seven person unilateral or bilateral pleural growths; in two persons spotty-striped shadings; in two persons unilateral enlarged hilus shadings (one worder from the coke batteries and one from CPCP). The enlarged unilateral hili with both roentgenographically positive workers suggested central lung carcinoma.

Among the total of 315 worders examined, 31 had comfirmed lung diagnoses (24 with chronic bronchitis, 1 with bronchial asthma, and six with restricted postpneumonic and metatuberculosis pneumofibrosis) and 64 with early and manifest obstructive changes in the small airways and the large bronchi without manifest clinical pulmonary symptoms. Five persons showed pleural accretion due to passed pleuritis or pleuropneumonia.

Clinical pulmonary symptoms were established which could not be directly connected with the duration of exposure, but which were predominantly in workers from the coke batteries, CPCP, benzene shop, and deep sulfur purification, where significant industrial risks were evident.

Specifically manifest were functional respiratory disorders, particularly early obstructive changes and obstruction of the small airways. Defects were especially in workers from the coke batteries, coal preparation, and CPCP. These were due to the irritative effects of dusts, gases, and vapors in the air of the work environment.

The 64 cases with early and manifest obstructive changes in the small and large bronchi suggest that particular efforts should be focused upon detecting chronic irritative bronchitis among those exposed to the harmful effects of aerosols in the air of the work environment.

Conclusions

1. The cases of confirmed chronic bronchitis and of early and manifest obstructive changes in the small and large bronchi were associated largely

with the irritative effects of the harmful aerosols of dusts, gases, and vapors. An allergenic effect of some benzene and naphthaline derivatives cannot be excluded, as well as the harmful influence of tobacco smoking.
2. Annual medical examinations must be performed for assessing the state of the respiratory system among those at risk, including clinical, functional, roentgenographic, and hygienic studies.
3. The considerable amount of pollutants involved in coke chemical production urgently requires sanitation of the air in the work environment and strict hygienic standard for reducing noxious factors to acceptable levels.

References

Bourilkov T, Dobreva M, St. Ivanova-Dzhubrilova (1983) Mineral dusts in the working environment. Medicina i Fizkultura, Sofia
Irmscher G (1961) Stanblungen Erkrankungen durch Koksstaube. In: Brand A (ed) Beiträge zur Silicose. Berlin, pp 52–58

Aerosol-Derived Airway Dimensions of Dog Lungs: Comparison of Bolus and Single-Breath Techniques

A. Rahmel[1], A. Schwalen[2], E. Calzia[2], A. Huber[2], H. Schulz[2],
and M. Meyer[2]

[1] MPI für Experimentelle Medizin, Abteilung Physiologie, Hermann-Rein-Straße 3
W-3400 Göttingen, FRG
Jetzt: Universitätskliniken, Innere Medizin C, Albert-Schweitzer-Straße 33 W-4400
Münster/Westf, FRG
[2] MPI für Experimentelle Medizin, Abteilung Physiologie, Hermann-Rein-Straße 3,
W-3400 Göttingen, FRG

Introduction

Changes in the diameter and cross-section of pulmonary airways and alveoli
constitute an important factor associated with many diseases of the lung
(Thurlbeck 1985). Diagnostic techniques for the assessment of airway
dimensions are restricted to larger airways (visualization by bronchoscopy or
radiographic techniques; Fraser and Pare 1977; Sackner 1980), to indirect
functional techniques (determination of airway resistance or closing volume;
Metzger et al. 1980), or for detecting changes in the late stage of the disease
when lung function is severely impaired. Analysis of the behavior of inhaled
1-µm monodisperse aerosol particles presents a novel noninvasive technique
for functional morphometric assessment of airway dimensions in vivo. Two
different techniques may be used: (a) inhalation of a bolus of monodisperse
particles at varying points of the inspired volume (Bolus technique; Palmes
et al. 1973; Heyder 1983) and (b) inhalation of a single breath with test
particles contained in the inspired tidal volume (single-breath technique;
Heyder 1989).

The purpose of the present study was (a) to determine the effective
airway dimensions of lungs in anesthetized, paralyzed, mechanically ventilated dogs using both the bolus and the single-breath recovery technique,
(b) to compare effective aerosol-derived airway diameters with morphometric estimates from lung models (Weibel 1963; Horsfield et al. 1982), and
(c) to assess the feasibility and reproducibility of the aerosol recovery
techniques from measurements of intra- and interindividual variability of
airway dimensions.

U. Mohr et al. (Eds.)
Advances in Controlled Clinical
Inhalation Studies
© Springer-Verlag Berlin Heidelberg 1993

Theory

The technique of determining aerosol-derived airway dimensions is based on the measurement of gravitational particle losses of inhaled monodisperse particles in the airways of the lung during breath holding (Palmes et al. 1967; Heyder 1975; Gebhart et al. 1981). If the lung is considered as a system of randomly oriented cylindrical tubes, with identical radius at a given volumetric depth, and particles are homogeneously distributed throughout the system at the end of inspiration, the number of particles recovered during expiration decreases exponentially with breath-holding time:

$$\frac{N_{(t)}}{N_{(0)}} = R_{(t)} = \exp\left[-\frac{2vt}{\pi r}\right] \tag{1}$$

(N = number of particles, $R_{(t)}$ = recovery function, v = terminal settling velocity of particles, r = airway radius, t = breath-holding time). The rate of decrease of aerosol concentration in the lung is inversely related to airway size because the average distance that aerosol particles must travel before settling is directly related to the airway radius. The effective aerosol-derived airway radius, defined as the equivalent radius of a system of randomly oriented cylindrical tubes of infinite length which would exhibit the same aerosol recovery function as that of the real lung, is calculated from the following relationship:

$$r = \frac{2v}{\pi d(\ln R)/dt} \tag{2}$$

Methods

Five beagle dogs (mean body weight, 13.6 ± 0.9 kg) were studied in supine position. They were intubated via the orotracheal route and mechanically ventilated using a computerized piston-type servo ventilator (Meyer and Slama 1983). Total lung capacity (TLC; 896 ± 113 ml BTPS) and functional residual capacity (FRC, 422 ± 52 ml BTPS) were determined by the helium dilution technique.

Monodisperse, nonhygroscopic di-(2-ethyl-hexyl) sebacate particles (density 0.912 g/cm^3, particle number concentration 10^6/cm^3) were produced by vapor condensation on NaCl nuclei using a modified Sinclair-LaMer aerosol generator (Sinclair and LaMer 1949) and were sized (mean aerodynamic particle diameter 0.89 ± 0.097 µm) in a convection-free sedimentation cell (Stahlhofen et al. 1975). For instantaneous monitoring of aerosol concentration at the airway opening, a miniaturized in-line light-scattering photometer was used. The optical system consists of a 2 mW laser diode ($\lambda = 820$ nm) and a photodiode arranged at an angle of 90°. Linearity

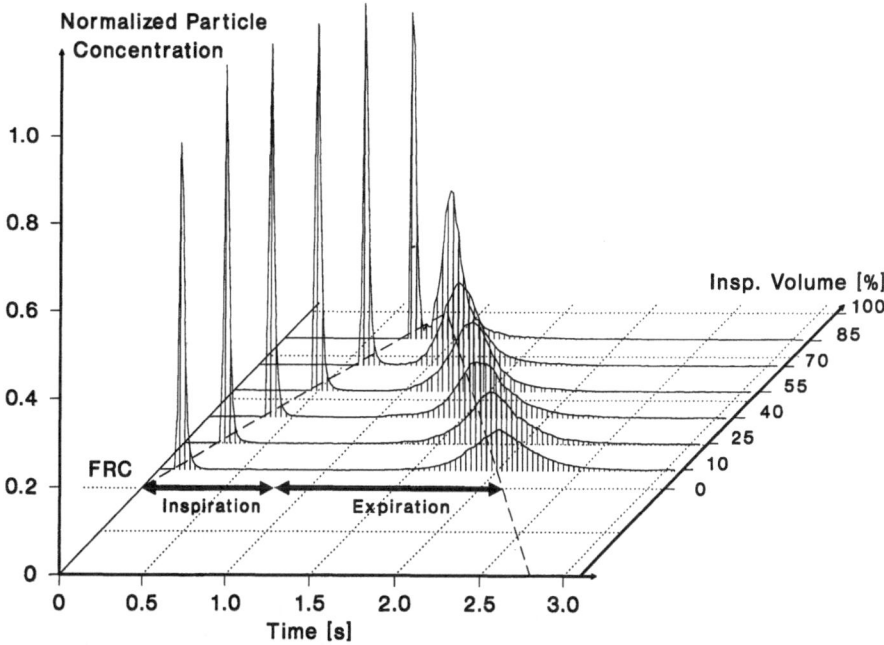

Fig. 1. Bolus technique. Superposition of inspiratory and expiratory aerosol concentration curves corresponding to volumetric penetration of inspired aerosol boli from 10%–85% (15% steps) of the normalized inspired volume. *x-Axis*, time; *y-axis*, normalized concentration (relative units); *z-axis*, normalized inspired volume. Symmetric distribution of the mode of the inspired and expired bolus within the respiratory cycle suggests that intrapulmonary penetration of tracer particles exhibits a "first-in/last-out" sequence

was tested with sebacate and latex particles of various sizes covering the range of particle concentrations encountered in determination of airway dimensions by the aerosol methods (Meyer et al. 1991). For the aerosol bolus technique, aerosol boli with a half-width of 8 ml were introduced into the main air stream at 10%–85% (step width 15%) of the inspired volume. Inspiratory and expiratory flow was constant at 0.5 l/s and 0.3 l/s, respectively, and expiration was terminated well below FRC level. For comparison between animals, i.e., to account for differences in lung size, the inspired volume was normalized to 50% of the individual's FRC. Breath-holding time was varied between 0 and 10 s at 2-s intervals.

Typical recordings of instantaneous particle concentration as a function of time are shown in Fig. 1 for the bolus technique. The aerosol recovery is calculated from the ratio of expired-to-inspired particle quantities (area under inspired and expired aerosol concentration curves, respectively). From the exponential slope of the aerosol versus breath-holding time relationship the effective airway dimensions were calculated according to Eq. 2 for any site of bolus penetration depths (Fig. 2). The airway radius

380   A. Rahmel et al.

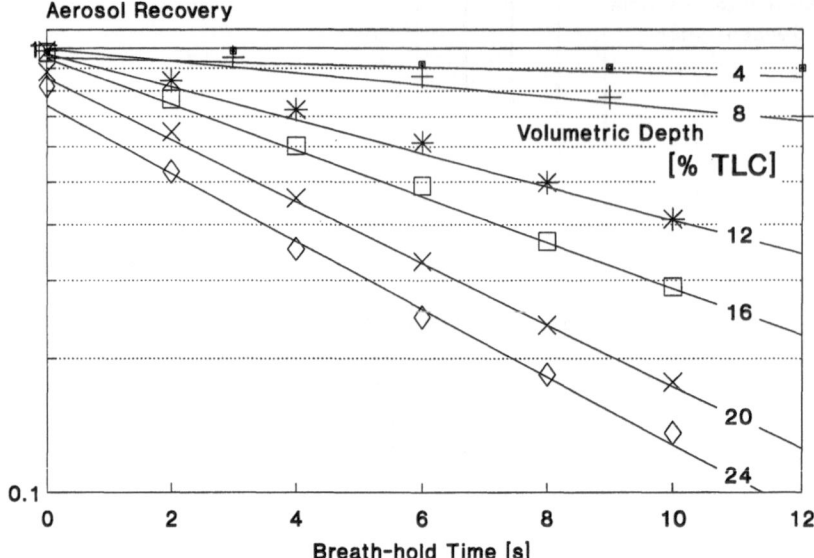

Fig. 2. Aerosol recovery (bolus technique). The aerosol recovery (ratio of expired-to-inspired particle number; *y-axis*) is plotted as a function of breath-holding time (*x-axis*) for different normalized volumetric lung depths (% TLC). The exponential regression of the recovery function is used to calculate the effective airway radius at the normalized volumetric location of the inspired tracer bolus

determined at a given volumetric penetration depth of the inspired bolus was expressed as a percentage of TLC, i.e., the site of determination of airway dimensions was normalized for varying body (lung) size of experimental animals.

Recordings by the single-breath aerosol recovery technique are shown in Fig. 3. The ratio of expired-to-inspired aerosol concentration at any point of expiration yields the local recovery which can be aligned with the individual's TLC for calculation of normalized volumetric depth. Therefore, a single set of aerosol single-breath curves obtained at different breath-holding times facilitates the calculation of an array of recovery functions (Fig. 4). Hence, effective dimensions of pulmonary airways along the bronchial tree can be determined for the range of volumetric depths covered by penetration of inspired aerosol particles.

Results

Effective aerosol-derived airway diameters as a function of normalized volumetric depth obtained by the bolus and the single-breath technique (mean values ±SD) are summarized in Fig. 5. In the proximal part of the lung airway diameters decrease rapidly from about 3000 µm at a volumetric

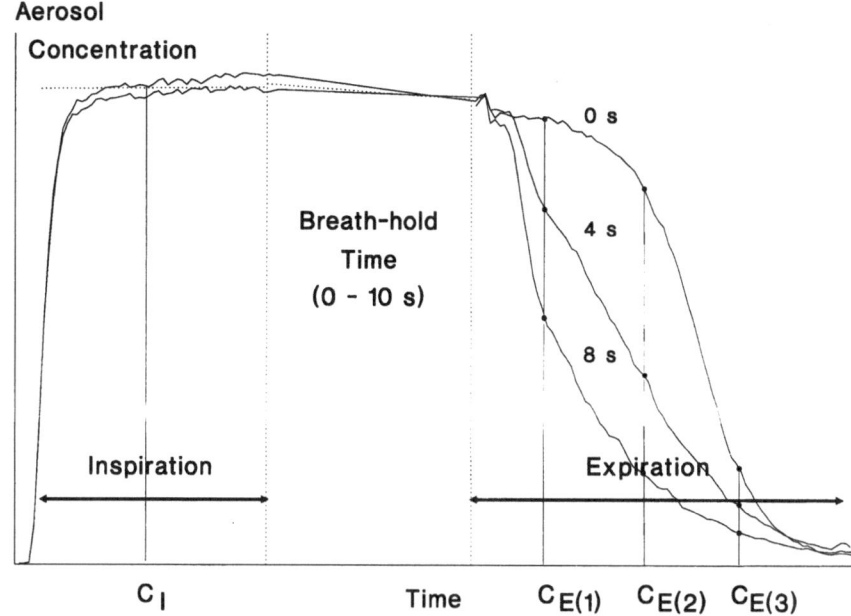

Fig. 3. Single-breath technique. Superimposed original tracings of instantaneous aerosol concentration for different breath-holding times. Inspiration and expiration is separated by varied breath-holding (0–10 s, 2-s intervals). The expiratory aerosol concentration depends on the duration of end-inspiratory breath-holding. The ratio of expiratory ($C_{E(n)}$) and (constant) inspiratory (C_I) aerosol concentration denotes the aerosol recovery. With constant respiratory airflow the aerosol recovery and hence airway dimensions can be calculated from the $C_{E(n)}/C_I$ ratio for any volumetric location (n) by transformation of expiratory time into expired volume

depth of 5% TLC toward more peripheral airways, and in the distal airways, beyond a volumetric depth of 15% TLC, effective airway diameters become almost constant at about 200 μm. While close agreement is obtained for medium-sized airways, for the most proximal and distal airways the single-breath technique yields insigificantly larger airway dimensions.

To analyze the intraindividual reproducibility of effective airway diameters, serial measurements (during an experimental session, short-term reproducibility, and after a period of 6 months, long-term reproducibility) were performed by both techniques and quantified by the coefficient of variation of mean airway diameters (CV = SD/mean) for different volumetric depths. Both techniques provided good short-term reproducibility with a CV of approximately 3% for the single-breath technique and approximately 10% for the bolus technique. Except for proximal airways, i.e., under 15% TLC volumetric depth, the long-term reproducibility was also below 10%. The interindividual variability of effective airway diameters was significantly larger (CV about 25%) than the intraindividual variability, and inter-

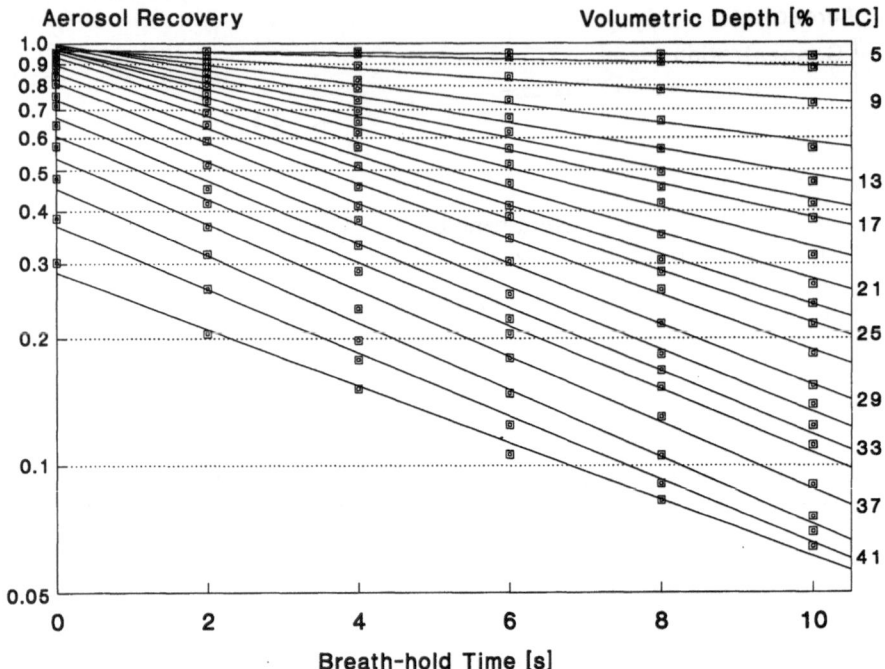

Fig. 4. Aerosol recovery (single-breath technique). The aerosol recovery (*y-axis*) is plotted as function of breath-holding time (*x-axis*) for volumetric depths ranging from 5% to 43% TLC (2% intervals). Effective airway diameters for different volumetric lung depths are calculated from the aerosol recovery function based on exponential regression of data points

individual differences were more pronounced for proximal airways compared to distal airways.

Discussion

The determination of airway dimensions by the aerosol recovery technique is based on a number of assumptions which is discussed in more detail below.

The decreasing number of particles recovered after increasing breath-holding periods should depend on a single mechanism, i.e., by gravitational particle sedimentation and deposition during these time intervals. Deposition by diffusion during breath-holding could be neglected because sufficiently large (approximately 1 μm) aerosol spheres were used (Gebhart et al. 1981; Heyder 1983). Particle deposition on airway walls during inspiration and expiration could be assumed to be constant for the present experimental series because a constant flow regime and constant intrapulmonary distribution of flow were achieved by the computer-controlled

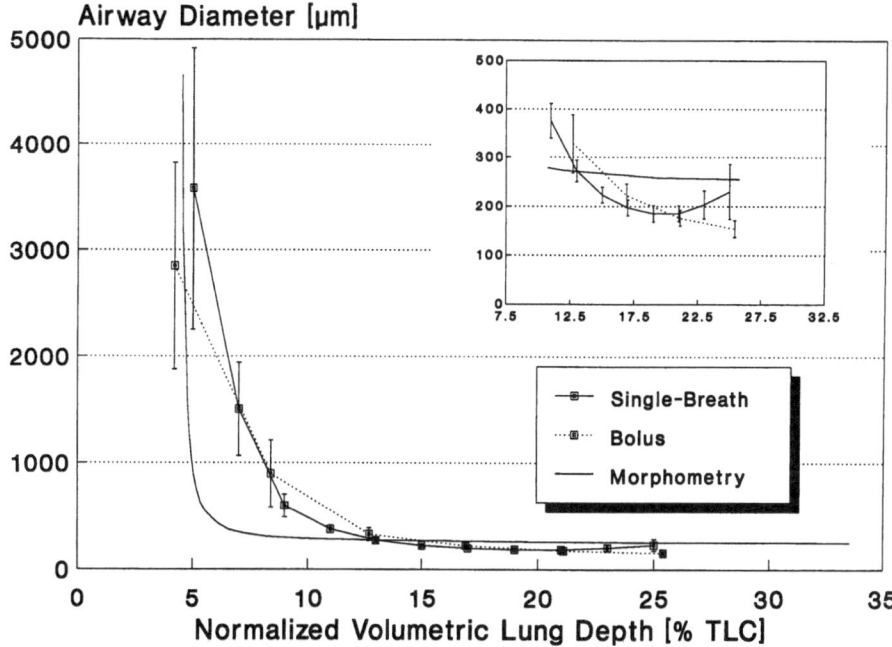

Fig. 5. Effective airway diameters of dog lungs by bolus and single-breath aerosol recovery techniques and by morphometric techniques. Airway diameters (*y-axis*) are displayed as function of normalized volumetric lung depth (*x-axis*). The window (*upper right*) shows the range of volumetric depths from 7.5% to 32.5% TLC. The morphometric data are based on the symmetric Weibel model A of the human lung isomorphically adjusted to the canine lung with a modified tracheal volume derived from the Horsfield lung model of the dog

servo ventilator. On the other hand, particle deposition during expiration could be affected by changes in the aerosol distribution over the cross-sectional area of airways as a result of varying breath-holding periods, but the effect is expected to be small (Gebhart et al. 1981).

For intrapulmonary localization of aerosol particles in terms of volumetric depth during breath-holding, aerosol transport by ventilation should proceed according to the "first-in/last-out" principle, i.e., particle-containing tidal volume fractions which enter the lung early in inspiration are exhaled late in expiration (Heyder and Davies 1971; Heyder 1983). Analysis of the position of the maximum aerosol concentration during inspiration and expiration has demonstrated that peak aerosol concentrations were in fact distributed symmetrically (in volumetric terms) within the ventilatory cycle (see Fig. 1).

Aerosol bolus dispersion is enhanced both by the duration of breath-holding and by volumetric penetration depth of the bolus. Theoretical analysis of bolus dispersion (Rosenthal 1985) and aerosol distribution during a single breath (Heyder et al. 1988) has demonstrated, however, that the effect of aerosol dispersion on effective airway dimensions is small provided dispersion occurs symmetrically around the particle-containing zone into both proximal and distal parts of the lung. However, even if no dispersion of the aerosol bolus would occur, aerosol particles are spread over a number of airway generations and would be located in airways with different diameters because the airways in real lungs branch in an asymmetric dichotomous pattern, particularly in dog lungs (Horsfield et al. 1982). The effects of small differences in the diameters of "parallel" airways, i.e., airways originating from different airway generations but located in the same volumetric depth, on calculated effective airway diameters are expected to be negligible (Gebhart et al. 1981).

The results from the present study demonstrate that the in vivo aerosol-derived airway diameters reveal close correspondence with morphometric data based on investigations of bronchial casts of excised human (Weibel 1963) and dog lungs (Horsfield et al. 1982). The discrepancies in the transition zone between the conducting and respiratory airways of the lung could be attributed to several factors: (a) limited spatial resolution of the aerosol technique, which is inversely related to the effectiveness of intrapulmonary mixing mechanisms leading to aerosol dispersion (Heyder 1989); (b) pronounced asymmetry of airway diameters (parallel inhomogeneity) in the transition zone of the lung; and (c) inappropropriate morphometric lung model. The importance of these factors remains to be determined.

The single-breath technique has several advantages over the bolus technique for the determination of aerosol-derived airway dimensions. It is less time-consuming because a single set of aerosol inhalation maneuvers with different breath-holding times is required for determination of airway dimensions in different regions of the lung. The tendency for larger effective airway diameters by the single-breath technique in proximal airways (see Fig. 5) is interpreted to reflect the superior spatial resolution of this technique. Finally, the better reproducibility along with less complex technical requirements favors the single-breath technique as method of choice. The high reproducibility in mechnically ventilated dogs may be attributed to constant ventilatory flow patterns, release of bronchomotor tone by paralysis, and by-passing the pharynx and larynx by oro-tracheal intubation, ultimately leading to reduced aerosol mixing in proximal airways. In human subjects breathing spontaneously through a mouthpiece the variability of airway dimensions was markedly larger than that observed in the present series in dogs (Lapp et al. 1975; Gebhart et al. 1981).

The magnitude of the interindividual variability of airway dimensions observed in dog lungs (about 20%) is similar to that reported for human subjects by both anatomical (Matsuba and Thurlbeck 1971) and aerosol recovery studies (Lapp et al. 1975; Gebhart et al. 1981; Heyder 1983). This finding would suggest two major implications for the application of the aerosol recovery technique in clinical and environmental health field studies. (a) Differences of airway diameters among individuals may be indicative for a varying degree of susceptibility of human subjects to lung diseases in adverse working environments (Palmes and Lippmann 1977; Hankinson et al. 1979; Kim et al. 1988). (b) Because of the high variability of airway diameters, identification of gold standards for "normal" effective airway diameters is rendered difficult, but the single-breath aerosol recovery technique could be used in follow-up studies because of its high long-term reproducibility.

References

Fraser RG, Paré JAP (1977) Diagnosis of diseases of the chest, vol I, 2nd edn Saunders, Philadelphia

Gebhart J, Heyder J, Stahlhofen W (1981) Use of aerosols to estimate pulmonary air-space dimensions. J Appl Physiol 51:465–476

Hankinson JL, Palmes ED, Lapp NL (1979) Pulmonary air space size in coal miners. Am Rev Respir Dis 119:391–397

Heyder J (1975) Gravitational deposition of aerosol particles within a system of randomly oriented tubes. Aerosol Sci 6:133–137

Heyder J (1983) Charting human thoracic airways by aerosols. Clin Phys Physiol Meas 4:29–37

Heyder J (1989) Assessment of airway geometry with inert aerosols. J Aerosol Sci 2:89–97

Heyder J, Davies CN (1971) The breathing of half micron aerosols: III. Dispersion of particles in the respiratory tract. Aerosol Sci 2:437–452

Heyder J, Blanchard JD, Brain JD (1988) Particle deposition in volumetric regions of the human respiratory tract. Ann Occup Hyg 32 [Suppl 1]:71–79

Horsfield K, Kemp W, Phillips S (1982) An asymmetrical model of the airways of the dog lung. J Appl Physiol 52:21–26

Kim CS, Lewars GA, Sackner MA (1988) Measurement of total lung aerosol deposition as an index of lung abnormality. J Appl Physiol 64:1527–1536

Lapp NL, Hankinson JL, Amandus H, Palmes ED (1975) Variability in the size of airspaces in normal human lungs as estimated by aerosols. Thorax 30:293–299

Matsuba K, Thurlbeck WM (1971) The number and dimensions of small airways in nonemphysematous lungs. Am Rev Respir Dis 104:516–524

Metzger LF, Altose MD, Fishman AP (1980) Evaluation of pulmonary performance. In: Fishman AP (ed) Assessment of pulmonary function. McGraw-Hill, New York, pp 211–237

Meyer M, Slama H (1983) A versatile hydraulically operated respiratory servo system for ventilation and lung function testing. J Appl Physiol 55:1023–1030

Meyer M, Rahmel A, Hahn G, Slama H (1991) A miniaturized aerosol photometer for particle inhalation experiments. J Aerosol Med 4 [Suppl 1]:44

Palmes ED, Lippmann M (1977) Influence of respiratory air space dimensions on aerosol deposition. In: Walton WH (ed) Inhaled particles and vapours IV. Pergamon, Oxford, pp 127–135

Palmes ED, Altshuler B, Nelson N (1967) Deposition of aerosols in the human respiratory tract during breath holding. In: Davies CN (ed) Inhaled particles and vapours II. Pergamon, London, pp 339–347

Palmes ED, Wang CS, Goldring RM, Altshuler B (1973) Effect of depth of inhalation on aerosol persistence during breath holding. J Appl Physiol 34:356–360

Rosenthal FS (1985) A model for determining alveolar and small airway dimensions from aerosol recovery data. J Appl Physiol 58:582–591

Sackner MA (1980) Bronchoscopy. In: Fishman AP (ed) Pulmonary diseases and disorders, vol 1. McGraw Hill, New York, pp 122–130

Sinclair D, LaMer VK (1949) Light scattering as a measure of particle size in aerosols. Chem Rev 44:245–267

Smaldone GC, Itoh H, Swift DL, Kaplan J, Florek R, Wells W, Wagner HN (1983) Production of pharmacologic monodisperse aerosols. J Appl Physiol 54:393–399

Stahlhofen W, Armbruster L, Gebhart J, Grein E (1975) Particle sizing of aerosols by single particle observation in a sedimentation cell. Atmos Environ 9:851–857

Thurlbeck WM (1985) Chronic airflow obstruction–correlation of structure and function. In: Petty TL (ed) Chronic obstructive pulmonary disease, 2nd edn Dekker, New York, pp 129–203

Weibel ER (1963) Morphometry of the human lung. Springer, Berlin Göttingen Heidelberg

Nonoccupational Exposure to Benzene

G. Scherer[1], C. Conze[1], J. Angerer[2], and F. Adlkofer[1]

[1] Analytisch-biologisches Forschungslabor Prof. Dr. med. F. Adlkofer,
Goethestraße 20, 8000 München 2, FRG
[2] Institut für Arbeitsund Sozialmedizin, Schillerstraße 25, W-8520 Erlangen, FRG

Introduction

Benzene has been identified as a human carcinogen. It occurs ubiquitously in the modern industrialized world, with automobile traffic being the most important source of nonoccupational benzene exposure (Fishbein 1988). Tobacco smoke (both active and passive smoking) and food intake are thought to be additional sources for benzene exposure. Whereas smoking leads to elevated benzene concentrations in blood and expired air, no conclusive results exist for the role of passive smoking and food intake on the total benzene body burden (Adlkofer et al. 1990).

The purpose of our investigations was to determine the possible contribution of passive smoking to everyday benzene exposure. The uptake of benzene was determined by biological monitoring after experimental exposure to environmental tobacco smoke (ETS) and after real-life passive smoking.

Methods

Design of Studies. Three controlled laboratory studies with healthy male volunteers were performed. During all studies the subjects stayed in the laboratory and were put on a defined diet low in polycyclic aromatic hydrocarbons. Experimental ETS exposures took place in a furnished room ($45 \, m^3$) with windows and door kept closed during the exposure sessions. The ETS was produced by smokers smoking their usual brands of cigarettes according to a prescribed schedule. Sham exposures were performed in an identical way without smoking. Blood and exhalate from all subjects were sampled immediately before and after each exposure and sham exposure session. Urine samples (24-h) were collected on each day of the studies starting at 8 a.m. When the subjects first reported to the laboratory on the eve of the first day of the study, blood and exhalate samples were drawn, and a 12-h urine collection was started. These samples together with a

U. Mohr et al. (Eds.)
Advances in Controlled Clinical
Inhalation Studies
© Springer-Verlag Berlin Heidelberg 1993

completed questionnaire on life-style and other factors were used for the investigation of real-life passive smoking as a potential source of benzene exposure. Self-reported passive smoking at home and at the workplace was classified as none (0), low (1), or strong (2). A score for total ETS exposure (home and workplace) was calculated by addition of the single scores.

Analytical Methods. For air monitoring, sampling tubes were installed at the breathing height of a seated person at the end of the room opposite to where the smokers sat. Carbon monoxide was measured continuously by an infrared CO monitor UNOR 6N (Maihak, Hamburg, FRG). Nicotine (Odgen 1989), respirable particles (Oldaker et al. 1990), and benzene (NIOSH 1984) were determined according to published methods. For biomonitoring, carboxyhemoglobin (COHb) was determined spectro-photometrically using a IL 282 CO oximeter (Instrumentation Laboratories, USA). Nicotine and continine in urine were determined by gas chromato-graphy (Hengen and Hengen 1978). Benzene in 2- to 5-ml blood samples was analyzed by dynamic head-space gas chromatography and flame ionisa-tion detection (Angerer et al. 1991). Exhalate sampling for benzene was performed with 60-l Tedlar bags according to the procedure of Pellizzari et al. (1988). A 30-l sample of the exhaled air was drawn through a charcoal tube and analyzed as described for ambient air samples (NIOSH 1984).

Results

The results obtained from the experimental ETS studies are summarized in Table 1. Benzene concentrations in room air ranged from 3 to $12\,\mu g/m^3$ on the control days and from 60 to $206\,\mu g/m^3$ on the exposure days. Benzene in blood increased from 167 ng/l (range: 80–220) to 320 ng/l (range: 210–470) after experimental ETS exposure. Concentrations of exhaled benzene increased from $1.8\,\mu g/m^3$ (range: 1.2–2.3) after sham exposure to $6.7\,\mu g/m^3$ on exposure to ETS at a concentration of 10 ppm CO (study 1) and to $6.0–9.3\,\mu g/m^3$ in the 20- to 30-ppm CO experiments (studies 2 and 3). The time course of the benzene levels in blood and exhalate of both smokers and nonsmokers for study 3 are shown in Fig. 1.

Subjects with higher real-life ETS exposure (based on both urinary nicotine metabolites and self-reported passive smoking) showed no signi-ficant increase in the concentrations of COHb or benzene in blood or exhalate (Table 2).

Discussion

The air monitoring results show that the experimental ETS exposure con-centrations were at the upper limit of real-life passive smoking situations in

Table 1. Room air concentrations and biomonitoring results of experimental ETS studies

Study number	Cigarettes smoked	Number of subjects	Air monitoring[a]				Biomonitoring[b]		
			CO (ppm)	Nicotine (µg/m³)	Particles (µg/m³)	Benzene (µg/m³)	COHb (%)	Benzene in blood (ng/l)	Benzene in exhalate (µg/m³)
1	–	8	0.4	1	25	5	0.8 (0.2)	160 (40)	1.9 (0.8)
1	–	8	0.6	7	52	3	0.7 (0.2)	180 (70)	1.9 (0.7)
2	–	5	1.4	4	77	8	0.6 (0.2)	190 (50)	ND
2	–	5	2.0	6	78	12	0.7 (0.2)	170 (30)	ND
3	–	5	1.3	2	35	8	0.5 (0.2)	220 (50)	2.3 (1.8)
3	–	5	1.3	6	69	9	0.5 (0.1)	80 (20)	1.2 (3.1)
1	102/9 h	8	9.5	67	1800	60	1.3 (0.2)	210 (40)	6.7 (0.7)
2	120/8 h	5	24	71	3180	190	2.8 (0.2)	470 (70)	ND
2	120/8 h	5	24	71	4090	206	3.6 (0.2)	370 (140)	ND
3	129/8 h	5	22	67	4290	123	2.4 (0.1)	260 (80)	9.3 (2.5)
3	122/8 h	5	31	53	2160	125	3.4 (0.3)	310 (100)	6.0 (1.8)

ND, Not determined.

[a] Values are time-integrated levels during the exposure and sham exposure sessions.

[b] Values are means (standard deviations) before and after the exposure sessions.

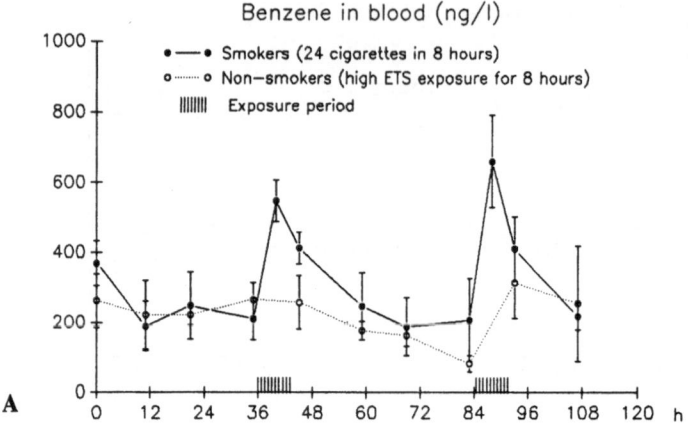

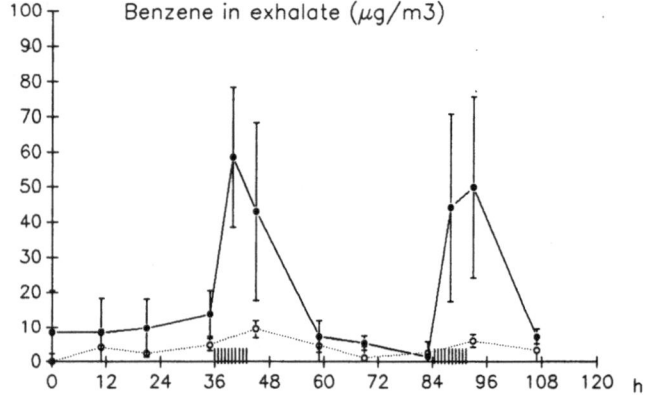

Fig. 1. Time course of benzene levels in blood (**A**) and exhalate (**B**) of smokers and nonsmokers in study 3

Table 2. Benzene levels in blood and exhalate after real-life passive smoking: means (standard deviations)

Nicotine + cotinine in urine (µg/g creatinine)	n	ETS score (0–4)	COHb (%)	Benzene in blood (ng/l)	Benzene in exhalate (µg/m³)
<5 (mean = 2.4)	13	0.69 (0.95)	0.53 (0.20)	250 (130)	1.84 (0.92)
≥5 (mean = 10.9)	7	1.14 (0.89)	0.61 (0.41)	250 (60)	2.77 (1.15)
p		0.32	0.54	0.98	0.15

the 10-ppm CO study (study 1) and far above realistic levels in studies 2 and 3. Under our experimental ETS exposure conditions only small but consistent elevations of benzene concentrations were observed in the blood and exhalate of the exposed nonsmokers.

Wallace and Pellizzari (1986) found that smoking at home may increase the indoor air concentration of benzene in winter by about $7\,\mu g/m^3$ but not in spring or summer. No increase in benzene breath levels of nonsmokers living with smokers were reported (Wallace et al. 1987). These results agree with our findings on benzene burden by real-life ETS exposures. The extent of benzene exposure by passive smoking as reported in the literature (Wallace and Pellizzari 1986; Wallace et al. 1987) and observed in our studies, together with the high background benzene exposure by other common sources such as automobile traffic (Adlkofer et al. 1990), cause doubt as to whether passive smoking in everyday life can measurably increase the benzene levels in blood and exhalate.

References

Adlkofer F, Scherer G, Conze C Angerer J, Lehnert G (1990) Significance of exposure to benzene and other toxic compounds through environmental tobacco smoke. J Cancer Res Clin Oncol 116:591–598

Angerer J, Scherer G, Schaller KH, Müller J (1991) The determination of benzene in human blood as an indicator of environmental exposure to volatile aromatic compounds. Fresenius J Anal Chem 339:740–742

Fishbein L (1988) Benzene. Uses, occurrences and exposure. IARC Sci Publ 85:67–96

Hengen N, Hengen M (1978) Gas-liquid chromatographic determination of nicotine and cotinine in plasma. Clin Chem 24:50–53

NIOSH – National Institute for Occupational Safety and Health (1984) Manual of analytical methods, method 1500/1501, vol 1. US Department of Health and Human Services Washington, pp 84–100

Odgen MW (1989) Gaschromatographic determination of nicotine in environmental tobacco smoke: collaborative study. J Assoc Off Anal Chem 72:1002–1006

Oldaker III GB, Perfetti PF, Conrad FC Jr, Conner JM (1990) Results from surveys of environmental tobacco smoke in offices and restaurants. In: Kasuga H (ed) Indoor air quality. Springer, Berlin Heidelberg New York, pp 99–104

Pellizzari ED, Zweidinger RA, Sheldon LS (1988) Breath sampling. IARC Sci Publ 85:255–266

Wallace LA, Pellizzari ED (1986) Personal air exposures and breath concentrations of benzene and other volatile hydrocarbons for smokers and non-smokers. Toxicol Lett 35:113–116

Wallace LA, Pellizzari ED, Martwell TD, Perritt R, Ziegenfus R (1987) Exposures to benzene and other volatile compounds from active and passive smoking. Arch Environ Health 42:272–279

Comparative Investigation of Genotoxic and Nongenotoxic Mechanisms and Their Relevance in Carcinogenesis Induced by Airborne Particulates and Automobile Exhaust Particulates

N.H. Seemayer, W. Hadnagy, and R. Tomingas

Medizinisches Institut für Umwelthygiene and der Heinrich-Heine-Universität, Gurlittstraße 53, W-4000 Düsseldorf 1, FRG

Introduction

The most important sources of air pollutants are industrial processes, power generation, traffic, waste incineration, and fuel or coal combustion for space heating (Fishbein 1990). Nearly 700 mostly organic compounds have been detected as air pollutants, among them potential and proven mutagens and carcinogens (Helmes et al. 1982; Schlipköter 1983). In addition to gaseous pollutants, airborne particulates are of special importance. Most organic substances are found in fine dust particles, which as respirable particulate matter with a particle diameter smaller than 3.5 µm can reach the bronchoalveolar space of the human lung (Hileman 1981). Genotoxic activity and rodent-derived airborne allergens are mostly associated with this fraction of fine particles (Talcott and Harger 1980; Corn et al. 1988). Genotoxic activity of airborne particulates leading to mutation and cancer has been well documented (Chrisp and Fisher 1980; Epstein et al. 1979; Hughes et al. 1980). Nongenotoxic or epigenetic effects have not been investigated thoroughly. To avoid an underestimation of the mutagenic and carcinogenic potential of airborne particulates, nongenotoxic or epigenetic effects leading to mutation and cancer must be considered (Williams 1983; ICPEMC 1984; Tennant 1988). In this study we report the genotoxic and nongenotoxic effects of two samples of airborne particulates collected in the highly industrialized Rhine-Ruhr district (FRG) and of two samples of exhaust particles from automobiles driven with leaded and unleaded gasoline, utilizing human and rodent tissue culture cells.

U. Mohr et al. (Eds.)
Advances in Controlled Clinical
Inhalation Studies
© Springer-Verlag Berlin Heidelberg 1993

Material and Methods

Samples of airborne particulates were collected utilizing a high-volume sampler HVS 150 (Ströhlein Instruments) equipped with glass fiber filters. Collection was performed at the end of the winter in 1987 in an urban area (Düsseldorf; global extract GEX 36) and in a highly industrialized area (Duisburg; GEX 37). Substances were extracted from filters with dichloromethane and quantitatively transferred to dimethyl sulfoxide (DMSO) as reported earlier (Seemayer et al. 1984, 1990). Samples of car exhaust particles were collected, extracted, and transferred to DMSO as previously described in detail (Hadnagy and Seemayer 1986, 1989).

For the detection of "sister chromatid exchanges" (SCEs), human lymphocytes were cultivated as whole blood cultures in chromosome medium 1A with phytohemagglutinin (Gibco) and 7.5 µg bromodeoxyuridine at 37°C for 72 h, the last 3 h in the presence of demecolcine (Colcemid; 0.2 µg/ml). Various concentrations of the test extracts were added at the beginning of cultivation. Hypotonic treatment of lymphocytes, fixation, slide preparation, and staining by the fluorescent plus Giemsa (FPG) technique has been described in detail previously (Hadnagy et al. 1986).

Cell transformation assay was outlined previously (Seemayer et al. 1984, 1986). Briefly, logarithmically growing cultures of Syrian hamster kidney (SHK) cells were exposed for 18 h to various concentrations of extracts. Thereafter, kidney cultures were infected with simian virus SV-40 (strain Rh 911) at a multiplicity of infection (MOI) of 300–500 ID_{50}, followed by a cultivation period of 4 weeks at 37°C. After fixation and staining the number of transformed colonies was determined macroscopically and verified microscopically.

Mitotic profile studies were conducted by determining the mitotic index scoring 1000 cells of logarithmically growing cultures of Chinese hamster lung cells (V79) treated with various concentrations of extracts for 16 h as described previously (Hadnagy and Seemayer 1988). Additionally, cell division disturbances were evaluated by scoring so-called "initial C metaphases" and "full C metaphases."

Aneuploidy assay was performed as described earlier (Hadnagy and Seemayer 1988). Briefly, after a treatment period with extracts of 16 h, V79 cell cultures were rinsed and incubated with fresh medium for further 26 h, the last 2 h in presence of demecolcine (0.2 µg/ml). Metaphase preparations were scored for numerical chromosome alterations such as hyperdiploidy and polyploidy.

Results

In our study we compared the genotoxic and nongenotoxic activity of two samples of airborne particulates from the atmosphere (Figs. 1, 2) with two

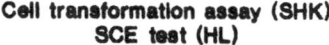

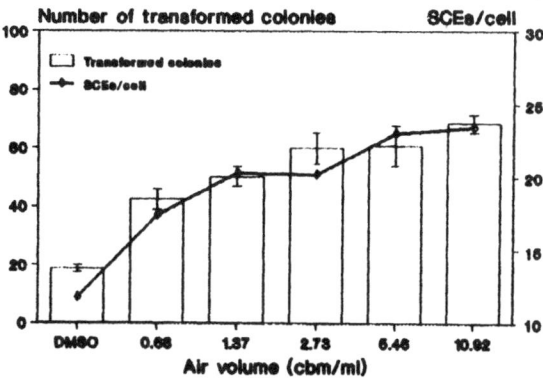

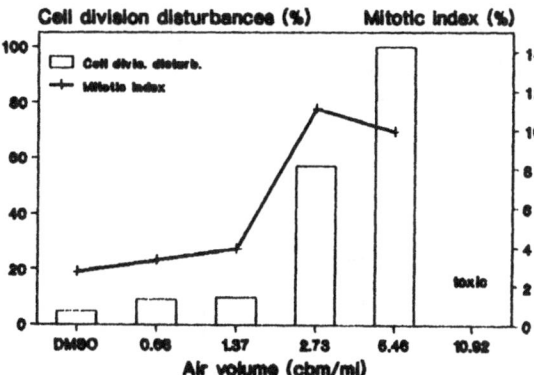

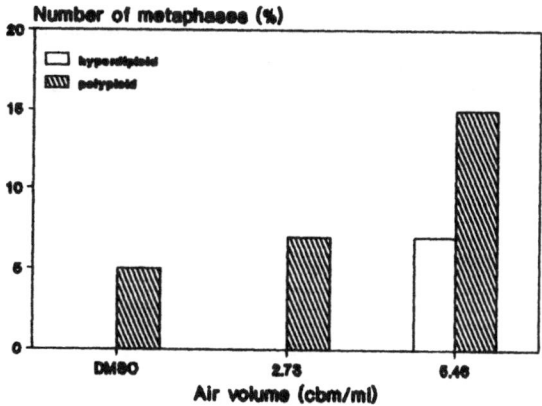

Fig. 1. Genotoxic and nongenotoxic effects induced by extract of airborne particulates (GEX 36)

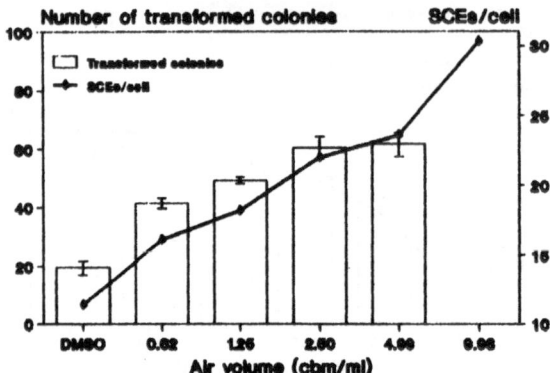

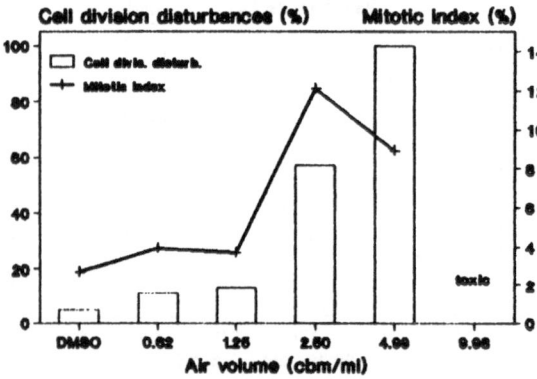

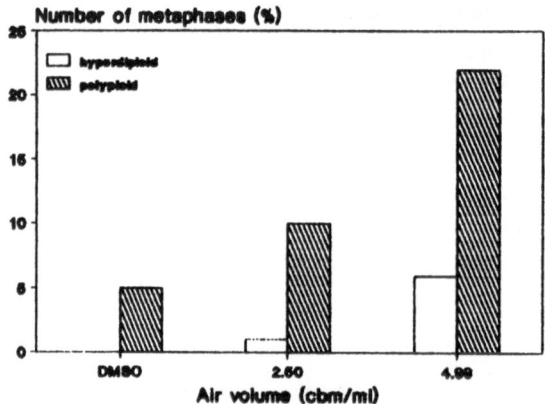

Fig. 2. Genotoxic and nongenotoxic effects induced by extract of airborne particulates (GEX 37)

samples of exhaust particles from automobiles driven with leaded and unleaded gasoline (Figs. 3, 4).

Extract of airborne particulates from the urban area (GEX 36) and from the highly industrialized area (GEX 37) led to genotoxic effects as shown by a dose-dependent induction of SCEs in human lymphocytes and the "enhancement" of malignant cell transformation of SHK cells. Significant effects were obtained with quantities of extractable substances corresponding to airborne particulates from approximately $0.6\,m^3$ air. Nongenotoxic effects were demonstrated by an increased mitotic index, cell division disturbances, and numerical chromosome alterations on V79 cells. In comparison to control (2.7%) the mitotic index increased to 11%–12% for GEX 36 and GEX 37. The effective dosage of extracts corresponded to particulates from air volumes of $2.5-5.5\,m^3$. In the same concentration range cell division disturbances were observed at frequencies from 60% to 100%. At lower concentrations "initial" and "full" C metaphases were observed. At higher concentrations almost only "full C-metaphases" were detected. As a consequence of cell division disturbances a dose-dependent increase in numerical chromosome alterations such as hyperdiploidy and polyploidy was found in subsequent cell divisions of V79 cells.

For the two samples of exhaust particles the SCE assay revealed no or a moderate increase in the SCE frequency. A significant increase was found only at the highest tested concentration of $10\,\mu g/ml$ for the sample obtained from the automobile driven with leaded gasoline. In the cell transformation assay a dose-dependent increase in transformed colonies was observed with both samples but was more pronounced for particles generated by the automobile driven with leaded gasoline. A strong increase in the mitotic index was observed at 5 and $10\,\mu g/ml$ (leaded gasoline) and at 40 and $60\mu g/ml$ (unleaded gasoline). In the same manner cell division disturbances increased from values of about 10% (control) to values of 80% to nearly 100%. These values remained unchanged for particulate exhaust from the automobile driven with unleaded gasoline at 80 and $100\,\mu g/ml$, whereas the mitotic index decreased due to cytotoxicity. The incidence of numerical chromosome alterations reflected the results of the mitotic profile studies. The induction of hyperdiploid and polyploid cells can be attributed to cell division disturbances.

Discussion

Airborne particulates by their mutagenic and carcinogenic activity pose a health risk for humans by inhalation (Fishbein 1990; Seemayer et al. 1990; Tomatis 1990). Employing the *Salmonella* microsome assay (Ames test), genotoxic activity of airborne particulates has been well documented (Dehnen et al. 1977; Krishna et al. 1983; Moller and Alfheim 1983; Talcot and Wei 1977). In vitro mammalian cell systems were utilized to determine

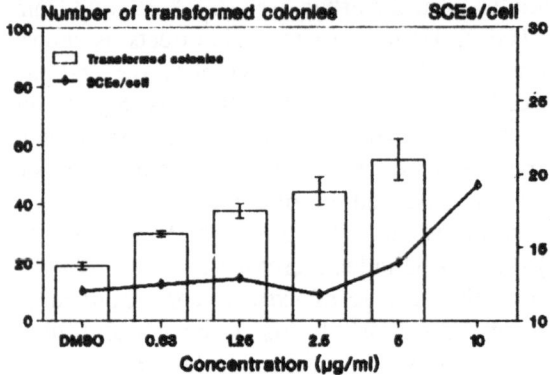

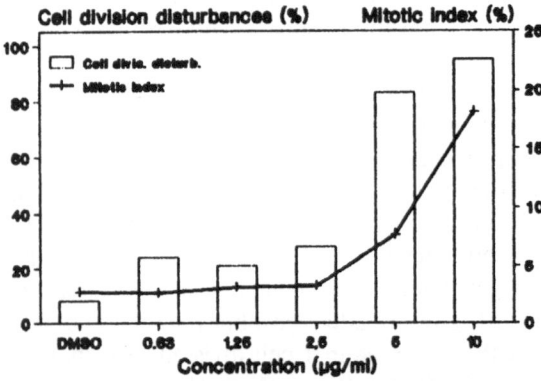

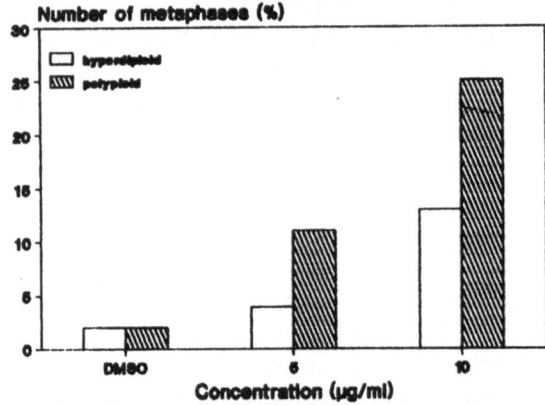

Fig. 3. Genotoxic and nongenotoxic effects caused by extract of exhaust particles from leaded gasoline powered engine

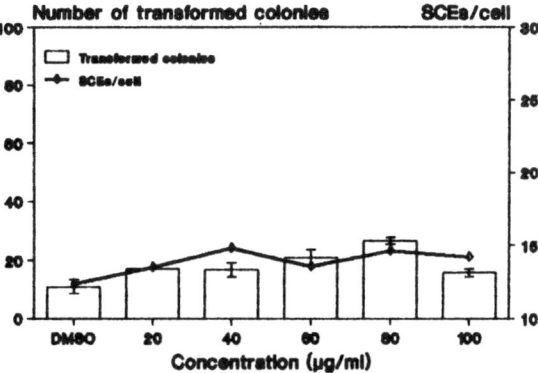

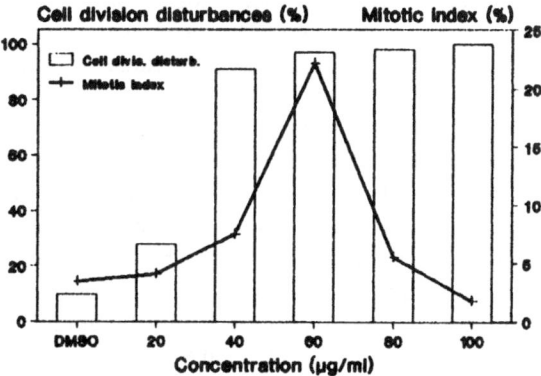

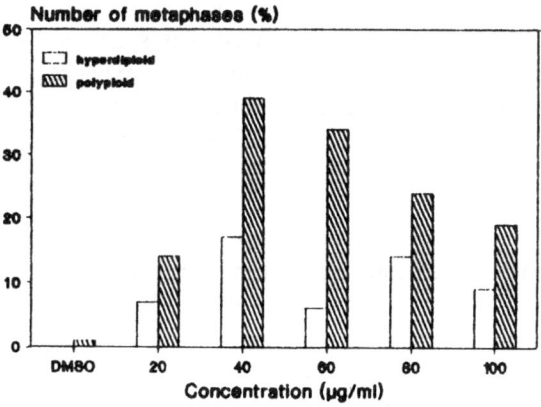

Fig. 4. Genotoxic and nongenotoxic effects caused by extract of exhaust particles from unleaded gasoline powered engine

genotoxicity of airborne particulates by diverse endpoints. Several authors reported induction of SCEs in rodent and human cells by extracts of airborne particulates (Alink et al. 1983; Hadnagy et al. 1986; van Houdt et al. 1984; Krishna et al. 1984; Lockhard et al. 1981; Motykiewicz et al. 1990; de Raat 1983; Schürer et al. 1980, 1983; Seemayer et al. 1984, 1990). Furthermore, gene mutations were demonstrated in mammalian cell cultures exposed to extracts of airborne particulates (Courtois et al. 1988; Seemayer et al. 1988). "Enhanced" malignant cell transformation was repeatedly reported with various samples of airborne particulates (Seemayer et al. 1984, 1986, 1990). Enhancement of viral transformation of SHK cells infected with simian adenovirus SA7 or simian virus SV40 was demonstrated with extracts of particulates of diesel and gasoline engine emissions (Casto et al. 1980; Hadnagy and Seemayer 1989; Lewtas 1983). Most short-term bioassays utilizing bacterial or mammalian cells are appropriate for the detection of genotoxic or mutagenic carcinogens (Dunkel and Williams 1981; Harnden 1978). Therefore, inadequate evidence was obtained with nonmutagenic, nongenotoxic, or epigenetic carcinogens (Barrett et al. 1985; von Borstel and Mehta 1982; ICPEMC 1984; Tennant et al. 1987; Tennant 1988). While genotoxic effects cause lesions of DNA, nongenotoxic or epigenetic effects can induce alterations of kinetochors, centromeres, and spindles affecting microtubule dynamics and chromosome movement leading to aneuploidy (Barrett et al. 1985; Hadnagy and Seemayer 1986, 1989; Motykiewicz 1990, 1991). Earlier reports (Hadnagy et al. 1986; Hadnagy and Seemayer 1987, 1989) and results presented here demonstrate that airborne particulates and exhaust particulates from automobiles driven with leaded or unleaded gasoline exert both a genotoxic and a remarkable nongenotoxic activity by affecting the spindle apparatus, with the result of cell division disturbances and aneuploidy. Recently Motykiewicz et al. (1991) reported strong cell division disturbances and numerical chromosome alterations in V79 cells exposed to organic extracts of airborne particulates, collected in the highly polluted industrial region of Silesia (Poland). Spindle poisons from airborne particulates acting by a nongenotoxic mechanism have so far not been identified. For exhaust particles from gasoline-powered engines suspected compounds may be trialkyl lead, the degradation product of the antiknock additive tetraalkyl lead, and benzene, especially its derivatives such as hydroquinone (Fishbein 1990; Hadnagy and Seemayer 1990).

Summarizing our results, complex chemical mixtures such as airborne particulates and exhaust particles from gasoline-powered engines act on mammalian cells by genotoxic and nongenotoxic or aneugenic mechanisms. Both mechanisms can lead to malignant cell transformation and cancer. To avoid an underestimation of carcinogenic risk to humans by airborne pollutants not only genotoxic but also nongenotoxic and aneugenic effects must be taken into consideration.

References

Alink GM, Smit HA, van Houdt JJ, Kolkman JR, Boley JSM (1983) Mutagenic activity of airborne particulates at non-industrial locations. Mutat Res 116: 21–34

Barrett JC, Oshimura M, Tanaka N, Tsutsui T (1985) Role of aneuploidy in early and late stages of neoplastic progression of Syrian hamster embryo cells in culture. In: Dellarco VL, Voytek PE, Hollaender A (eds) Aneuploidy. Plenum, New York, pp 523–538

Casto B, Hatch GG, Huang SL, Huisingh JL, Nesnow S, Waters MD (1980) Mutagenic and carcinogenic potency of extracts of diesel and related environmental emissions: in vitro mutagenesis and oncogenic transformation. In: Pepelko WE, Danner RM, Clarke NA (eds) Health effects of diesel engine emissions. US Environmental Protection Agency, Cincinnati, pp 843–860

Chrisp CE, Fisher GL (1980) Mutagenicity of airborne particles. Mutat Res 76:143–164

Corn M, Koegel A, Hall T, Scott A, Newill C, Evans R (1988) Characteristics of airborne particles associated with animal allergy in laboratory workers. Ann Occup. Hyg 32:435–446

Courtois YA, Min S, Lachenal C, Jacquot-Deschamps JM, Callais F, Festy B (1988) Genotoxicity of organic extracts from atmospheric particles. Ann. NY Acad Sci 534:724–740

Dehnen W, Pitz N, Tomingas R (1977) The mutagenicity of airborne particulate pollutants. Cancer Lett 4:5–12

de Raat WK (1983) Genotoxicity of aerosol extracts: some methodological aspects and the contribution of urban and industrial locations. Mutat Res 116:47–63

Dunkel VC, Williams GM (1981) End points in in vitro test systems for carcinogenicity and mutagenicity. In: Richmond CR, Walsh P, Copenhaver ED (eds) 3rd Health Risk Anal Proc Life Sci Symp Franklin Institute, Philadelphia, pp 237–248

Epstein SS, Fuji K, Asahina S (1979) Carcinogenicty of a composite organic extract of urban particulate atmospheric pollutants following subcutaneous injection into infant mice. Environ Res 19:163–176

Fishbein L (1990) Sources, nature and levels of air pollutants. In: Tomatis L (ed) Air pollution and human cancer. Springer, Berlin Heidelberg New York, pp 9–34

Hadnagy W, Seemayer NH (1986) Induction of C-type metaphases and aneuploidy in cultures of V79 cells exposed to extract of automobile exhaust particulates. Mutagenesis 1:445–448

Hadnagy W, Seemayer NH (1987) Comparative investigation on the genotoxicity of city smog and automobile exhaust particulates. J Aerosol Sci 18:697–699

Hadnagy W, Seemayer NH (1988) Cytotoxic and genotoxic effects of extract of particulate emissions from a gasoline-powered engine. Environ Mol Mutagen 12:385–396

Hadnagy W, Seemayer NH (1989) Genotoxicity of particulate emissions from gasoline-powered engines evaluated by short-term bioassays. Exp Pathol 37: 43–50

Hadnagy W, Seemayer NH (1990) The role of nongenotoxic mechanisms in carcinogenicity by airborne particulate pollutants. In: Seemayer NH, Hadnagy W (eds) Environmental hygiene II. Spinger, Berlin Heidelberg New York, pp 11–16

Hadnagy W, Seemayer NH, Tomingas R (1986) Cytogenetic effects of airborne particulate matter on human lymphocytes in vitro. Mutat Res 175:97–101

Harnden DG (1978) Relevance of short-terme carcinogenicity tests to the study of the carcinogenic potential of urban air. Environ Health Perspect 22:67–70

Helmes et al. (1982) Evaluation and classification of the potential carcinogenicity of organic air pollutants. J Environ Sci Health [A] 17/3:321–389

Hileman B (1981) Particulate matter: the inhalable variety. Environ Sci Technol 15:981–986

Hughes TJ, Pellizzari E, Little L, Sparacino C, Kobler A (1980) Ambient air pollutants: collection chemical characterization and mutagenic testing. Mutat Res 76:51–83

ICPEMC (1984) Report of ICPEMC Task Group on the differentiation between genotoxic and non-genotoxic carcinogens. Mutat Res 133:1–49

Krishna G, Ong T, Whong WZ, Nath J (1983) Mutagenicity studies with ambient airborne particles: I. Comparison of solvent systems. Mutat Res 12:113–120

Krishna G, Nath J, Ong T (1984) Correlative genotoxicity studies of airborne particles in Salmonella typhimurium and cultured human lymphocytes. Environ Mutagen 6:585–592

Lewtas J (1983) Evaluation of the mutagenicity and carcinogenicity of motor vehicle emissions in short-term bioassays. Environ Health Perspect 47:141–152

Lockard JM, Viau CJ, Lee-Stephens C, Caldwell JC, Wojciechowski JP, Enoch HG, Sabharwal PS (1981) Induction of sister chromatid exchanges and bacterial revertants by organic extracts of airborne particles. Environ Mutagen 3:671–681

Moller M, Alfheim I (1983) Mutagenicity of air samples from various combustion sources, Mutat Res 116:35–46

Motykiewicz G, Michalska J, Szeliga J, Konopacka M, Tkocz A, Hadnagy W, Chorazy M, Seemayer NH (1990) Genotoxicity of airborne suspended matter determined by in vitro and in vivo short-term assays. In: Seemayer NH, Hadnagy W (eds) Environmental hygiene II. Springer, Berlin Heidelberg New York, pp 17–21

Motykiewicz G, Hadnagy W, Seemayer NH, Szeliga J, Tkocz A, Chorazy M (1991) Influence of airborne suspended matter on mitotic cell division. Mutat Res 260:195–202

Schlipköter H-W (1983) Lufthygienische Probleme der Großstadt. Arcus 5:244–250

Schürer CC, Manojlovic N, Seemayer NH (1980) Induction of "sister chromatid exchanges" in human cells in vitro by the mutagenic effect of city-smog extract. Mutat Res 74:164–165

Schürer CC, Seemayer NH, Manojlovic N (1983) Induction of "sister chromatid exchanges" in human lympocytes in vitro by extracts of airborne particulate matter: comparison of samples from highly industrialized area followed up for several years. Mutat Res 113:347

Seemayer NH, Manojlovic N, Schürer CC, Tomingas R (1984) Cell cultures as a tool for detection of cytotoxic, mutagenic and carcinogenic activity of airborne particulate matter. J Aerosol Sci 15:426–439

Seemayer NH, Manojlovic N, Tomingas R (1986) Induction of malignant cell transformation in vitro by extract and fractions of airborne particulate matter. J Aerosol Sci 17:356–360

Seemayer NH, Manojlovic N, König H, Tomingas R (1988) Comparative investigation of carcinogenic and mutagenic activity of airborne particulate matter from polluted areas using human and rodent tissue culture cells. Ann Occup Hyg 32:247–256

Seemayer NH, Hadnagy W, Tomingas R (1990) Evaluation of health risks by airborne particulates from in vitro cyto- and genotoxicity testing on human rodent tissue culture cells: a longitudinal study from 1975 until now. J Aerosol Sci 21:501–504

Talcot R, Harger W (1980) Airborne mutagens from particles of respirable size. Mutat Res 79:177–186

Talcot R, Wei E (1977) Airborne mutagens bioassayed in Salmonella typhimurium. J Natl Cancer Inst 58:449–451

Tennant R (1988) Relationship between in vitro genetic toxicity and carcinogenicity studies in animals. Ann NY Acad Sci 534:127–132

Tennant R, Margolin BH, Shelby MD et al. (1987) Prediction of chemical carcinogenicity in rodents from in vitro genetic toxicity assays. Science 236:933–944

Tomatis L (1990) Air pollution and cancer: an old and new problem. In: Tomatis L (ed) Air pollution and human cancer. Springer, Berlin Heidelberg New York, pp 1–7

van Houdt JJ, Jongen WMF, Alink GM, Bolej JSM (1984) Mutagenic activity of airborne particulates inside and outside homes. Environ Mutagen 6:861–869

von Borstel RC, Mehta RD (1982) Nonmutagenic carcinogens. In: Mutagens in our environment. Liss, New York, pp 47–57

Williams GM (1983) Genotoxic and epigenetic carcinogens: their identification and significance. Ann NY Acad Sci 407:328–333

Gestational Inhalation of Indoor Air Pollution Alters Neonatal Reflex Development and Fetal Hematology

J. SINGH

Stillman College, Department of Biology, P.O. Box 1430, Tuscaloosa, AL 35403, USA

Introduction

Although most studies have traditionally focused on the health effects of outdoor air, it is now apparent that elevated air pollution of carbon monoxide (CO) and nitrogen dioxide (NO_2) are common in indoor air. Carbon monoxide has numerous sources in the home and the office (Caceres et al. 1983; Cox and Wichelow 1985; Nagda and Koontz 1985; Samet et al. 1987; Sterling et al. 1981). Offices may be contaminated by outdoor CO because of building design problems (Wallace 1983). Furthermore, indoor CO levels in buildings are usually related to nearby outdoor CO levels (Yocom 1982); they increase more slowly than outdoor levels, but once built up, they remain higher for longer periods (Yocom 1982).

Numerous studies have reported elevated indoor levels of NO_2 in homes with unvented gas appliances (Chan et al. 1990; Melia et al. 1978; Spengler and Sexton 1983; Sterling et al. 1981; Wade et al. 1975). Exposure to NO_2 from gas cooking stoves and ovens is widespread (Samet et al. 1987; Yocom 1982). About 50% of homes in the United States have gas cooking stoves and in some urban areas more than 90% of homes are equipped with gas appliances (US Department of Commerce 1983).

Indoor air quality is not directly regulated, and use of some sources of indoor air pollution, such as wood stoves and kerosene heaters, is rapidly increasing. The present study was carried out to assess the effect of gestational inhalation of CO and NO_2 on neonatal reflex development and fetal hematology.

Materials and Methods

Adult female albino mice of the CD-1 strain (Charles River, Wilmington, MA) were maintained with continuous access to food and water, on a 12/12 h light/dark cycle, and at a room temperature of 23 ± 2°C. Females

U. Mohr et al. (Eds.)
Advances in Controlled Clinical
Inhalation Studies
© Springer-Verlag Berlin Heidelberg 1993

were bred overnight and the day on which a copulation plug was found was designated day 1 of gestation. The pregnant dams were exposed to 0 (control), 65, or 125 ppm CO in air in Plexiglas environmental chambers from gestation days 7–18 in the first experiment; to 0 (control), 22, or 45 ppm of NO_2 in air in the second experiment; and to 0 (control) and 250 ppm of CO in air in the third experiment. The controls were also exposed to the chamber environment and compressed air flows. The gas-air mixture flows were set at 450 ml per minute. The concentrations of CO were monitored by the Non-Dispersive Infrared Analyzer, Model 870 (Beckman Instruments, La Habra, CA) and that of NO_2 by the Saltzman and Wartburg method (Saltzman and Wartburg 1965).

The animals of the first two experiments were taken out of the chamber environment on the 18th gestation day and allowed to deliver. The number of live pups and their weight were recorded on day of birth. In order to assess the effect of CO and NO_2 exposure on neonatal development, the righting reflex, negative geotaxis, and aerial righting tests were carried out (Singh 1986, 1988).

Animals of the third experiment were killed on gestation day 18, and 44.7 µl blood samples were collected from the mothers and fetuses. The samples were dissolved in 10 ml isoton, and the quantities of white blood cells (WBC), red blood cells (RBC), hemoglobin (HGB), and hematocrit (HCT) were determined by the use of a Coulter Counter, Model ZBI.

All data were analyzed using the litter as the sampling unit. Analysis of variance was used for comparison between control and test groups for all data (Steel and Torrie 1980). The coefficient of correlation between birth weight and righting reflex time, negative geotaxis time, and aerial righting scores were calculated. Results reported are based on data from 12 litters in each concentration of each air pollutant gas for the first two experiments and 10 litters each for the control and CO concentration in the third experiment.

Results

Exposure to CO did not have significant effect on the birth weight of pups; however, dose-dependent birth weight deficits were apparent (Fig. 1). NO_2 exposure at both levels significantly reduced the birth weight of pups (Fig. 2).

The correlation between birth weight and surface righting time on postnatal day (PND) 1 of pups from CO-exposed dams was $r = -0.930$ (Fig. 1). The correlation between birth weight and negative geotaxis time on PND 10 of the pups was $r = -0.869$. That between birth weight and aerial righting score on PND 12 of the pups was $r = +0.968$ (Fig. 1).

The correlation between birth weight and surface righting time on PND 1 of pups from NO_2-exposed animals was $r = -0.733$ (Fig. 2) and that

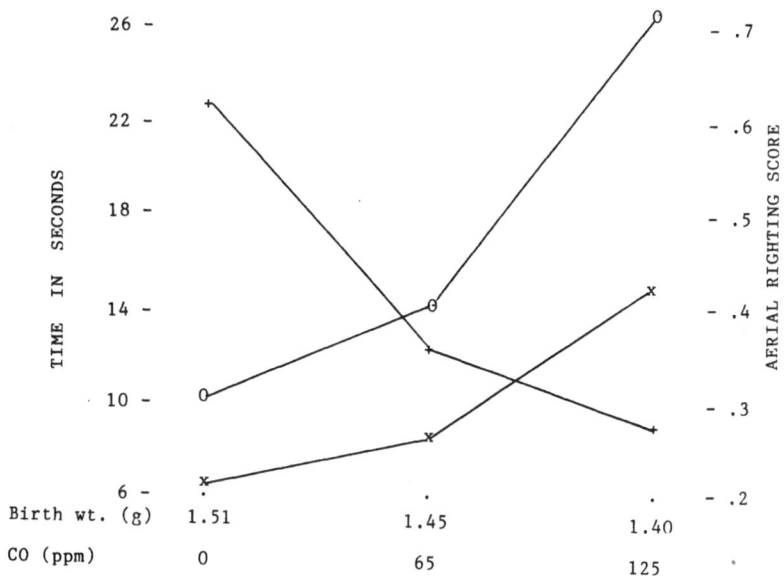

Fig. 1. Relationship between birth weight and aerial righting score (+---+; $r = +0.968$), surface righting time (0---0; $r = -0.930$), and negative geotaxis time (×---×; $r = -0.869$). Statistical significance for each: $p \leqslant 0.01$

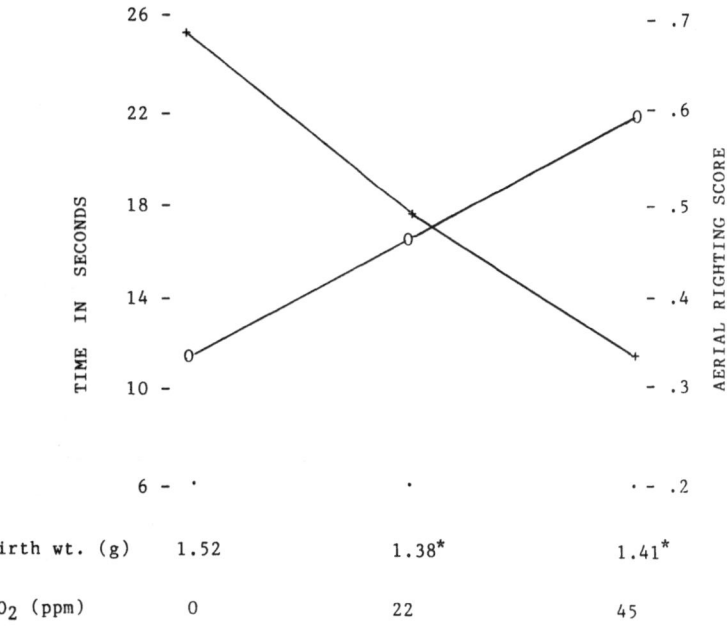

Fig. 2. Relationship between birth weight and aerial righting score (+---+; $r = 0.660$) and surface righting time (0---0; $r = -0.733$). Statistical significance for each: $p \leqslant 0.05$

Table 1. Effect of gestational inhalation of carbon monoxide on the mean (±SE) parameters of maternal and fetal blood

	WBC (10³)	RBC (10⁶)	HCT (%)	HGB (%)
Maternal				
0 ppm CO	5.53 ± 0.45	5.86 ± 0.33	43.10 ± 2.61	14.29 ± 0.90
250 ppm CO	7.32 ± 0.63*	5.07 ± 0.32	38.82 ± 2.82*	14.11 ± 0.63
Fetal				
0 ppm CO	6.65 ± 0.37	6.69 ± 0.37	49.27 ± 3.08	15.53 ± 0.72
250 ppm CO	7.56 ± 0.86	5.49 ± 0.44	39.56 ± 3.57	14.32 ± 1.00

* Significantly different from control at $p \leqslant 0.05$.

between birth weight and aerial righting score on PND 12 of the pups was $r = +0.660$ (Fig. 2).

The data indicate that the quantities of WBC, RBC, HCT, and HGB were higher in the fetal blood than that of the maternal blood at the control as well as at the 250-ppm CO exposure level (Table 1). The quantities of WBC and HCT in the maternal blood were significantly increased and decreased respectively, by the CO exposure.

Discussion

The results of the present study indicate that gestational inhalation of CO or NO_2 produces birth weight deficits in pups, delayed neonatal reflex development of pups, and altered maternal and fetal hematology. This finding is important because it may be symptomatic of an alteration in the neuromuscular coordination and immune system of the developing offspring as a result of early indoor pollution exposure.

The results also indicate that the birth weight deficits produced by the CO or NO_2 exposure may be a key indicator of neonatal reflex development. The birth weight deficits may mean fewer or smaller cells in the organs of the developing offspring. Smaller or fewer cells in the neuro-muscular organs of the offspring may result in delayed reflex development.

The results reported here are similar to those reported by other studies on CO (Singh 1984, 1986; Tachi and Aoyama 1990) and NO_2 (Singh 1988) exposures. These studies reported that prenatal exposure to CO or NO_2 reduces the fetal weight; and functional deficits in the neonate (Singh 1986, 1988) may accompany the birth weight deficits. However, none of the studies has reported a strong relationship between birth weight deficits due to air pollution and delays in reflex development.

The energy requirements of the brain are among the highest in the body, and the brain needs one fifth of the oxygen consumed by the entire body at rest (Ketty 1979). Therefore, the central nervous system may be one of the most sensitive systems to hypoxia (Towbin 1969). The chronic CO exposure in the present study may have reduced the oxygen supply to the developing brain, which manifests as delayed reflex development in the offspring.

The results of the present study also indicate that the quantities of WBC, RBC, HCT, and HGB were higher in the fetal blood from CO-exposed mothers. This may be a quantitative adaptation by the developing fetus which compensates for alterations in oxygen availability in the fetal environment (Hochachka and Somero 1973).

The data suggest that gestational inhalation of indoor air pollutants can result in functional deficits in the offspring and alters fetal hematology. The clinical implication of the results suggest the monitoring of children potentially exposed to indoor air pollution containing CO or NO_2.

Acknowledgement. This work was supported by NIH grant no. 5 S14 RR02867.

References

Caceres T, Soto H, Lissi E (1983) Indoor house pollution: appliance emissions and indoor ambient concentrations. Atmos Environ 17:1009–1013

Chan CC, Yanagisawa Y, Spengler JD (1990) Personal and indoor/outdoor nitrogen dioxide exposure assessment of 23 homes in Taiwan. Toxicol Ind Health 6:173–182

Cox BD, Wichelow MJ (1985) Carbon monoxide levels in the breath of smokers and nonsmokers: effect of domestic heating systems. J Epidemiol Community Health 39:75–78

Hochachka PW, Somero GN (1973) The basic strategies of biochemical adaptation. In: Strategies of biochemical adaptation. Saunders, Philadelphia, pp 332–333

Ketty SS (1979) Disorders of human brain. In: Flanagan D (ed) The brain. Freeman, San Francisco, pp 120–127

Melia RJW, Florey CDuV, Darby SC, Palmes ED, Goldstein BD (1978) Differences in NO_2 levels in kitchens with gas or electric cookers. Atmos Environ 12:1379–1381

Nagda NL, Koontz MD (1985) Microenvironmental and total exposure to carbon monoxide for three pollution subgroups. JAPCA 35:134–137

Saltzman BE, Wartburg AF (1965) Precision flow dilution system for standard low concentrations of nitrogen dioxide. Anal Chem 37:1261–1265

Samet JM, Marbury MC, Spengler JD (1987) Health effects and sources of indoor air pollution: I. Am Rev Respir Dis 136:1486–1508

Singh J (1984) Postnatal behavioral alteration by prenatal carbon monoxide exposure at low concentrations. Teratology 29:8B

Singh J (1986) Early behavioral alteration in mice following prenatal carbon monoxide exposure. Neurotoxicology 7:475–482

Singh J (1988) Nitrogen dioxide exposure alters neonatal development. Neurotoxicology 9:545–550

Spengler JD, Sexton K (1983) Indoor air pollution: a public health perspective. Science 221:9–17

Steel RGD, Torrie JH (1980) Analysis of variance: III. Factorial experiments. In: Napier C, Maisel JW (eds) Principles and procedures of statistics. McGraw Hill, New York, pp 336–347

Sterling TD, Dimich H, Kobayashi D (1981) Use of gas ranges for cooking and heating in urban dwellings. JAPCA 32:162–165

Tachi N, Aoyama M (1990) Postnatal growth in rats prenatally exposed to cigarette smoke or carbon monoxide. Bull Environ Contam Toxicol 45:641–648

Towbin A (1969) Cerebral hypoxic damage in fetus and newborn: basic pattern and their clinical significance. Arch Neurol 20:35–43

US Department of Commerce, Bureau of Census (1983) 1980 census of housing, vol I. Characteristics of housing units. Chap. B. Detailed housing characteristics. United States Summary. US government printing office, Washington, DC, T.82–T.153, HC80-1-B1

Wade WA, Cote WA, Yocom JE (1975) A study of indoor air quality. JAPCA 25:933–939

Wallace LA (1983) Carbon monoxide in air and breath of employees in an under ground office. JAPCA 33:678–682

Yocom JE (1982) Indoor-outdoor air quality relationships – a critical review. JAPCA 35:500–520

Aerosol Deposition Pattern of Technetium-99m-Labeled Fenoterol After Inhalation from Three Devices in Healthy Volunteers

J. Waitzinger[1], T. Zimmermann[2], A. Hammermaier[1], W. Fleischer[2], G. Pabst[3], and H. Jaeger[4]

[1] Klinische Leitung Nuklearpharmakologie, L.A.B. GmbH & Co, Wegener Straße 13, W-7910 Neu-Ulm, FRG
[2] Boehringer Ingelheim KG, Abteilung Medizin, Fachbereich Pneumologie, Binger Straße 173, W-6507 Ingelheim, FRG
[3] Leitung Biometries, L.A.B. GmbH & Co, Wegener Straße 13, W-7910 Neu-Ulm, FRG
[4] Wissenschaftlicher Direktor, L.A.B. GmbH & Co, Wegener Straße 13, W-7910 Neu-Ulm, FRG

Introduction

For drugs administered by inhalation, the site of deposition of aerosol drops has a crucial bearing on its effect. If it is possible to produce a picture of the site of deposition, the possibility exists to correlate these results with clinical experience and therefore to reduce clinical investigations with patients in the future. Using a simple procedure, it is possible to label a β_2-agonist with the gamma emitter technetium-99 m (^{99m}Tc). A study using radioactive labeling was planned as a nonradioactive study; this was not suitable for the investigation of the lung deposition pattern. Now, in this study the lung deposition pattern of ^{99m}Tc-labeled fenoterol (Berotec) was investigated after aerosol inhalation from a metered dose inhaler (MDI), from an MDI with spacer, and from an ultrasonic nebulizer.

Material and Methods

Selection of Volunteers. Twelve healthy male volunteers aged over 50 years and within ±15% of the weight limits of the Metropolitan Life Insurance tables were included in this study. Subjects were not allowed to participate in the study if functional vital capacity was lower than 3.7 l and/or forced expiration volume was lower than 3.0 l. Before being entered into the study all volunteers underwent a medical examination including 12-lead ECG and clinical laboratory screening and lung function test. The clinical and

U. Mohr et al. (Eds.)
Advances in Controlled Clinical
Inhalation Studies
© Springer-Verlag Berlin Heidelberg 1993

analytical tests performed showed good health status at the time of prestudy screening. The subjects gave their informed consent.

Study Design. The open, nonrandomized, non-placebo-controlled study was conducted with a three-way design and a wash-out phase of 1 week between treatments. An aerosol puff or ultrasonic nebulized drop of fenoterol solution of approximately 0.2 mg ^{99m}Tc-labeled fenoterol hydrobromide with a single radioactivity dose lower than 200 µCi was administered by inhalation. Labeling of fenoterol with ^{99m}Tc was performed by qualified staff. After drug administration a gamma camera acquisition of radioactive decay was performed from the posterior position.

Study Structure. The study was divided into three treatments (treatments A, B, and C) with similar structure. Fenoterol in the MDI and fenoterol in the solution used for the ultrasonic nebulizer (piezoelectric inhalation device, PID; Respimat, Boehringer Ingelheim; Lang 1962; Mercer et al. 1968) was labeled by a specific procedure in a controlled access area. Each subject was administered one of the test preparations once per treatment. The test preparations were administered by aerosol inhalation in a dose of 0.2 mg fenoterol. The following breathing maneuver was observed: Slow, deep inhalation by the mouthpiece (reaching vital capacity), holding breath for 5–10 s and afterwards forced expiration. Breathing in for treatment A started together with release of one aerosol puff and for treatment C together with initiating the PID. In treatment B the spacer was closed with a lid, one aerosol puff was released into the closed spacer, and breathing in started immediately after removal of the lid.

Determination of Radioactivity in the Body. The emitted counts were recorded from the dorsal position with a high-sensitive collimator in the energy window of 126–155 keV (the photopeak for ^{99m}Tc is at 140 keV). A 64 × 64 image matrix was used. Acquisition was started 1–5 min after application, continued for 20 min, and then stopped manually.

Evaluation. A quantitative evaluation was carried out by the regions-of-interest (ROI) method. The contour of the organ or device (spacer or mouthpiece) was marked with a paddle and integrated automatically to give total counts for each region. The ^{99m}Tc radioactivity distribution was printed on a color plotter. The following ROI were selected: treatment A (MDI): lungs, oropharynx and esophagus and stomach if visible, background; treatment B (MDI with spacer): lungs, oropharynx and esophagus and stomach if visible, spacer used; treatment C (PID): lungs, oropharynx and esophagus and stomach if visible, mouthpiece used.

Data Calculation and Statistical Procedures. The amounts of radioactivity administered in treatments were corrected for radioactive decay of [99m]Tc (half-life = 6.02 h). The measured radioactivity levels in the ROI were corrected for background. The background-corrected counts were then corrected for relative absorption in different tissues (factor 1.35 for oropharynx and esophagus, factor 1.91 for lung (Köhler et al. 1988). Relative deposition in whole lung (percentage) was compared between treatments by analysis of variance. Factors separated in the analysis of variance were subject and treatment effects.

Results

The test preparations were tolerated very well. No adverse events or adverse drug reactions occurred. The volunteers' state of health was not impaired by the study.

Gamma Scintigraphy. The proportion of counts after correction in whole lung versus the sum of whole lung, oropharynx, and esophagus represents the amount of fenoterol reaching its place of action relative to the body, and these percentages may be compared statistically between the treatments. The three treatments differed significantly with respect to the relative deposition pattern.

Mean relative ^{99m}Tc radioactivity deposition levels after correction by the absorption factors, not considering radioactivity found in the mouth-piece, were calculated as follows: treatment A: whole lung = 27.1%, oropharynx and esophagus = 72.9%; treatment B: whole lung = 29.9%, oropharynx and esophagus = 2.9%, spacer 67.2%; treatment C: whole lung = 23.3%, oropharynx and esophagus = 76.7% (Table 1). These results show a comparable relative drug deposition in the lung after inhalation from three different devices. The best relative lung deposition was seen using the MDI with spacer device. The results accord well with the pharmaceutical in vitro measurements of the different treatments and correspond with the results from therapeutic equivalence studies using the MDI versus the PID.

Table 1. Relative ^{99m}Tc radioactivity (mean levels) leaving the device used (excluding mouthpiece), corrected for background and normalized for relative absorption

	Treatment		
	A	B	C
Lung (factor 1.91)	27.1%	29.9%	23.3%
Oropharynx/esophagus (factor 1.35)	72.9%	2.9%	76.7%
Mean spacer	–	67.2%	–

Discussion

With respect to the relative radioactivity deposition pattern the deposition in the lung proved similar for the ultrasonic nebulizer (PID) and the MDI without spacer. The ultrasonic nebulizer therefore seems to be an alternative to the MDI containing chlorofluorocarbon propellant. The results for MDI without spacer are comparable to those reported by other authors (Köhler et al. 1988; Newman 1983).

The MDI with spacer proved best (a) comparing the relative deposition in the lung with the relative deposition in the body and (b) comparing the relative deposition in the lung with the relative deposition in the body and spacer, because the relative deposition in oropharynx and esophagus was reduced (Vidgren et al. 1987). This may be of clinical relevance, for example, for the administration of corticosteroids to reduce local side effects.

References

Köhler D, Fleischer W, Matthys H (1988) New method for easy labeling of beta-2-agonists in the metered dose inhaler with technetium 99m. Respiration 53:65

Lang RJ (1962) Ultrasonic atomization of liquids. J Acoust Soc Am 34:16

Mercer TT, Goddard RF, Fiores RL (1968) Output characteristics of three ultrasonic nebulizers. Ann Allergy 26:18

Newman SP (1983) Deposition and effects of inhalation aerosols, Draco, Lund, Sweden

Vidgren MT, Paronen TP, Karkainen A, Karjalainen P (1987) Effect of extension devices on the drug deposition from inhalation aerosols. Int J Pharmacol 39:107

Comparison of Bronchospasmolytic Effects of 200 µg Fenoterol After Inhalation with Respimat and Metered Dose Inhaler

T. Zimmermann[1], R. Stechert[2], H. Schweisfurth[3], and R. Wettengel[4]

[1] Boehringer Ingelheim KG, Abteilung Medizin, Fachbereich Pneumologie, Binger Straße 173, W-6507 Ingelheim, FRG
Jetzt: c/o G. POHL-BOSKAMP GmbH & Co., Med.-wiss. Abteilung, Kieler Straße 11, W-2214 Hohenlockstedt, FRG
[2] Boehringer Ingelheim, Klinische Entwicklung, Binger Straße 173, W-6507 Ingelheim, FRG
[3] Michelsberg Hospital, W-8732 Münnerstadt, FRG
[4] Karl-Hansen-Hospital, W-4792 Bad Lippspringe, FRG

Introduction

The piezoelectric inhalation device (PID, Respimat) is a pocket-sized ultrasonic nebulizer run on accumulators. A charger is provided. A compatible liquid metering cartridge has been developed specially for this device which releases metered amounts of medicinal solutions onto the atomizer plate, which oscillates in the ultrasonic zone. The conversion of mechanical deformation force to electric signals and vice versa is used in the PID to generate microfine liquid mist without pressure. The device is therefore a propellant-free alternative to the metered dose inhaler (MDI), reflecting the newest technology. Generation of the liquid mist uses the reverse piezoelectric effect. The atomization process takes approximately 1 s. By releasing the button on the PID, the compliant patient is able to coordinate triggering and inhalation. The range of particles produced by the Respimat corresponds to that of an MDI; 50% of the particles produced are less than 10 µm in diameter, the most common particle size being $d_t = 2.1$ µm.

This study compared the bronchodilator effect of inhaling 0.2 mg fenoterol hydrobromide (Berotec) over 6 h from the PID with that from the MDI.

Materials and Method

A total of 24 patients (13 women, 11 men) took part in the study. They were diagnosed as having stable obstructive airways disease and were aged

U. Mohr et al. (Eds.)
Advances in Controlled Clinical
Inhalation Studies
© Springer-Verlag Berlin Heidelberg 1993

between 28 and 76 years (median 56.5). All patients met the criteria for selection: at least 15% increase in forced expiratory volume in 1 s (FEV_1) 15 min after inhalation of one puff from the fenoterol MDI. The precise diagnosis was bronchial asthma with perennial symptoms in 15 patients, intrinsic asthma in 9, and mixed bronchial asthma in 6. In three cases the symptoms were described as mild, in eight as moderate, and in four as severe. Bronchitis was diagnosed in 12 patients, three of whom also had emphysema; thus three patients were suffering from both bronchial asthma and chronic obstructive bronchitis.

The trial protocol was observed at all times, and all patients completed the study in accordance with the trial protocol. This was a randomized, double-blind, crossover study with a double-dummy design, carried out at two centers, each with 12 patients. Treatment consisted of one actuation from the PID and one puff from the MDI. The dose on each administration was 0.2 mg fenoterol hydrobromide.

The principal parameters measured were maximum increase in FEV_1 and area under the time profile curve and maximum fall in total resistance (R_t) and area under the time profile curve. Other parameters included: resting vital capacity (VC), forced expiratory vital capacity (FVC), FEV_1, R_t, intrathoracic gas volume (IGV), and specific conductance (sG_{aw}). All parameters were calculated by means of whole-body plethysmography. Extrapulmonary parameters included blood pressure (systolic/diastolic, seated), adverse events (fine finger tremor with arms outstretched, etc.), handling, preference.

Patients were selected according to reversibility of their airways obstruction (at least 15% increase in FEV_1) following inhalation of one puff of Berotec, corresponding to 0.2 mg fenoterol. On 2 examination days lung function, blood pressure, and pulse rate were measured 15 min before administration of the allocated test drugs and 15, 30, 60, 120, 240, and 360 min after inhalation. A tremor score was also recorded.

Results

Results of the examination of data from all 24 patients are presented in Table 1. Following statistical examination to investigate the bioequivalence of the two dosage forms, the confidence interval was not completely within

Table 1. Maximum increase in FEV_1 as a percentage of baseline

Order of use	PID	MID
PID, MDI	54.1 ± 34.0	53.2 ± 23.5
MDI, PID	56.0 ± 29.2	48.1 ± 18.8
	55.0 ± 31.0 (Av.)	50.6 ± 27.0 (Av.)

Table 2. Area under the FEV_1/time (min) profile curve as a percentage of baseline

Order of use	PID	MID
PID, MDI	47 518 ± 8663	47 164 ± 7019
MDI, PID	49 747 ± 9295	47 927 ± 6934
	48 632 ± 8861 (Av.)	47 542 ± 6834 (Av.)

Table 3. Maximum relative decrease in R_t as a percentage off baseline

Order of use	PID	MID
PID, MDI	65.3 ± 13.1	60.7 ± 12.4
MDI, PID	53.1 ± 13.9	57.2 ± 11.0
	59.2 ± 14.6 (Av.)	59.0 ± 11.6 (Av.)

Table 4. Area under the R_t/time profile curve as a percentage of baseline

Order of use	PID	MID
MDI, PID	20 686 ± 6805	21 064 ± 5731
PID, MDI	23 798 ± 7245	21 923 ± 6922
	22 242 ± 7055 (Av.)	21 494 ± 6230 (Av.)

the range of equivalence. The equivalence of the two products could therefore not be confirmed. However, as the upper confidence interval was within the range of equivalence, it can be concluded that inhalation with the PID is at least equally as effective as that with MDI. The trend in favor of the PID was not significant ($p = 0.35$).

For the area under the FEV_1/time profile curve as a percentage of the baseline, the confidence interval was completely within the range of equivalence. Therapeutic equivalence of the two dosage forms was confirmed for this parameter at a multiple level ($N = 0.05$; see Table 2).

The maximum relative decrease in R_t as a percentage of the baseline was 59.2% on average for the PID and 59% for the MDI. The confidence interval was completely within the range of equivalence. Consequently, therapeutic equivalence was confirmed for this parameter (Table 3).

Regarding the area under the R_t/time profile curve the confidence interval was also completely within the range of equivalence. The therapeutic equivalence of the two dosage forms in respect of this parameter was thereby confirmed. Table 4 gives the data for the 24 patients examined.

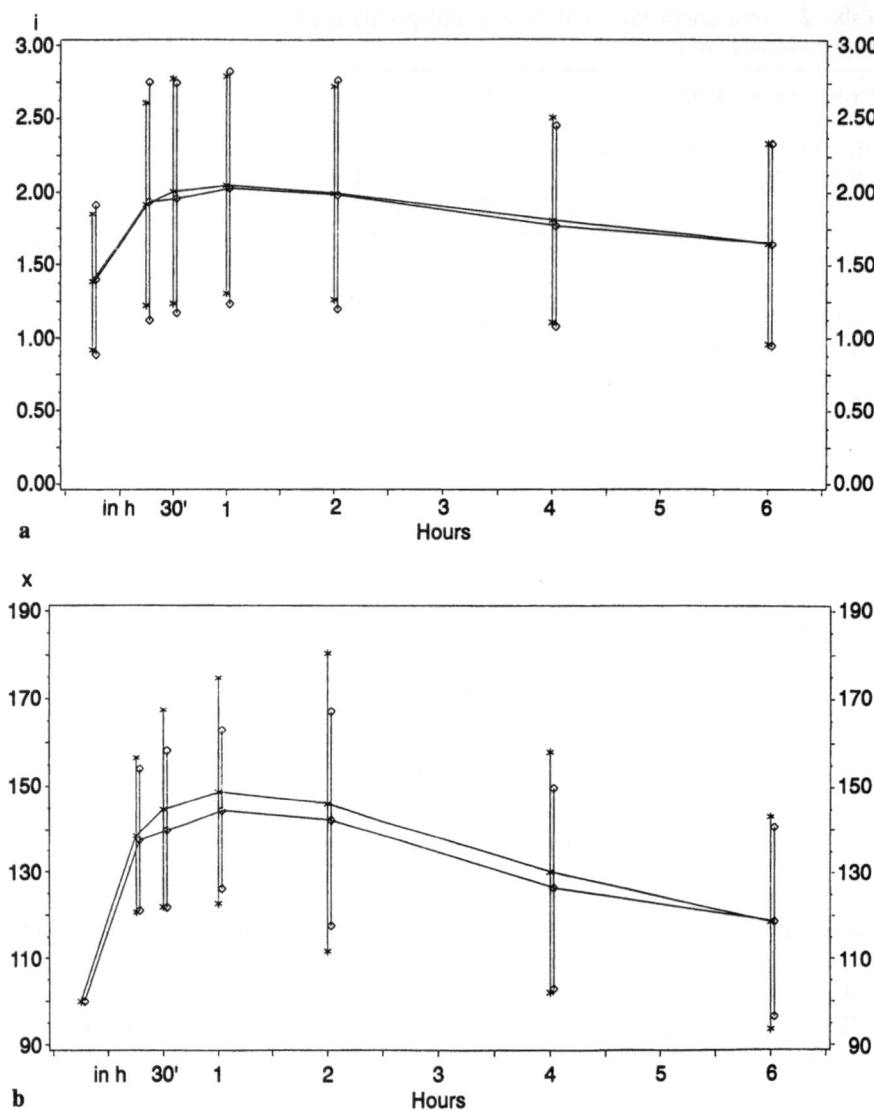

Fig. 1. FEV$_1$ (**a**) and FEV$_1$ as a percentage of baseline (**b**). *Crosses*, PID; *squares*, MID

The time courses of the lung function parameters are presented for FEV$_1$ in liters (Fig. 1a), FEV$_1$ as a percentage of the baseline (Fig. 1b), R$_t$ in millibars per liter per second (Fig. 2a) and R$_t$ as a percentage of the baseline (Fig. 2b). There were no striking differences between the two dosage forms for these lung function parameters or any of the other parameters measured (VC, FVC, IGV, SG$_{aw}$).

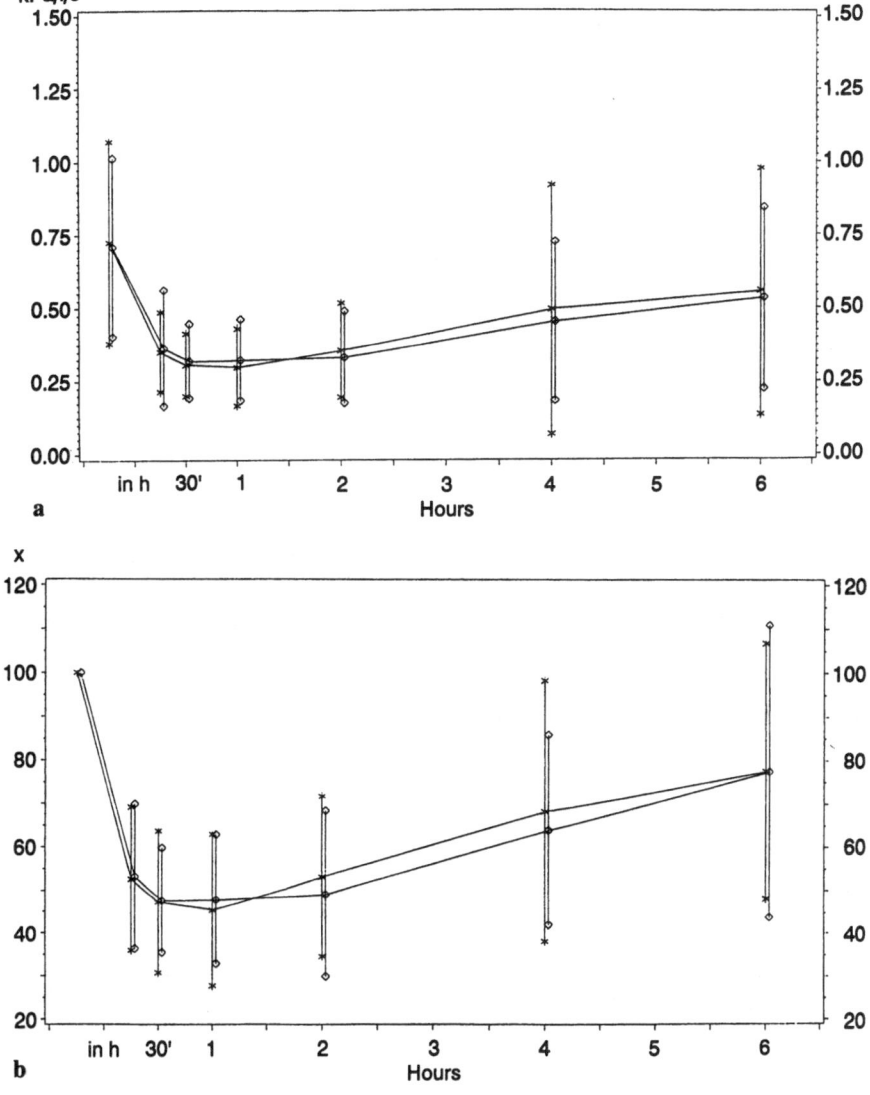

Fig. 2. R_t ($kPa\,l^{-1}s^{-1}$; **a**) and R_t as a percentage of baseline (**b**). *Crosses*, PID; *squares*, MID

There were no major differences between the two dosage forms on comparison of the incidence/intensity of tremor. The time courses of pulse rate and blood pressure measurements did not reveal any differences between inhalation of fenoterol using the PID or the MDI.

No serious adverse events related to the test medication were observed or reported spontaneously by the patients during the study.

Discussion

The present study is part of a wider study to compare the effect of inhalable therapeutic agents for the treatment of chronic obstructive airways disease after using two different dosage forms. The same dose of therapeutic agent is administered once with the PID and once with the MDI.

The data showed equivalence of therapeutic effect using MDI and PID on three of the four parameters: maximum decrease in R_t, area under the FEV_1/time profile curve as a percentage of the baseline, and area under the R_t/time profile curve as a percentage of the baseline.

These results correspond to those of studies in which 0.1 mg fenoterol hydrobromide using the PID was compared with the same dose administered from the Berotec 100 MDI (Fischer et al. 1990). Here, again, no differences in therapeutic effect were established between the two dosage forms. Ipratropium bromide was also found to be therapeutically equivalent after administration with the MDI and the PID (Fleischer et al. 1990).

All studies carried out so far with the new inhalation system indicate that the PID meets the requirements of a propellant-free alternative to the MDI. From a technical point of view the conditions are fulfilled in the form of particle size and reliable nebulization of precisely metered amounts of inhalant solution. This is further supplemented by the results of bio-equivalence studies. Not only are the pharmacodynamic effects comparable, but there is also evidence to confirm comparable tolerance after inhalation using the PID or the MDI.

Conclusions

The results of the present study comparing the therapeutic effects of inhaling 0.2 mg fenoterol hydrobromide as a single actuation from the PID or as a single puff from the MDI confirm the therapeutic equivalence of the two dosage forms in the dose examined. From a medical point of view, previous bioequivalence studies with various bronchospasmolytic substances and the data from the present study confirm the comparable therapeutic effect of inhalation with the PID and that with the MDI. On the basis of this and previous studies, there are no signs to suggest differences in efficacy, tolerance, or the incidence of adverse events between the MDI and the PID. The PID functioned reliably in this and other studies. On the whole, the PID is a forward-looking alternative to the chlorofluorocarbon-containing MDI.

References

Fischer J, Köhler D, Morr H, Wettengel R, Mütterlein R, Fleischer W, Rauber G, Stechert R (1990) Neue Techniken zur Erzeugung inhalierbarer Aerosole – Erste Erfahrungen mit dem piezoelektrischen Inhalationsgerät. Pneumologie 44:275–276

Fleischer W, Stechert R, Rauber G, Zimmermann T (1990) New technology of generation inhalation aerosols: preliminary results with the piezoelectric inhaler. Eur Respir J 3/10:232s

References

Subject Index

Springer-Verlag
and the Environment

We at Springer-Verlag firmly believe that an international science publisher has a special obligation to the environment, and our corporate policies consistently reflect this conviction.

We also expect our business partners – paper mills, printers, packaging manufacturers, etc. – to commit themselves to using environmentally friendly materials and production processes.

The paper in this book is made from low- or no-chlorine pulp and is acid free, in conformance with international standards for paper permanency.